Coloproctology and the Pelvic Floor

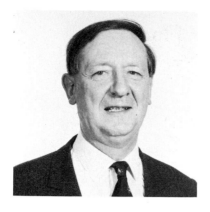

Sir Alan Parks
1920–1982

This book represents the ideas and concepts elaborated during several years of friendship and collaboration with Alan Parks. These ideas have been redefined since his death by studies in our laboratory that have taken advantage of new electrophysiological techniques that have allowed us to look at the problem of pelvic floor function and its disorders in new ways. The collaboration that developed between a surgeon and his research fellows, and a neurologist, was conceived in response to a shared problem that required the common experience of the two disciplines to allow its solution. Weakness of the pelvic floor muscles was shown, in histological studies, to be due to denervation of these muscles. This first step in understanding led directly to the development of electrophysiological techniques to investigate the underlying pathogenesis of this abnormality. The application of these methods, first into research, and secondly into clinical practice, was enthusiastically taken on by a series of young surgical research fellows from many different countries. We cannot praise their hard work and determination too highly, and Alan Parks would have been the first to acknowledge them. However, it was his own enthusiasm and delight in the results of the work, and in keeping the problem to the forefront of attention, that made these studies possible in the early days. We have been fortunate in having the opportunity, provided by the St. Mark's Hospital Research Foundation, and by St. Mark's Hospital itself, to continue these ideas and, indeed, to develop them. These advances are described in the pages of this book. Lately, a research fellowship has been established by the Royal College of Surgeons of England, in conjunction with the two hospitals with which Alan Parks was associated, St. Mark's Hospital and The London Hospital, to provide resources to enable young surgeons to work in this general field, so carrying on one of Alan Parks's main aims, the training and firing with enthusiasm of the next generation of surgeons, not only in practical surgical technique, but also in research methods. We hope that some of these ideas will be apparent in this book; and in this hope we dedicate it to his memory.

Michael Swash
Michael M. Henry

Coloproctology and the Pelvic Floor
PATHOPHYSIOLOGY AND MANAGEMENT

M. M. Henry MB, FRCS
Consultant Surgeon, Central Middlesex Hospital, London;
Honorary Consultant in Physiology, St. Mark's Hospital, London

M. Swash MD, FRCP, MRCPath
Consultant Neurologist, The London Hospital;
Honorary Consultant Neurologist, St. Mark's Hospital, London

Butterworths
London   Boston   Durban   Singapore   Sydney   Toronto   Wellington

First published, 1985

© Butterworth & Co. (Publishers) Ltd, 1985

British Library Cataloguing in Publication Data
Coloproctology and the pelvic floor:
  pathophysiology and management.
  1. Pelvis—Diseases
  I. Henry, M. M.   II. Swash, Michael
  617'.55   RC946

  ISBN 0-407-00352-5

Library of Congress Cataloging in Publication Data
Main entry under title:

Coloproctology and the pelvic floor.

  Bibliography: p.
  Includes index.
  1. Colon (Anatomy)—Surgery. 2. Rectum—Surgery.
3. Pelvis—Anatomy. 4. Proctology. I. Henry, M. M.
(Michael M.)   II. Swash, Michael.
  RD544.C646 1985   617'.555   85–380
  ISBN 0-407-00352-5

Filmset by Mid-County Press, London SW15
Printed and bound in Great Britain at the University Press, Cambridge

Foreword

For many readers the question that will immediately arise on first contemplating this book is exactly what is meant by the term 'pelvic floor'. Clearly in this text the expression has been given a wider connotation than usual, for it has been made to include not only the levatores ani muscles or pelvic diaphragm, but also the external and internal anal sphincters, attention in fact being directed mainly to the sphincters and to the puborectalis parts of the levators.

The objective of the editors in producing the volume has been essentially threefold: first, to assemble the now considerable body of information available on the normal anatomy and physiology of these structures (and also to a minor extent of the rectum and colon), special consideration naturally being devoted to the paramount functions of continence and defaecation; secondly, to describe the structural and functional abnormalities that are known to be associated with certain diseased conditions, believed to be attributable in greater or lesser part to defects of the sphincters and levators, notably anal incontinence and prolapse, and, perhaps less appropriately, complaints such as haemorrhoids and anal fissures; and thirdly, to discuss the treatment of these ailments partly in the light of this new knowledge.

To these ends the editors have enlisted the aid of a group of co-authors who are already distinguished for their contributions to this field. Between them they have been able to bring readers up to date with the latest advances in their respective subjects by means of a series of excellent chapters, which include among their references— incidentally recorded in what I consider to be the much more interesting Harvard nominal system than in the now almost obligatory much duller Vancouver numerical system—many papers that appeared as recently as 6–9 months ago.

Admittedly, despite the wealth of information provided, there is still some uncertainty regarding accepted concepts on several issues, even major ones, such as the precise mechanisms of anal continence, defaecation and colonic propulsion. There is also still some dubiety as to the relative importance of the various abnormal findings in several of the diseased conditions mentioned. But no one reading this text can fail to be enlightened as to both the extent and the limitations of our knowledge and as to the directions in which progress is being made. Particularly useful to the practising clinician, it seems to me, are the sections indicating how best to assess the state of patients presenting with abnormalities connected with the pelvic floor, using the various methods of investigation now available.

Altogether I have no doubt of the great value of this work and I offer my warmest congratulations to Michael Henry and Michael Swash and their collaborators on a very timely publication, which will assuredly earn them the deep gratitude of their colleagues who have to deal with patients suffering from colorectal disease. From no other current treatise will they be able to obtain such detailed and relevant information on the physiological aspects of the anorectum and pelvic musculature.

John Goligher
Emeritus Professor of Surgery, University of Leeds

Preface

The study of pelvic floor disorders has only recently emerged from obscurity. The acceleration of interest in this group of disorders owes much to the work of the late Sir Alan Parks and this book has developed from the stimulating and close association of the two editors with Sir Alan at St. Mark's Hospital, London, during the last ten years of his life. The starting point of the studies described here was the problem posed by the misery of the patient with anorectal incontinence. Recognition of the neurogenic aetiology of this disorder by a combination of clinical, pathological and, later, electrophysiological studies has led to a better understanding of the causation and treatment of related disorders, especially rectal prolapse, descending perineum syndrome, solitary ulcer syndrome and constipation. Recent work has permitted fresh understanding of the role of occult obstetric injury in the pathogenesis of incontinence, rectal prolapse and descending perineum syndrome.

The studies described in this book represent a multidisciplinary approach to pelvic floor disorders, with collaboration between laboratory workers and clinicians. New concepts of the anatomy and physiology of pelvic floor musculature and of the smooth muscle of the rectum and anal canal are described. Functional tests of the pelvic floor muscles, including anal manometry, conventional EMG, single fibre EMG, and pudendal and spinal motor latencies, are described in practical terms. These methods are fully documented, with normal data, and the abnormalities in various pelvic floor disorders are described by experts in this field. The more practical aspects of clinical management of pelvic floor disorders, including faecal incontinence, rectal prolapse, haemorrhoids, descending perineum syndrome, constipation, solitary ulcer syndrome, fissure and perineal pain, occupy two-thirds of the book. For each of these disorders pathophysiological mechanisms are discussed and a critical review of approaches to treatment is provided. The chapters are fully referenced so that the book forms a basis for detailed reference and for practical guidance in the management of patients.

It is a happy coincidence that publication of the book coincides with the 150th Anniversary Year of the foundation of St. Mark's Hospital. The hospital was founded by Frederick Salmon for the special purpose of treating patients afflicted by many of the disorders which are considered in this book.

M. M. Henry and M. Swash

Acknowledgements

It is a great pleasure to acknowledge the assistance of Miss Jill Maybee, who has prepared many of the illustrations, and Miss Nicola Knight, who has assisted with the typing of the manuscript. We have received generous financial support from the St. Mark's Hospital Research Foundation and from a number of other sources. We thank our patients without whose co-operation and assistance these studies would not have been possible. We are grateful to the surgeons of St. Mark's Hospital, who have been most stimulating in their encouragement of our work, and thank them for referring their patients. Finally, we acknowledge with particular pleasure the contribution to our work made during recent years by our Research Fellows: P. Barnes, F. Beersiek, G. Browning, E. S. Kiff, M. E. Neill, J. Percy, M. Pescatori, S. J. Snooks, T. Teramoto and M. Wunderlich.

Contributors

J. J. Bannister, MA FRCS
Surgical Research Fellow, Royal Hallamshire Hospital, Glossop Rd., Sheffield, UK

C. I. Bartram, MB MRCP FRCR
Consultant Radiologist, St. Mark's Hospital, City Rd., London EC1, UK; Consultant Radiologist, St. Bartholomew's Hospital, London EC1, UK

R. W. Beart, Jr, MD
Head, Section of Colon and Rectal Surgery, Mayo Clinic and Mayo Foundation; Assistant Professor of Surgery, Mayo Medical School, Rochester, Minnesota, USA

M. Burke, MS FRCS
Senior Surgical Registrar, St. Mark's Hospital, City Rd., London EC1, UK

D. E. Burleigh, PhD
Lecturer in Pharmacology, The London Hospital Medical College, London E1, UK

M. A. Clifton, MS FRCS
Consultant Surgeon, Princess Alexandra Hospital, Harlow, Essex, UK; Consultant Surgeon, St. Margaret's Hospital, Epping, Essex, UK (formerly Senior Registrar, The London Hospital, UK)

R. C. M. Cook, FRCS
Consultant Paediatric Surgeon, Alder Hey Children's Hospital, Liverpool, UK

M. L. Corman, MD
Surgeon, Section of Colon and Rectal Surgery, Sansum Medical Clinic, Santa Barbara, California, USA

A. D'Mello, MSc PhD
Senior Lecturer and Head, Department of Pharmacology, The London Hospital Medical College, London E1, UK

S. M. Goldberg, MD FACS
Clinical Professor of Surgery, Division of Colon and Rectal Surgery, University of Minnesota, Minneapolis, Minnesota, USA

J. C. Goligher, ChM FRCS
Emeritus Professor of Surgery, University of Leeds, Leeds, UK; Consulting Surgeon, St. Mark's Hospital, City Rd, London EC1, UK

L. Hakelius, MD
Professor of Plastic Surgery, University Hospital, Uppsala, Sweden

P. R. Hawley, MS FRCS
Consultant Surgeon, St. Mark's Hospital, City Rd., London EC1, UK; Civilian Consultant in Colorectal Surgery to the Army

M. M. Henry, MB FRCS
Consultant Surgeon, Central Middlesex Hospital, Acton Lane, London NW1, UK; Hon. Consultant Surgeon, Sir Alan Parks Physiology Unit, St. Mark's Hospital, City Rd., London EC1, UK

D. Kumar, MB FRCS
Beecham Clinical Research Fellow, The London Hospital Medical College Research Unit in Gastroenterology, London E1, UK

R. J. Leicester, FRCS RN
Consultant Surgeon and Head of Surgical Division, Royal Naval Hospital, Haslar, Gosport, Hampshire, UK (formerly Research Fellow, St. Mark's Hospital, City Rd., London EC1, UK)

J. E. Lennard-Jones, MD FRCS
Consultant Gastroenterologist, St. Mark's Hospital, City Rd., London EC1, UK; Professor of Gastroenterology, The London Hospital Medical College, London E1, UK; Consultant Gastroenterologist, The London Hospital, London E1, UK

P. H. G. Mahieu, MD
Professor, Department of Radiology, Institut Chirurgical de Bruxelles, Université Catholique de Louvin (en Woluwe), Square Marie-Louise 59, 1040-Bruxelles, Belgium

D. A. Mandelstam, MCSP DipSocSc
Incontinence Adviser, Disabled Living Foundation, 380 Harrow Rd., London W14, UK, and Royal Free Hospital, Pond St., London NW3, UK

P. A. Merton, MA MD FRS
Professor in Human Physiology, The Physiological Laboratory, Cambridge, UK

R. W. Motson, MS FRCS
Consultant Surgeon, Colchester General Hospital, Colchester, Essex, UK (formerly Senior Registrar, The London Hospital, UK)

R. J. Nicholls, BA MChir FRCS
Consultant Surgeon, St. Mark's Hospital, City Rd., London EC1, UK; Consultant Surgeon, St. Thomas's Hospital, Lambeth Palace Rd., London SE1, UK

E. Pedersen, MD
Chief Neurologist, Aarhus Kommunehospital, DK-8000, Aarhus C, Denmark

N. W. Read, MA MD MRCP
Reader, Department of Physiology, and Honorary Consultant Gastroenterologist, Royal Hallamshire Hospital, Sheffield, UK

D. A. Rothenberger, MD FACS
Clinical Assistant Professor, Division of Colon and Rectal Surgery, University of Minnesota, Minneapolis, Minnesota, USA

K. R. P. Rutter, MA FRCS
Consultant Surgeon, Frimley Park Hospital, Portsmouth Rd., Frimley, Surrey, UK

D. J. Schoetz, Jr, MD
Staff Surgeon, Section of Colon and Rectal Surgery, Lahey Clinic Medical Center, Burlington, Massachusetts, USA; Assistant Clinical Professor of Surgery, Boston University School of Medicine, Boston, Massachusetts, USA

M. M. Schuster, MD FACP FAPA
Chief, Division of Digestive Diseases, Francis Scott Keys Medical Center, Baltimore, Maryland, USA; Professor of Medicine and Psychiatry, Johns Hopkins School of Medicine, Baltimore, Maryland, USA

S. J. Snooks, MB FRCS
Sir Alan Parks Research Fellow, St. Mark's Hospital, City Rd., London EC1, UK

M. Swash, MD FRCP MRCPath
Consultant Neurologist, The London Hospital, London E1, UK, and Newham Hospital, London E13, UK; Hon. Consultant Neurologist and Director, Sir Alan Parks Physiology Unit, St. Mark's Hospital, City Rd., London EC1, UK; Senior Lecturer in Neuropathology, The London Hospital Medical College, London E1, UK

J. P. S. Thomson, MS FRCS
Consultant Surgeon, St. Mark's Hospital, City Rd., London EC1, UK; Consultant Surgeon, Hackney Hospital, London; Hon. Consultant Surgeon, St. Mary's Hospital, London; Hon. Lecturer in Surgery, The Medical College of St. Bartholomew, London; Civil Consultant in Surgery (Rectal) to The Royal Air Force

I. P. Todd, MS MD FRCS
Consultant Surgeon, St. Mark's Hospital, City Rd., London EC1, UK; Consulting Surgeon, St. Bartholomew's Hospital, London EC1, UK; Civil Consultant in Surgery to The Royal Navy; Consultant to King Edward VII Hospital for Officers, London, UK

M. C. Veidenheimer, MD
Head, Section of Colon and Rectal Surgery, Lahey Clinic Medical Center, Burlington, Massachusetts, USA; Lecturer in Surgery, Harvard Medical School, Boston, Massachusetts, USA

J. D. Watts, MD FACS
Head, Division of Colon and Rectal Surgery, Scripps Clinic and Research Foundation, La Jolla, California, USA

D. L. Wingate, DM FRCP
Reader in Gastroenterology, The London Hospital Medical College, London E1, UK; Honorary Consultant Gastroenterologist, The London Hospital, UK

B. A. Wood, BSc MB PhD
S.A. Courtauld Professor of Anatomy, The Middlesex Hospital Medical School, Cleveland St., London W1, UK

Contents

Part I

Anatomy and physiology

Chapter 1

Anatomy of the anal sphincters and pelvic floor

B. A. Wood

Introduction

The anal canal, the pelvic floor and, to a lesser extent, the rectum are structures which have been sadly neglected by non-clinical anatomists. In spite of the important contributions of clinicians, our ignorance of the region is still profound, and this is attested to by the often widely differing morphological interpretations of what must be the same structures.

Several factors contribute to this state of affairs. The region is inaccessible, difficult to fix and bony reference points are few. The 'normal' relationships between its components are in part maintained by muscle tone so that its appearance *post mortem* may not reflect *in vivo* relationships. There are also well-recorded morphological differences between the neonate and the adult. Nevertheless, the results of conventional dissection and histological studies, together with those of histochemical, ultrastructural and comparative anatomical investigations, are helping to repair these deficiencies in our knowledge.

What follows in this chapter is a survey of our present understanding of this region. This review does not pretend to be comprehensive and is idiosyncratic to the extent that it emphasizes information about comparative anatomy and development. This reflects the author's particular interest and his belief that sound comparative anatomical evidence is more likely to throw light on the complexities of the pelvic floor than studies which are restricted to modern human material. Although this review has attempted to present the most recent research results, this should not by any means be taken as indicating that apparently accurate and reliable observations are limited to the recent literature. Much of our fundamental understanding of the region comes from the efforts of the researchers of the nineteenth and early twentieth centuries. Space prevents these authors from being cited, where appropriate, but the works of Holl (1881, 1896, 1897), Thompson (1899) and Paramore (1910) are particularly valuable contributions to our understanding of the pelvic floor musculature. The studies of Herrmann (1880), Robin and Cadiat (1874), Symington (1889), Stroud (1896) and Milligan and Morgan (1934) are similarly seminal contributions to our knowledge of the anal canal. Of the more recent studies, the work of Wendell-Smith (1967) deserves special mention. Apart from two abstracts (Wendell-Smith, 1963, 1964) and a review (Wendell-Smith and Wilson,

1977), the bulk of the thesis remains unpublished. The present author is indebted to the author of that thesis.

The chapter is divided into two parts: the first describes the pelvic floor and the second considers the rectum and anal canal together. Any scheme has its disadvantages, and dealing separately with the muscles of the pelvic floor and the striated sphincter of the anal canal artificially separates what many consider to be a functional unit made up of puborectalis and the deep part of the external sphincter (see below). However, the advantage of the present treatment is that it emphasizes the continuity between the anal canal and the rectum, and reminds us that the region now known as the anal canal was, until relatively recently, thought of as the third, or anal, part of the rectum.

Pelvic floor

The major component of the pelvic floor is a pair of symmetrical compound muscular sheets, composed of predominantly striated muscle; these are usually referred to as the levator ani muscles or pelvic diaphragm. The sheet is defective in the midline in those places where viscera pass through it, but, as will be seen later in this discussion, the muscle sheet is intimately related to the striated muscle associated with the anal canal, vagina and urethra. Loose connective tissue and vessels occupy the midline ventral to the urethra, but the remainder of the midline pelvic floor ventral and dorsal to the recto-anal flexure is made up, respectively, of the perineal body and the postanal plate (Wendell-Smith, 1967). They are both complex in form and character, the former being a fibromuscular 'wedge' between the urogenital viscera and the anal canal. The postanal plate is a laminated musculotendinous structure situated between the anal canal and the caudal part of the vertebral column. From deep to superficial the component layers are the presacral fascia, the tendinous plate-like insertion of pubococcygeus, which blends with the ventral sacrococcygeal ligament (sometimes referred to as the anococcygeal ligament), the midline attachment of the iliococcygeus component of levator ani as the anococcygeal raphe and, most superficially, fibres of puborectalis intermingled with that part of the external anal sphincter which attaches to the coccyx.

Most surgical and anatomical textbook descriptions of the levator ani are usually modifications of that of Thompson (1899) who recognized three parts, each corresponding to a component of the innominate, and thus referred to as pubo-, ilio- and ischiococcygeus. The peripheral attachment of the levator is a linear one and extends from the body of the pubis to the ischial spine. There is direct attachment to bone on the body of the pubis just lateral to the symphysis and to the ischial spine, but between these sites the muscle originates from a condensation of the obturator fascia which is often referred to as the arcus tendineus.

It is now more conventional to divide the muscle into four parts, one of which, the pubococcygeus, is usually further subdivided. The puborectalis and pubococcygeus components are both attached to the pubic bone, but differ in their distribution. The puborectalis is a muscular loop which runs around the recto-anal flexure. The extent to which it merges or mingles with the external anal sphincter will be referred to later. It is generally agreed that it has no significant attachment to the vertebral column. The fibres of the pubococcygeus arise from the pubic bone in continuity with those of the puborectalis, but unlike the latter its attachment also extends laterally so that it arises from that part of the arcus which is related to the pubic bone. The main body of the fibres of the pubococcygeus attach to a flattened tendon which inserts behind the rectum, via the postanal plate, onto the ventral surface of the coccyx as the ventral sacrococcygeal ligament. The medial part of the pubococcygeus is often further subdivided to recognize those fibres which merge with the musculature of prostate, vagina and perineal body; levator prostatae, pubo-urethralis and pubovaginalis are just three of the many names which have been given to such fibres. Most workers acknowledge that some of its fibres enter the wall of the anal canal medial to the puborectalis, and thus reinforce the smooth muscle of the longitudinal coat; in the orang-utan and the gorilla these fibres are also distinct (Elftman, 1932).

The third part of the levator ani is the iliococcygeus. Its origin is contiguous with that of the pubococcygeus, and is from that part of the arcus tendineus which overlies the ileum, and the medial surface of the ischial spine. It partly overlaps the pubococcygeus (on the latter's perineal surface) to insert below it onto the lateral surfaces of the terminal pieces of coccyx, the tip of the coccyx and the anococcygeal raphe. The fourth component is usually referred to as either the ischiococcygeus, or simply coccygeus. It arises from the tip and posterior surface of the ischial spine and is inserted into the lateral surface of the caudal part of the sacrum and the upper coccygeal vertebrae. In the human it is often rudimentary and represented by a few muscle fibres on the surface of the sacrospinous ligament; the development of the coccygeus varies reciprocally with that of the ligament (Wendell-Smith, 1967). The functions of the components of the levator ani complex, to maintain the anorectal angle and relax, to depress, and then contract to elevate the pelvic floor during defaecation, are well reviewed in Wilson (1973a) and Wendell-Smith (1967).

The description of the levator ani given above is the conventional one, but workers who have made a special study of the muscle have come to a variety of different interpretations of its form. Nevertheless, if one ignores the differences in nomenclature, there is a consensus that the complex of muscles called the levator ani can be subdivided into a posterior group of 'somatic', diaphragmatic' or 'obturator' muscles, and an anterior group of 'visceral' fibres, the latter being intimately linked to, if not actually continuous with, the deep part of the striated external anal sphincter (Wilson, 1973a; Lawson, 1974a). Holl (1881) was one of the earliest workers to stress the effective fusion between the external anal sphincter and the anterior fibres of the levator ani complex. Although they differ in their detailed interpretation, the same general conclusion has been reached by Thompson (1899), Courtney (1950), Goligher, Leacock and Brossy (1955), Gorsch (1955), Hughes (1957), Oh and Kark (1972), Wilson (1973a, 1973b), Lawson (1974a, 1974b), Shafik (1975), Ayoub (1979a) (but see Ayoub, 1979b) and Beersiek, Parks and Swash (1979), and the author believes we must accept that such a relationship, at least on the dorsal and lateral aspects of the anal canal, has been convincingly demonstrated. Porter (1962) has also stressed the functional integration of this striated muscle complex. Thus, whether the muscle loop behind the recto-anal flexure is referred to as the pubo-anal sphincteric sling (Lawson, 1974a), the puborectalis (Gorsch, 1955) or merely a component of the puborectalis (Uhlenhuth, 1953), we are faced with the problem of deciding whether the external anal sphincter and the puborectalis part of levator ani form a homogeneous unit, or whether they are phylogenetically and ontogenetically distinct parts of a heterogeneous muscle complex. Taking, for example, the former hypothesis, is puborectalis a pelvicaudal muscle which has secondarily lost most of its caudal attachment, or is it a subset of sphincter fibres which have become secondarily tethered to the pubis? Evidence from developmental and comparative studies, the pattern of innervation and the results of histological and histochemical investigations are all relevant to substantiating or refuting these hypotheses, and the results of pertinent studies are presented below.

Developmental and comparative evidence

There is very little information in the literature about the ontogeny of the external anal sphincter (EAS) and the levator ani. The EAS appears in human embryos of about 30 mm crown rump length (CRL), a size which corresponds to a gestation age of approximately 8 weeks (Johnson, 1914; Nobles, 1984). It, together with the levator ani, is believed to originate from hypaxial myotomes (Hamilton and Mossman, 1972). Johnson (1914) describes the EAS lying 'just below its (levator ani's) inferior extremity' and goes on to point out that even at that stage 'its fibers are not distinctly marked off from those of levator ani' (Johnson, 1914, p. 19). Thus, what published evidence of normal development as exists suggests that the EAS and the adjacent levator ani have a common developmental origin, but this will have to be confirmed by studies of pelvic floor development. Stephens and Durham-Smith (1971) have interpreted the distribution of striated muscle in cases of recto-urethral fistula and anal agenesis as suggesting that the levator ani and the external sphincter arise separately, but no special mention is made of the puborectalis.

The first systematic treatises on comparative anatomy date from the latter part of the seventeenth century, but it was not until the middle of the eighteenth century that investigators applied this type of study to the pelvic musculature. Straus-Durckheim (1845) was the first to demonstrate the link between the human levator ani and the tail muscles of lower animals, and Paulet (1876, 1877) extended this work to include a wider sample of animals, including, among others, non-human primates. Thompson (1899), and particularly Paramore (1910), pursued their own comparative studies, and the latter was one of the few workers who extended their scope beyond mammals. The most comprehensive review of the morphology and comparative context of the sphincter/ levator complex of muscles was undertaken by Wendell-Smith (1967), and it is a pity that this excellent source (which should be consulted for an exhaustive bibliography of comparative studies) has been neglected by most contemporary workers.

Wendell-Smith (1967) traces the phylogeny of the sphincter and pelvic musculature back through reptiles, fish and lampreys to the simple *Amphioxus*. He uses this series to establish the presence of two muscle groups related to the cloaca which are apparently ontogenetically and phylogenetically distinct. They are a 'sphincter' group and a 'lateral compressor' group. The former are found in most, but not all, of the animals investigated. The latter connect the rudimentary pelvis to the caudal end of the vertebral column, and thus are called 'pelvicaudal' muscles. Cartilaginous and bony fish have a well-developed, but apparently single, set of pelvicaudal muscles, whereas in reptiles and mammals these muscles are usually separated into a lateral and a medial group. In monkeys and the apes, the mammals most closely related to modern humans, the homologue of the lateral pelvicaudal group is the ischiococcygeus muscle. Primates show considerable species differences in the extent to which pubo- and iliococcygeus can be separated, but whether or not the two muscles can be distinguished, it is apparent that in monkeys and apes this part of the levator complex is derived from the medial group of pelvicaudal muscles (*Figure 1.1*). In higher mammals, the sphincter or cloacal musculature is divided into a ventral, or urogenital, and a dorsal, or anal, group of muscles; in primates, the latter make up the external anal sphincter. However, in addition, primates possess a variable-sized group of striated muscle fibres which virtually encircle the rectum, and then pass forwards, parallel with and closely applied to the inner border of the medial pelvicaudal muscles, to attach to the symphysis pubis. Elftman (1932) makes it clear that these fibres are present in the orang-utan and gorilla, but they are lacking in the chimpanzee; in man, these fibres are well developed and

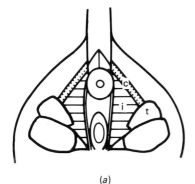

(a)

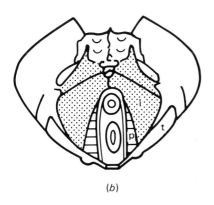

(b)

Figure 1.1. Diagrammatic inferior view of the pelvic diaphragm in (a) *Macaca* (rhesus monkey) and (b) modern man. The stippled areas are the lateral pelvicaudal muscles and the hatched ones the medial pelvicaudal muscles. Sphincter cloacae muscles are unshaded. Note that the different phylogenetic origin of the pubo- and iliococcygeus in man would help to explain their overlap. Puborectalis is the unshaded loop within the medial pelvicaudal musculature. c, Coccygeus; i, iliococcygeus; p, pubococcygeus; t, ischial tuberosity (After Wendell-Smith, 1967)

known as the puborectalis. In the female, other fibres run in a figure-of-eight pattern around the rectum and vagina to reach the pubis.

On the basis of his comparative evidence, Wendell-Smith (1967) comes down firmly in favour of the interpretation that the puborectalis, and its homologues in non-human primates (Wendell-Smith, 1964; Wilson, 1973b; Oelrich, 1978), are ventrally tethered parts of the sphincter cloacae complex. Wendell-Smith (1967) concludes that it is the intimate relationship of the puborectalis to the medial pelvicaudal muscle group, and its secondary pubic attachment, which has led to its erroneous classification as a pelvicaudal muscle. Incidentally, Wendell-Smith (1967) does not consider the ilio-coccygeus of man and monkey to be homologues, but instead regards the human iliococcygeus as a member of the lateral pelvicaudal group; this would help to explain the lamination and overlap of the pubo- and iliococcygeus muscles in man. A separation between the medial pelvicaudal and sphincter muscles is also implicit in Lawson (1974a), who shows clearly that the puborectalis, or what he calls the 'puboanal sphincteric sling', is separate from, and outside the plane of, what he refers to as the pubo-analis/iliococcygeus muscle layer.

Innervation

Innervation is both ontogenetically and phylogenetically conservative, and thus the nerve supply of the human puborectalis should provide some clue about its derivation, for comparative evidence shows that 'sphincter cloacae derivatives are generally supplied by the pudendal nerve from their perineal aspect and the pelvicaudal muscles by branches from the sacral plexus on their pelvic surface' (Wendell-Smith, 1967, p. 210).

The same worker reviews the early literature on innervation and has made his own dissection study of human cadavers. Of the 16 cadavers in his own series, in 13 the puborectalis was innervated from below by the pudendal nerve, while in three it enjoyed a joint innervation from the inferior rectal and perineal branches of the pudendal nerve on its undersurface, and from branches of the sacral plexus on its pelvic surface. The observations of Stelzner (1960), Wilson (1973a) and Lawson (1974a), who examined 13 infant and neonatal pelves, also bear out such an arrangement and a careful and detailed microdissection study of 17 human hemipelves was clear in its conclusion that 'the rectal attachment of the levator ani (presumably the puborectalis) is always innervated by the perineal and inferior rectal nerves' suggesting that 'this muscular portion has been derived not from the primitive mass of the levator ani but from a portion of the primitive sphincter ani externus or the sphincter cloacae' (Sato, 1980, p. 222). It is important to note that the latter author came to this conclusion quite independently of Wendell-Smith (1967), who is not cited in his references. However, the electrophysiological study of Percy et al. (1981) concluded that in 19 out of 20 of their preoperative experiments, stimulation of sacral nerves above the pelvic floor resulted in EMG activity in the ipsilateral puborectalis, but not in the external anal sphincter. Their use of needle electrodes should have prevented any contraction of pelvicaudal muscles being confused with activity in the puborectalis.

Clearly the weight of evidence in favour of a pudendal nerve supply for the puborectalis has now been challenged by recent *in vivo* findings, and further investigations are required to clarify this important point of anatomy.

Histological and histochemical studies of fibre types

Light and electron microscopy, and techniques of enzyme histochemical analysis (Padykula and Herman, 1955), now allow muscles to be characterized according to both the size and morphology of the fibres and by the type of intracellular enzyme system. How do the results of applying these techniques to pelvic musculature bear on the hypothesis of a 'sphincteric' derivation and classification of the puborectalis? Wilson (1973a) reported on her own morphological and histochemical analysis and concluded that 'very large numbers' of the fibres of the puborectalis were 'small tonic Type 1 fibres' with a lesser number of phasic Type II fibres, and went on to comment that there were more fibres in a similar-sized fascicle in the puborectalis than in the main levator muscle (186 vs. 120) (Wilson, 1973a, pp. 1157–1158). No mention was made of the fibre population of the external anal sphincter.

Wendell-Smith and Wilson (1977) refer to a similar pattern of fibre distribution for both the deep external sphincter and the puborectalis, but do not make it clear whether these are their own, independent, observations or a report of the work of others. However, the observations of Wilson (1973a) are given independent confirmation by Parks, Swash and Urich (1977), Beersiek, Parks and Swash (1979) and Critchley, Dixon and Gosling (1980). The latter authors also demonstrated that the fibre populations in the perianal (sling) and periurethral parts of the levator ani were different, with a greater percentage of Type II fibres and a smaller mean fibre diameter (45.8 vs. 59.5 μm) in the perianal part. Beersiek, Parks and Swash (1979) provide good evidence that the diameter of fibres in the external anal sphincter and puborectalis is smaller than that in the 'diaphragmatic' part of levator ani, but their implication that the patterns of Type I fibre dominance are different in the puborectalis and levator ani are not borne out by their data. Mannen *et al.* (1982) and Schrøder and Reske-Nielsen (1983) have subsequently confirmed the fibre pattern in the deep part of the external sphincter.

Thus, the balance of the comparative and morphological evidence does support the hypothesis that the puborectalis should be set apart from the majority of the levator ani, and treated as part of the complex of striated sphincter muscles. However, for a problem such as this the results of studies of development and innervation are crucial. Evidence about the ontogeny of the striated musculature of the pelvis is too meagre to be counted as supporting the hypothesis. The *post mortem* innervation studies are strongly in favour of a perineal nerve supply to the puborectalis, and before their evidence can be judged to have been superseded by the results of the *in vivo* innervation experiments, the precision of the latter needs to be confirmed, and the conclusions need to be verified. Thus, the hypothesis, although supported by much of the foregoing evidence, still awaits its two most thorough tests.

Rectum and anal canal

Definitions and topography

Merkel (1900) reports that early accounts of the rectum (e.g. those of Sanson and Treves) regarded its origin as lying in the plane of the pelvic brim, and proposed that it was divisible into three sections. The first part of this 'oldest' rectum is the terminal part of what is now regarded as the sigmoid colon; the second, the rectum of the current Nomina Anatomica; and the third, the part of the gut presently referred to as the anal canal. According to Symington (1889) it was Treves who, in 1885, excluded the sigmoid colon component and thus introduced the definition of what is referred to here as the 'old' rectum. It was Symington himself, in 1889, who is usually given the credit for applying the term 'anal canal' to the terminal, or caudal, part of the alimentary tract. Prior to and indeed for some time subsequent to Symington's report, the anal canal was simply regarded as the distal, or terminal, portion of the rectum, and referred to as the 'pars analis recti'. Gray (1858) suggests that the rectum received its name 'from being somewhat less flexuous than any other part of the intestinal canal' (Gray, 1858, p. 611) yet, despite its name, it is S-shaped, or doubly-curved, in the sagittal plane, and has three flexures, an upper and a lower one convex to the right, and a middle one convex to the left, in the coronal plane.

The 'old' rectum is about 15–20 cm long and was said to extend from the junction with the sigmoid colon to the anal orifice. Both termini are ill-defined. The proximal junction is usually level with the third piece of the sacrum, and corresponds to the caudal end of the sigmoid mesocolon and the disappearance of appendices epiploicae and sacculations. The exact site of the anal orifice depends on the state of contraction of the external sphincter. The proximal of the two sagittal curves of the rectum is called the sacral flexure, and the backward curve as the rectum passes through the pelvic diaphragm in the sagittal plane is called the perineal flexure. One reason for reverting to the scheme of the 'old' rectum for this review is the apparent confusion in the literature about where the 'new' rectum ends and the 'anal canal' begins. It is clear from the literature that there are two anal canals; a longer (approximately 4.0–4.5 cm) 'surgical' or 'clinical' one, and a shorter (approximately 2.0 cm) 'anatomical' or 'embryological' one (Nivatvongs, Stern and Fryd, 1981). The 'short' canal is said to extend from the anal valves to the anal margin and is regarded as an entity on what, as argued here, is a misapprehension, notably that the anal valves mark the site of the embryonic cloacal membrane (Milligan *et al.*, 1937; Gorsch, 1955). Gray (1858) describes the 'third portion' of the rectum as being an inch (2.5 cm) long, so we must conclude that the 'anal part' of the rectum referred to in older descriptions corresponds to the 'anatomical' or 'short' canal of today.

Milligan and Morgan (1934) are credited with being the first to describe the 'long' canal, and its proximal terminus is usually put at the level of the anorectal ring (Milligan *et al.*, 1937; Gabriel, 1945) or the levator ani (Walls, 1958; Nivatvongs, Stern and Fryd, 1981). This corresponds to the distal end of the dilated, or ampullary, part of the rectum, and the acute angle of the perineal flexure, and it is also nearest the centre of the region of highest intraluminal pressure (Bennett and Duthie, 1964). The angle between the rectum and anal canal is maintained by the active contraction of the puborectalis loop. Thus, these factors lend support to the claim that the 'long' canal is a useful physiological concept, even though its proximal limit is not marked by any apparent epithelial or developmental boundary. Other definitions of the anal canal are to be found in the literature (e.g. that part of the alimentary tract limited by the upper and lower borders of the internal sphincters (Fenger, 1974, 1979)), but mercifully they have attracted few adherents.

At the proximal boundary of the rectum, the transverse, crescentic, folds of the mucous membrane of the sigmoid colon give way to the smoother rectal lining. This thin, pink, mucosa lines the sacral and the perineal flexures and extends into the upper part of the anal canal. When the rectum is empty its mucosal lining is folded longitudinally, but these disappear when the rectum is distended. Three transverse folds (the valves of Houston) partly encircle the upper part of the rectum. The middle is the least variable and the most substantial. It projects from the anterior and right walls of the rectum and contains more smooth muscle than the other two.

The anal canal is an anteroposterior slit, with its lateral walls in close contact. In the upper part of the anal canal, the mucosa is thrown into another series of longitudinal folds, known as the anal columns, or columns of Morgagni. These vary in number (6–12), and are more marked in the neonate. The distal ends of the columns lie about midway down the internal sphincter and at this level adjacent columns are joined together by folds of mucous membrane; these are the anal valves, or the valves of Ball. A little below the valves, smooth, paler, mucosa is replaced by hairy anal skin.

Nature of the epithelium and its correlation with developmental history

In a region where confusion abounds, this is nowhere more apparent than in the literature describing the landmarks and the nature of the epithelial lining of the anal canal.

Epithelium

Between the anal margin and a line corresponding to the lower border of the internal sphincter, the anal canal is lined with hairy skin containing sebaceous and sweat glands and large apocrine glands, the circumanal glands of Gay. The next 10–15 mm of the canal is lined by thicker stratified squamous epithelium, largely devoid of hairs and glands, but with a thin horny layer and retaining some pigment; Stroud (1896) called this zone the 'pecten' and cited Hilton's 'white line' as its distal boundary, but Ewing (1954) has cast doubt on its reliability as a landmark. At or, more usually, below the level of the anal valves the nature of the epithelium changes; Robin and Cadiat (1874) called this boundary the 'ligne sinueuse cutanee', and Herrmann (1880) used the term 'ligne ano-cutanee'. Here the epithelium changes to a stratified columnar epithelium or retains its stratified squamous character, but reduces in thickness with surface cells that are less flattened than those in the pecten (Goligher, Leacock and Brossy, 1955). It is not unusual to find islands of columnar epithelium within it, and Herrmann (1880) suggested that columnar epithelium is more commonly found between the anal columns, while the columns themselves are more often covered with stratified squamous epithelium (Johnson, 1914). The thinned stratified squamous, or columnar, epithelium extends up a variable distance (5–10 mm) above the anal valves and has a sinuous, but fairly abrupt, junction with rectal-type mucosa; Herrmann (1880) called this is the 'ligne ano-rectale'. The cell type in this rectal-type columnar epithelium is mucus-secreting (or goblet) cells, and the epithelium is invaginated to form multiple, tubular glands. In summary, the valves lie about half-way along a 40 mm canal. The proximal 10 mm, or so, of the canal is lined by a rectal-type mucosa, with the next 15 mm (which includes the valves) being lined by stratified, or a modified columnar, epithelium. Distal to that is about 10 mm of thick, non-hairy, stratified epithelium (the pecten), below which there is about 5–10 mm of hairy skin.

The terminology used to describe the junctions of epithelial types in the wall of the anal canal is, to say the least, very confused. Some confusion is due to justified attempts to integrate histological findings with macroscopic appearances, but the residue is either due to use of terms which are inadequately defined in the literature, or to the erroneous use of established terms. Although the anal valves and columns are not always very obvious in the adult, they are almost the only unambiguous landmarks. The original description of the pecten by Stroud (1896) quite clearly implies that the 'pectinate' or 'dentate' line is the lower of the two irregular mucosal boundaries, equivalent to the 'ligne sinueuse cutanee' or 'ligne ano-cutanee', a boundary which usually lies at, or just distal to, the anal valves. Without any detailed qualification, terms such as 'anocutaneous' or 'mucocutaneous' to describe lines or junctions are best abandoned. Likewise, authors should be discouraged from apparently arbitrarily redefining the pectinate line, e.g. to refer to the proximal boundary of the transitional zone of epithelium (Wilde, 1949; Parks, 1956). In a review of 20 dissections, Walls (1958) makes the point that none of these mucosal boundaries is at the same level at all places around the circumference of the canal wall. As a result, longitudinal sections through the same canal often show different epithelial relationships, and this may account for much of the confusion in the literature.

Development

The rectum/anal canal develops in part from the posterior section of the endodermal cloaca, and partly from the anal pit, which is ectodermal in origin. The cloaca and pit are separated by the posterior part of the cloacal membrane, and much has been written about the fate of the anal membrane. Ball (1894) clearly regarded the anal valves as vestigial remnants of the anal membrane, and wrote 'I think it may, with tolerable confidence, be asserted that the anal valves are vestigial remains of the anal plate, the rest of which has disappeared in the process of development'. Milligan *et al.* (1937) are emphatic in adopting the anal valves as the adult site of the anal membrane. Henrich (1980) regards it as 'probable' that the two germ layers meet at the proctodeal membrane, whereas Johnson admits that the line of demarcation in the adult 'cannot be definitely located', but claims that it is 'undoubtedly somewhere in the neighbourhood of the linea ano-cutanea' (Johnson, 1914, p. 40), a boundary which is often distal to the anal valves.

Nobles (1984) has recently reviewed the development of the anal canal and the fate of the anal membrane in a series of 29 human embryos ranging from 13.5 to 135 mm CRL. This study confirmed that the anal membrane broke down at a stage when the epithelial lining of the developing canal was homomorphic and thus before there were any signs of anal valves or columns. The anatomical relationships that these early stages bear to the adult form is only approximate because the sphincters appear to migrate through the region during their development; the external growing upwards, and the internal sphincter moving distally. The anal columns make their first appearance at about 30 mm, and, together with the valves, are well developed by 45 mm CRL. At the 35 mm stage there is already admixture of epithelial types, and this area of admixture gradually expands to occupy about 15 mm of the canal lining, to run from the upper boundary of the pecten to the junction with rectal-type mucosa. There was no evidence that islands of squamous epithelium in this region are due to stratified epithelium creeping proximally (Krafka, 1940; Jit, 1975). Instead, Nobles (1984) suggests that the attachment of the anal membrane undergoes differentially rapid growth and enlarges in area to become, in the adult, the whole of the 15 mm, or so, of the anal transitional zone (ATZ). That the zone is the site of overlapping distributions of endocrine cells from above (Fenger and Lyon, 1982), and melanin-containing cells from below (Duthie and Gairns, 1960; Fenger and Lyon, 1982) also lends some support to the suggestion that the whole of the ATZ represents the endoderm–ectoderm boundary. A recent light and electron microscopic analysis of a more restricted definition of the 'transitional zone', in this case a band of epithelium situated well above the level of the anal valves, has concluded that the ultrastructural characteristics of the area are closest to cloacal epithelium (Devaux et al., 1982). However, this does not necessarily contradict the suggestions cited above, for the area analysed may well be at the proximal limit of the epithelium which most authors consider to make up the transitional band of epithelium.

Musculature

Smooth

The general distribution of smooth muscle in the rectum is typical for the gut; that is, there is a modest muscularis mucosae, and inner circular and outer longitudinal layers of muscle.

In the rectum, the circular muscle takes part in the formation of the folds, or valves, of Houston. At the perineal flexure of the rectum, the thickness of circular muscle increases to form the internal sphincter which extends distally for about 30 mm, so that this makes up the innermost layer of the muscular wall of the anal canal for the proximal 30 mm of its 40 mm long course. The sphincter is up to 5 mm wide (Wilde, 1949) and is made up of dense bundles of smooth muscle fibres which are separated by fascicles which run obliquely at the proximal and distal ends of the muscle, and horizontally in its middle part. Lawson claims that the shape and orientation of the bundles changes at the level of the pelvic floor, so that the junction between the internal sphincter and the rectal muscle can be 'readily distinguished' (Lawson, 1974b, p. 292). Most authors regard the internal sphincter as a homogeneous structure, but Lawson (1974b) sees it as being divided into a proximal and a distal part by a fibromuscular bundle containing both smooth and striated muscle.

The junction between the sigmoid colon and the rectum is marked by rearrangement of the longitudinal muscle. Although the sigmoid colon is completely clothed in longitudinal muscle, on its anterior, posterolateral and posteromedial aspects the longitudinal muscle is particularly thick, where it is known as the taenia coli. As the junction with the rectum is approached, the muscle becomes more diffuse and, around the rectum, the longitudinal layer is concentrated into broad bands situated on the anterior and posterior walls of the rectum, and strands of fibres connect these bands with the perineal body and the coccyx (Wesson, 1951). At the anorectal junction the longitudinal muscle blends with inferiorly directed fibres of the pubococcygeus (not the puborectalis) to form a conjoined longitudinal muscle layer which splits to pass both sides of the external sphincter, but it is the deeper of the two layers, the one in the plane between it and the internal sphincter, which is the more substantial; this is the so-called intersphincteric plane. The striated fibres contributed by the pubococcygeus rapidly thin out, so that few travel distal to the pectinate line (Wilde, 1949).

Milligan and Morgan (1934) made a special study of the fate of the longitudinal muscle, and concluded that it was concentrated into lateral and medial fasciculi. They called the more substantial medial one the 'anal intermuscular septum' because of its course between the internal sphincter and superficial part of the external sphincter to the mucosal lining. They claimed that this attachment helped to produce the intersphincteric groove which is palpable in the wall of the distal canal in a conscious patient. More recent investigators have been less impressed with the significance of these two particular muscle fascicles, and instead have claimed that the longitudinal muscle ends by dividing into numerous bundles which fan out and pass through both the internal and the external sphincters (Wilde, 1949; Goligher, Leacock and Brossy, 1955; Hughes, 1957). Other workers have made different interpretations of the arrangement of smooth muscle in the subepithelial space. Several authors (Harris, 1928; Fine and Lawes, 1940; Hughes, 1957) have drawn attention to the existence and arrangement of the muscularis mucosae in the middle and distal part of the canal; Harris (1928) claims that the density of the muscularis mucosae increases as the amount of longitudinal muscle in the subepithelial space becomes attenuated. Fine and Lawes (1940) claim that the muscularis mucosae is especially concentrated beneath the pecten and at the level of the anal valves, where it is identified as a separate muscle, the 'muscularis mucosae ani'. Parks (1956) offers yet a different interpretation and terminology, and calls the smooth muscle fibres inserted at the valvular level the 'mucosal suspensory ligament' and claims that the muscularis mucosae is reinforced by smooth muscle fibres and fascia from the internal sphincter: Hughes (1957) and Parks (1956) should be consulted for useful reviews.

Striated

The external sphincter complex of muscles is phylogenetically derived from the posterior part of the cloacal sphincter. The division of the external anal sphincter into three layers, or bundles, of circumferentially arranged fibres can be traced back to Santorini in 1715, and this has become the conventional classification (Thompson, 1899; Milligan and Morgan, 1934; Milligan *et al.*, 1937; Gabriel, 1945; Gorsch, 1955; Hughes, 1957). The subcutaneous part of the sphincter is classically regarded as a multifascicular ring of muscle which has no distinct ventral or dorsal attachments. The superficial part is an elliptical muscle, attached posteriorly to the coccyx, and helping to form the most superficial layer of the postanal plate (Wendell-Smith, 1967). The deep part of the sphincter is regarded by many authors as being intimately related to the puborectalis (see above), and there is general agreement that while its fibres usually fail to make contact with the coccyx, they do decussate anteriorly to blend with the perineal muscles.

Many recent investigators have, however, abandoned the trilaminar classification in favour of a scheme which regards the external sphincter as basically divided into superficial and deep compartments; the superficial incorporating the old 'sub-cutaneous' and 'superficial' components, and the deep combining the old 'deep' part with puborectalis (Courtney, 1950; Goligher, Leacock and Brossy, 1955; Walls, 1963; Oh and Kark, 1972; Lawson, 1974b). Oh and Kark (1972), who provide a balanced and useful review of this debate, also stress, as did Gabriel (1945), that there are sex differences in the form of the external sphincter, and the former authors emphasize that the form of the sphincter varies from one aspect of the wall of the anal canal to another.

Of more recent reviews of the external sphincter, those of Shafik (1975) and Ayoub (1979b) are the most idiosyncratic in their interpretation. Shafik (1975) based his conclusions on a histological and dissection study of 18 cadavers, and rejects the description of the sphincter as predominantly circumferential, in favour of regarding it as a series of three loops. The top loop, he proposed, is made up of the deep part of the external sphincter and the puborectalis, and its limbs are attached to the pubis; the middle one is made of the 'midportion' of the sphincter and is attached to the coccyx, and the base loop comprises the lower portion of the sphincter, and, while its limbs are shown attached to the perineal body, the base loop is acknowledged to include some circumferential fibres. Ayoub commented on the 'great degree of variation' between specimens, but differs from other authors by rejecting *any* subdivision of the external sphincter into component parts, and by claiming that at all levels the fibres of the sphincter 'run transversely and terminate posteriorly at the anococcygeal ligament to the coccyx' (Ayoub, 1979b, p. 33).

Several conclusions emerge from this review of what seems at first glance to be a series of irreconcilable descriptions of the same structures. First, there are the effects of differences in age and sex, and the extent of individual variation. Secondly, there is the realization that a single diagram of structures seen in one plane only cannot hope to represent the complexity of the striated muscle around the terminal part of the alimentary tract.

The functional integration of the smooth and striated muscle of the anal canal will be dealt with in Chapters 2 and 3, but Schuster (1975) and Duthie (1982) provide excellent reviews of the reflex connections of the muscles, as well as of their roles in maintaining continence and in defaecation.

Innervation

Sensory

Knowledge about the nature and functional correlations of the nerve endings in the human anal canal and rectum comes from a series of investigations which have been well reviewed as part of a major study by Duthie and Gairns (1960); Gould (1960) and Kadanoff and Cuckov (1965) have also provided important evidence.

In the rectal mucosa there are abundant beaded, non-myelinated, nerve fibres, but only one recognizable intra-epithelial receptor ending was identified (Duthie and Gairns, 1960), and this pattern of nerve supply persists down to about 10 or 15 mm above the anal valves. It has always been tacitly assumed that the receptors responsible for detecting rectal distension lie in the rectal wall. However, experiments in patients who had undergone colo-anal anastomosis showed that internal sphincter reflexes were intact, thus suggesting that the receptors must lie outside the rectal wall, perhaps in the pelvic fascia or musculature (Scharli and Kiesewetter, 1970; Lane and Parks, 1977). Textbooks are unanimous that whereas the sensation of rectal distension travels with the pelvic splanchic nerves to S2 and S3, nociceptive information travels in both the parasympathetic and the sympathetic systems. The pathway for the latter is via the inferior and superior hypogastric plexuses, and the network around the inferior mesenteric artery to the sympathetic chain; the ganglion cells lie at L1 and L2. However, it must be said that there is little evidence in the literature to substantiate such confident statements about the pathways of the two modalities.

From about 10–15 mm above the valves, down to the boundary with hairy skin, the epithelium has a rich sensory nerve supply made up of both free and organized nerve endings. Some of these are recognizable as Meissner's corpuscles, genital corpuscles, Golgi–Mazzoni bodies and Krause end-bulbs, but many others are present which cannot be readily allocated to these categories (Duthie and Gairns, 1960; Gould, 1960). A few large Pacinian corpuscles have been identified, but these are found deeper in the wall, close to the smooth muscle of the internal sphincter (Walls, 1958; Gould, 1960). There is some disagreement about the relative concentration of the endings in different parts of the canal. Duthie and Gairns (1960) and Gould (1960) found that free and encapsulated nerve endings were more numerous in the region of the valves, yet Kadanoff and Cuckov (1965) report that two-thirds of the receptors they recorded lay in the region of the pecten. The sensory endings in the hairy perianal skin are similar to those in hairy skin elsewhere.

Duthie and Gairns (1960) were able to correlate their histological findings with sensory stimulation experiments, and showed that touch, pin-prick and heat and cold stimuli were readily perceived in the anal canal to a level 2.5–15 mm above the anal valves. The level of the demarcation line varied from one aspect of the canal to another, and for different modalities. The extension of this somatic-type sensitivity above the valves has already been referred to in connection with proposals that the valves mark the limit of the ectodermal contribution to the anal canal. The sensitivity of this region of the canal had been postulated as a mechanism to aid continence by discriminating between fluid, faeces, etc. (Duthie and Bennett, 1963), but recent studies have shown that application of surface anaesthetic agents to this area did not interfere with patients' ability to retain fluid in the rectum (Read and Read, 1982).

The constant tonic contraction of the external sphincter, and its integrated response to raised intra-abdominal pressure, imply that it must possess a mechanism for measuring muscle length and, indeed, Gould (1960) has reported the presence of a sparse population of muscle spindles, but Schrøder and Reske-Nielsen (1983) were unable to identify spindles in their study of seven sphincters (see Chapter 8).

Motor

It is customary to regard the autonomic and somatic nervous systems as separate entities, and their respective connections with the rectum and anal canal will be discussed separately in this review. However, note should be taken of evidence which suggests that structures in this region may have central connections in both major subdivisions of the nervous system. Laux, Marchal and Thevenet (1955) reported that, in their study of the chimpanzee, the nervi erigentes gave a constant branch to supply the external anal sphincter, and studies in the rat suggest that striated cloacal musculature may be under the control of two populations of neurons in the lumbar cord (Schrøder, 1980).

Functionally, the most important part of the smooth musculature of the rectum and anal canal is the internal sphincter, for it is apparently responsible for about 85 per cent of the resting pressure in the lumen of the canal (Frenckner and Euler, 1975). The classical studies of Denny-Brown and Robertson (1935) showed that the sphincter was under inhibitory as well as positive motor control. Frenckner and Ihre (1976) considered that internal sphincter tone is controlled only by sympathetic, i.e. hypogastric, pathways, but Meunier and Mollard (1977) have shown that sacral parasympathetic pathways are also involved, and clinical evidence supports this (Gunterberg et al., 1976). A dual excitatory pathway for the internal sphincter has also been demonstrated in the vervet monkey (Rayner, 1979), but comparative studies suggest that there is considerable species variation in the location of the ganglion cells in the sympathetic pathway (Costa and Furness, 1973). The inhibition brought about by rectal distension (the recto-anal inhibitory reflex) was previously regarded as being under exclusively parasympathetic control via the sacral nerves. However, more recent evidence from both physiological studies and studies of the function of patients with congenital abnormalities suggests that the reflex is predominantly an intramural one (Meunier and Mollard, 1977), although it is subject to some sacral control (Shepherd and Wright, 1968).

The cell bodies of the neurons controlling the striated muscle in the external anal sphincter lie at S2 in the ventral horn of the spinal cord (Onuf, 1901; Mannen et al., 1977; Schrøder, 1981; Mannen et al., 1982). These neurons (known eponymously as Onuf's nucleus) have been most extensively studied in the rat, cat and dog where there is evidence of topographical localization (Schrøder, 1980; Kuzuhara, Kanazawa and Nakanishi, 1980), and in man and the monkey there is evidence that there is cross-over of fibres so that unilateral transection of the motor fibres does not abolish tonic discharge (Wunderlich and Swash, 1983).

The motor fibres to the human external sphincter travel in the pudendal nerve (S2 and S3) and the perineal branch of S4; Shafik (1975) claims that the latter innervates the fibres he includes in his 'intermediate' loop.

Vasculature

The major arterial blood supply to the rectum and anal canal is provided by the superior and inferior rectal arteries. The middle rectal artery also supplies this part of the bowel, but the extent and significance of its contribution has been a matter of debate, some authors regarding it as relatively insignificant (Drummond, 1913; Steward and Rankin, 1933; Gabriel, 1945; Michels et al., 1965), while others consider that it plays a more important role in the blood supply of this region (Griffiths, 1956; Morgan and Griffiths, 1959; Griffiths, 1961; Thomson, 1975).

The superior rectal artery is the direct continuation of the inferior mesenteric artery and it begins as that artery passes over the left common iliac vessel. It travels in the root of the sigmoid mesocolon, and gives off sigmoid, rectosigmoid and upper rectal branches before it divides at the level of S3 into right and left branches which descend on either side of the distal part of the rectum. Each vessel breaks up into a series of smaller arteries which extend down beyond the level of the anorectal ring approximately to the level of the valves; an average of five branches of the superior rectal artery reach to this level (Thomson, 1975). Foster, Lancaster and Leaper (1984) report that the two collateral vessels each give off an anterior and a posterior branch. Ayoub (1978) claims that there are no extramural anastomoses between the two collateral branches of the superior rectal vessel, and the paucity of vessels on the anterior and posterior walls has been advanced as the reason for the high leak rate of low anterior resections (Lancaster, Foster and Leaper, in press). In a *post mortem* injection study, a paucity of midline vessels was demonstrated in seven out of 12 specimens; three showed the anterior wall to be deficient, and in four specimens it was the posterior wall (Foster, Lancaster and Leaper, 1984). Mucosal branches of the superior rectal arteries are said to run in the columns of Morgagni, with those vessels in the left lateral and the right posterior and right anterior quadrants being particularly well developed (Gabriel, 1945) (see below).

The most recent detailed study of the incidence of the middle rectal artery (Ayoub, 1978) showed that a vessel of 'appreciable diameter (1–2 mm)' (Ayoub, 1978, p. 322) was found bilaterally in 5 per cent of 42 cadavers investigated, with such a vessel being present on one side only in a further 7 per cent of specimens. In these cases there was an inverse relationship between the size of the superior and middle rectal vessels. However, in 70 per cent of a similar-sized injection series (50 adult cadavers) 'substantial branches of one or both middle rectal arteries could also be traced into the anal submucosa' (Thomson, 1975, p. 545).

The inferior rectal arteries are branches of the internal pudendal artery, which cross the ischiorectal fossa, divide, and then send their branches through the external anal sphincter to reach the distal part of the canal. The branches then run proximally in the submucosa.

Reports about the extent of anastomoses between the arterial supply to the rectum and anal canal vary in their conclusions; Ayoub (1978) discounts the presence of extramural connections, which have been reported by others (Michels *et al.*, 1965), but Moiseev and Prokhorova (1983) support Ayoub (1978) in his conclusion that there are relatively rich intramural anastomoses between the superior and inferior rectal vessels. Neither study could demonstrate the sort of rich anastomoses with the middle rectal artery that Morgan and Griffiths (1959) reported. Other vessels, such as the median sacral and the inferior vesical arteries, take part in the supply of the rectum, but their contribution is small and variable. Whatever the anatomical arrangement of the vasculature, there is abundant clinical evidence that much of the rectum and the anal canal can survive the division of both the superior and middle rectal arteries (e.g. Goligher, 1949).

The venous drainage of the rectum and anal canal is via veins that run with the main arterial supply. There is no evidence that the submucous veins of the distal part of the anal canal have any special connection with the portal circulation via the superior rectal vein and there appears to be free anastomosis between the venous channels.

Important advances in our understanding of the clinical anatomy of haemorrhoids have been made in the past decade or so. There is now good clinical data to confirm that there is no association between haemorrhoids and portal hypertension (Hunt, 1958; Johansen, Bardin and Orloff, 1980; Bernstein, 1983), and Thomson (1975) has demonstrated that there is free communication between the main veins draining the anal canal. However, an important step towards understanding the pathophysiology of haemorrhoids came when Stelzner and his colleagues demonstrated the presence of cavernous vascular tissue, rich in arteriovenous anastomoses, in the submucosa of the anal canal (Stelzner, Staubesand and Machleidt, 1962; Stelzner, 1963); they called this tissue the corpus cavernosum recti. This, they claimed, would explain the bleeding of bright red blood which is seen in patients with haemorrhoids. Bernstein (1983) has emphasized that the concept of vascular tissue in the wall of the anal canal is not a new one, and he shows that reference was made to it in the anatomical literature as long ago as 1826. Nevertheless, Thomson (1975) must be credited with providing the most detailed and painstaking study of this unusual vascular tissue, and others have confirmed its cavernous nature (Guntz *et al.*, 1976), its location around the level of the anal valves and its presence at an early stage in development (Datsun, 1983). Thomson (1975) showed that the vascular tissue (which he termed 'vascular cushions') was concentrated in the '4, 7 and 11' positions in the canal at, or above, the level of the anal valves. Thomson (1975) interprets the columns of Morgagni as being the products of longitudinal clefts in the anal cushions. The cushions are submucosal, and comprise dilated blood vessels (mainly veins), smooth muscle and connective tissue. Thus, the current hypothesis is that haemorrhoids are due to a breakdown in the connective tissue and smooth muscle (Treitz's muscle) which provides support for these cushions. This results in their prolapsing into the lumen of the distal canal (Thomson, 1975, 1981). Further research is required to find out whether the cushions are enlarged prior to, or as a result of, their displacement; however, it is likely that a combination of displacement and enlargements is responsible for raised intra-anal pressure in patients with internal haemorrhoids (Hancock, 1977).

Acknowledgements

I am most grateful to Diane Marson for her help with the preparation of this review, and to Paula Smith for typing the manuscript.

References

AYOUB, S. F. (1978). Arterial supply to the human rectum. *Acta Anatomica*, **100**, 317–327

AYOUB, S. F. (1979a). The anterior fibres of the levator ani muscle in man. *Journal of Anatomy*, **128**, 571–580

AYOUB, S. F. (1979b). Anatomy of the external anal sphincter in man. *Acta Anatomica*, **105**, 25–36

BALL, C. B. (1894). The anal valves, their origin and pathogenic significance. *Matthews Medical Quarterly*, **1**, 191–198

BEERSIEK, F., PARKS, A. G. and SWASH, M. (1979). Pathogenesis of anorectal incontinence. A histometric study of the anal sphincter musculature. *Journal of the Neurological Sciences*, **42**, 111–127

BENNETT, R. C. and DUTHIE, H. L. (1964). The functional importance of the internal anal sphincter. *British Journal of Surgery*, **51**, 355–357

BERNSTEIN, W. C. (1983). What are hemorrhoids and what is their relationship to the portal venous system? *Diseases of the Colon and Rectum*, **26**, 829–834

COSTA, M. and FURNESS, J. B. (1973). The origins of the adrenergic fibres which innervate the internal anal sphincter, the rectum, and other tissues of the pelvic region in the guinea-pig. *Zeitschrift für Anatomie und Entwicklungs-geschichte*, **140**, 129–142

COURTNEY, H. (1950). Anatomy of the pelvic diaphragm and anorectal musculature as related to sphincter preservation in ano-rectal surgery. *American Journal of Surgery*, **79**, 155–173

CRITCHLEY, H. O. D., DIXON, J. S. and GOSLING, J. A. (1980). Comparative study of the periurethral and perianal parts of the human levator ani muscle. *Urologia Internationalis*, **35**, 226–232

DATSUN, I. G. (1983). Construction of the cavernous structures in the human rectum. *Anatomii Gistologii*, **84**, 41–48

DENNY-BROWN, D. and ROBERTSON, G. E. (1935). An investigation of the nervous control of defaecation. *Brain*, **58**, 256–310

DEVAUX, A., LECOMTE, D., PARNAUD, E., BRULE, J., ZEMOUCA, L. and BAUER, P. (1982). Étude en microscopie optique et électronique de la zone transitionelle ana-rectale chez l'homme (a propos de 107 observations). *Gastroenterology and Clinical Biology*, **6**, 177–182

DRUMMOND, H. (1913). The arterial supply of the rectum and pelvic colon. *British Journal of Surgery*, **1**, 677–685

DUTHIE, H. L. (1982). Defaecation and the anal sphincters. *Clinics in Gastroenterology*, **11**, 621–631

DUTHIE, H. L. and BENNETT, R. C. (1963). The relation of the sensation in the anal canal to the functional anal sphincter: a possible factor in anal continence. *Gut*, **4**, 179–182

DUTHIE, H. L. and GAIRNS, F. W. (1960). Sensory nerve endings and sensation in the anal region of man. *British Journal of Surgery*, **47**, 585–595

ELFTMAN, H. O. (1932). The evolution of the pelvic floor of primates. *American Journal of Anatomy*, **51**, 307–346

EWING, M. R. (1954). The white line of Hilton. *Proceedings of the Royal Society of Medicine*, **47**, 525–530

FENGER, C. (1974). The anal epithelium: a review. *Scandinavian Journal of Gastroenterology*, **14**, 114–117

FENGER, C. (1979). The anal transitional zone. *Acta pathologica et microbiologica scandinavica*, Sect. A, **87**, 379–386

FENGER, C. and LYON, H. (1982). Endocrine cells and melanin containing cells in anal canal. *Histochemical Journal*, **14**, 631–639

FINE, J. and LAWES, C. H. W. (1940). On the muscle fibres of the anal submucosa with special reference to the pecten band. *British Journal of Surgery*, **27**, 723–727

FOSTER, M. E., LANCASTER, J. B. and LEAPER, D. J. (1984). Leakage of low rectal anastomosis. An anatomic explanation? *Diseases of the Colon and Rectum*, **27**(3), 157–158

FRENCKNER, B. and EULER, Chr.v. (1975). Influence of pudendal block on the function of the anal sphincters. *Gut*, **16**, 482–489

FRENCKNER, B. and IHRE, T. (1976). Influence of autonomic nerves on the internal anal sphincter. *Gut*, **17**, 306–312

GABRIEL, W. B. (1945). *The Principles and Practices of Rectal Surgery*, 3rd edn. London; H. K. Lewis

GOLIGHER, J. C. (1949). The blood supply to the sigmoid colon and rectum with reference to the technique of rectal resection with restoration of continuity. *British Journal of Surgery*, **37**, 157–162

GOLIGHER, J. C., LEACOCK, A. G. and BROSSY, J.-J. (1955). The surgical anatomy of the anal canal. *British Journal of Surgery*, **43**, 51–61

GORSCH, R. V. (1955). *Proctologic Anatomy*, 2nd edn. Baltimore; Williams and Wilkins

GOULD, R. P. (1960). Sensory innervation of the anal canal. *Nature*, **187**, 337–338

GRAY, H. (1858). *Anatomy Descriptive and Surgical*. London; Parker and Son

GRIFFITHS, J. D. (1956). Surgical anatomy of the blood supply of the distal colon. *Annals of the Royal College of Surgeons of England*, **19**, 241–256

GRIFFITHS, J. D. (1961). Extramural and intramural blood supply of the colon. *British Medical Journal*, **1**, 323–326

GUNTERBERG, B., KEWENTER, J., PETERSEN, I. and STENER, B. (1976). Anorectal function after major resections of the sacrum with bilateral or unilateral sacrifice of sacral nerves. *British Journal of Surgery*, **63**, 546–554

GUNTZ, M., PARNAUD, E., BERNARD, A., CHOME, J., REGNIER, J. and TOULEMONDE, J. L. (1976). Vascularization sanguine du anal canal. *Bulletin d l'Association anatomistes*, **60**, 527–538

HAMILTON, W. J. and MOSSMAN, H. W. (1972). *Hamilton, Boyd and Mossman's Human Embryology*, 4th edn. Cambridge; Heffer

HANCOCK, B. D. (1977). Internal sphincter and the nature of haemorrhoids. *Gut*, **18**, 651–655

HARRIS, H. A. (1928). Discussion of fistula-in-ano. Some embryological aspects of the problem involved. *Proceedings of the Royal Society of Medicine*, **22**, 1341–1350

HENRICH, M. (1980). Clinical topography of the proctodeum. *Acta Anatomica*, **106**, 161–170

HERRMANN, G. (1880). Sur la structure et le développment de la muqueuse anale. *Journal de l'anatomie et de la physiologie normales et pathologiques de l'homme et des animaux*, **16**, 434–472

HOLL, M. (1881). Uber den Verschluss des männlichen Beckens. *Archiv für Anatomie und Physiologie*, Leipzig, Anat. Abt., 225–271

HOLL, M. (1896). Zur Homologie und Phylogenese der Muskeln des Beckenausgangs des Menschen. *Anatomischer Anzeiger*, **12**, 57–71

HOLL, M. (1897). Die Muskeln und Fascien des Beckenausganges, in *Handbuch der Anatomie des Menschen* (*von Bardeleben*). Jena; Justav Fischer

HUGHES, E. S. R. (1957). Surgical anatomy of the anal canal. *Australian and New Zealand Journal of Surgery*, **26**, 48–55

HUNT, A. H. (1958). *A Contribution to the Study of Portal Hypertension*. Edinburgh; Livingstone

JIT, I. (1975). Creeping epithelium of the human anal canal. *Indian Journal of Medical Research*, **63**, 411–416

JOHANSEN, K., BARDIN, J. and ORLOFF, M. J. (1980). Massive bleeding from hemorrhoidal varices in portal hypertension. *Journal of the American Medical Association*, **244**, 2084–2085

JOHNSON, F. P. (1914). The development of the rectum in the human embryo. *American Journal of Anatomy*, **16**, 1–57

KADANOFF, D. and CUCKOV, C. (1965). Uber die afferente Innervation des canalis (Pars) analis beim menschen. *Zeitschrift für microskopisch-anatomische Forschung*, **73**, 117–144

KRAFKA, J. (1940). The creeping epithelium of the human anal canal. *American Journal of Surgery*, **49**, 42–68

KUZUHARA, S., KANAZAWA, I. and NAKANISHI, T. (1980). Topographical localisation of the Onuf's nuclear neurons innervating the rectal and vescical striated sphincter muscles: a retrograde fluorescent double labeling in cat and dog. *Neuroscience Letters*, **16**, 125–130

LANCASTER, J. F., FOSTER, M. E. and LEAPER, D. J. (in press). Clinical implications of rectal arterial blood supply. *Annals of the Royal College of Surgeons of England*

LANE, R. H. S. and PARKS, A. G. (1977). Function of the anal sphincter following colo-anal anastomosis. *British Journal of Surgery*, **64**, 596–599

LAUX, G., MARCHAL, G. and THEVENET, A. (1955). Constance sur quatre preparations chez le chimpanze du remeau, du sphincter anal provenant des nerfs erecteurs. *Compte rendu de l'Association des anatomistes*, **42**, 874–878

LAWSON, J. O. N. (1974a). Pelvic anatomy. I Pelvic floor muscles. *Annals of the Royal College of Surgeons*, **54**, 244–252

LAWSON, J. O. N. (1974b). Pelvic anatomy. II Anal canal and associated sphincters. *Annals of the Royal College of Surgeons of England*, **54**, 288–300

MANNEN, T., IWATA, M., TOYOKURA, Y. and NAGASHIMA, K. (1977). Preservation of a certain motoneuron group of the sacral cord in amyotrophic lateral sclerosis: its clinical significance. *Journal of Neurology, Neurosurgery and Psychiatry*, **40**, 464–469

MANNEN, T., IWATA, M., TOYOKURA, Y. and NAGASHIMA, K. (1982). The Onuf's nucleus and the external anal sphincter muscles in amyotrophic lateral sclerosis and Shy–Drager syndrome. *Acta Neuropathologica*, Berlin, **58**, 255–260

MERKEL, F. (1900). Pars ampullaris recti. *Ergebnisse der Anatomie und Entwicklungsgeschichte*, **10**, 524–546

MEUNIER, P. and MOLLARD, P. (1977). Control of the internal anal sphincter (manometric study with human subjects). *Pflügers Archiv*, **370**, 233–239

MICHELS, N. A., SIDDARTH, P., KORNBLITH, P. L. and PARK, W. W. (1965). The variant blood supply to the descending colon, rectosigmoid and rectum based on 400 dissections. Its importance in regional dissections: a review of medical literature. *Diseases of the Colon and Rectum*, **8**, 251–278

MILLIGAN, E. T. C. and MORGAN, C. N. (1934). Surgical anatomy of the anal canal. *Lancet*, **2**, 1150–1156; 1213–1217

MILLIGAN, E. T. C., MORGAN, C. N., JONES, L. E. and OFFICER, R. (1937). Surgical anatomy of the anal canal and the operative treatment of haemorrhoids. *Lancet*, **2**, 1119–1124

MOISEEV, A. Yu and PROKHOROVA, T. P. (1983). Sources of blood supply to the rectum after ligation of the superior rectal artery. *Vêstnik khirurgii*, **130**, 64–66

MORGAN, C. N. and GRIFFITHS, J. D. (1959). High ligation of the inferior mesenteric artery during operations for carcinoma of the distal colon and rectum. *Surgery, Gynecology and Obstetrics*, **108**, 641–650

NIVATVONGS, S., STERN, H. S. and FRYD, D. S. (1981). The length of the anal canal. *Diseases of the Colon and Rectum*, **24**, 600–601

NOBLES, V. P. (1984). The development of the human anal canal. *Journal of Anatomy*, **138**, 575

OELRICH, T. M. (1978). Pelvic and perineal anatomy of the male gorilla: selected observations. *Anatomical Record*, **191**, 433–446

OH, C. and KARK, A. E. (1972). Anatomy of the external anal sphincter. *British Journal of Surgery*, **59**, 717–723

ONUF, B. (1901). On the arrangement and function of the cell groups of the sacral region of the spinal cord in man. *Archives of Neurology and Psychopathology*, Chicago, **3**, 387–412

PADYKULA, H. A. and HERMAN, A. (1955). The specificity of the histochemical method for adenosine triphosphatase. *Journal of Histochemistry and Cytochemistry*, **3**, 170–195

PARAMORE, R. H. (1910). The Hunterian lectures on the evolution of the pelvic floor in non-mammalian vertebrates and pronograde mammals. *Lancet*, **1**, 1393–1399; 1459–1467

PARKS, A. G. (1956). The surgical treatment of haemorrhoids. *British Journal of Surgery*, **43**, 337–351

PARKS, A. G., SWASH, M. and URICH, H. (1977). Sphincter denervation in anorectal incontinence and rectal prolapse. *Gut*, **18**, 656–665

PAULET, M. (1876). Conclusions d'un mémoire sur l'anatomie comparée du perinée. *J. Zool. P. Gervais* (cited by Holl, 1897)

PAULET, M. (1877). Recherches sur l'anatomie comparée du perinée. *Journal of Anatomy*, Paris, **13**, 144–180

PERCY, J. P., NEILL, M. E., SWASH, M. and PARKS, A. (1981). Electrophysiological study of motor nerve supply of pelvic floor. *Lancet*, **1**, 16–17

PORTER, N. H. (1962). A physiological study of the pelvic floor in rectal prolapse. *Annals of the Royel College of Surgeons of England*, **31**, 379–404

RAYNER, V. (1979). Characteristics of the internal anal sphincter and the rectum of the vervet monkey. *Journal of Physiology*, **286**, 383–399

READ, M. G. and READ, N. W. (1982). The role of anorectal sensation in preserving continence. *Gut*, **23**, 345–347

ROBIN and CADIAT (1874). Sur la structure et les rapports des téguments au niveau de leur jonction dans les régions anale, vulvaire et du col utérin. *Journal de l'anatomie et de la physiologie normales et pathologiques de l'homme et des animaux*, **16**, 434–472

SATO, K. (1980). A morphological analysis of the nerve supply of the sphincter ani externus, levator ani and coccygeus. *Acta anatomica nipponica*, **55**, 187–223

SCHARLI, A. F. and KIESEWETTER, W. B. (1970). Defecation and continence: some new concepts. *Diseases of the Colon and Rectum*, **13**, 81–107

SCHRØDER, H. D. (1980). Organisation of the motor neurons innervating the pelvic muscles of the male rat. *Journal of Comparative Neurology*, **192**, 567–587

SCHRØDER, H. D. (1981). Onuf's nucleus X: a morphological study of a human spinal nucleus. *Anatomy and Embryology*, **162**, 443–453

SCHRØDER, H. D. and RESKE-NIELSEN, E. (1983). Fiber types in the striated urethral and anal sphincters. *Acta Neuropathologica*, Berlin, **60**, 278–282

SCHUSTER, M. M. (1975). The riddle of the sphincters. *Gastroenterology*, **69**, 249–262

SHAFIK, A. (1975). A new concept of the anatomy of the anal sphincter mechanism and the physiology of defecation. The external anal sphincter: a triple-loop system. *Investigative Urology*, **12**, 412–419

SHEPHERD, J. J. and WRIGHT, P. J. (1968). The response of the internal anal sphincter in man to stimulation of the presacral nerve. *American Journal of Digestive Diseases*, **13**, 421–427

STELZNER, F. (1960). Uber die Anatomie des analen sphincterorgans wie sie der Chirurg sieht. *Zeitschrift für Anatomie und Entwicklungs-geschicht*, **121**, 525–535

STELZNER, F. (1963). Die Hamorrhoiden und andere Krankheiten des corpus cavernosum recti und des anal Kanals. *Deutsche medizinische Wochenschrift*, **88**, 689–696

STELZNER, F., STAUBESAND, J. and MACHLEIDT, H. (1962). Das corpus cavernosum recti: die grundlate der inneren hammorrhoiden. *Archiv für Klinische Chirurgia*, **299**, 302–312

STEPHENS, F. D. and DURHAM-SMITH, E. (1971). *Ano-rectal Malformations in Children*. Chicago; Year Book Medical Publishers

STEWARD, J. A. and RANKIN, F. W. (1933). Blood supply of the large intestine: its surgical consideration. *Archives of Surgery*, Chicago, **26**, 843–891

STRAUS-DURCKHEIM, H. (1845). *Anatomie descriptive et comparative du chat*. Paris (cited by Wendell-Smith, 1967)

STROUD, B. B. (1896). On the anatomy of the anus. *Annals of Surgery*, **24**, 1–15

SYMINGTON, J. (1889). The rectum and anus. *Journal of Anatomy*, London, **23**, 106–115

THOMPSON, P. (1899). *The Myology of the Pelvic Floor: A Contribution to Human and Comparative Anatomy*. London; McCorquodale

THOMSON, W. H. (1975). The nature of haemorrhoids. *British Journal of Surgery*, **62**, 542–552

THOMSON, W. H. (1981). The anatomy and nature of piles, in *The Haemorrhoid Syndrome*, pp. 15–33 (H. D. Kaufman, Ed.). Tunbridge Wells; Abacus

UHLENHUTH, E. (1953). *Problems in the Anatomy of the Pelvis*. Philadelphia; Lippincott

WALLS, E. W. (1958). Observations on the microscopic anatomy of the human anal canal. *British Journal of Surgery*, **45**, 504–512

WALLS, E. W. (1963). Anorectal anatomy, in *The Scientific Basis of Medicine—Annual Reviews*, pp. 113–124. London; Athlone Press

WENDELL-SMITH, C. P. (1963). Adaptions of anal musculature. *Journal of Anatomy*, London, **97**, 489

WENDELL-SMITH, C. P. (1964). The homologues of the puborectalis muscle. *Journal of Anatomy*, London, **98**, 489

WENDELL-SMITH, C. P. (1967). Studies on the morphology of the pelvic floor. *Ph.D. thesis*, University of London

WENDELL-SMITH, G. P. and WILSON, P. M. (1977). In *Scientific Foundations of Obstetrics and Gynaecology*, pp. 78–84 (E. E. Philipp, J. Barnes and M. Newton, Eds). London; Heinemann

WESSON, M. B. (1951). Rationale of prostactectomy. *American Journal of Surgery*, **82**, 714–719

WILDE, F. R. (1949). The anal intermuscular septum. *British Journal of Surgery*, **36**, 279–285

WILSON, P. M. (1973a). Understanding the pelvic floor. *South African Medical Journal*, **47**, 1150–1167

WILSON, P. M. (1973b). Some observations on pelvic floor evolution in primates. *South African Medical Journal*, **47**, 1203–1209

WUNDERLICH, M. and SWASH, M. (1983). The overlapping innervation of the two sides of the external anal sphincter by the pudendal nerves. *Journal of the Neurological Sciences*, **59**, 97–109

Chapter 2

Physiology and pharmacology of the internal anal sphincter

D. E. Burleigh and A. D'Mello

Introduction

Faecal incontinence causes social and medical problems (Parks, 1975; *Lancet*, 1977). There have been many investigations of mechanisms causing anal continence (Schuster, 1968; Duthie, 1971; Stelzner, Baumgarten and Holstein, 1974). A region of high intraluminal pressure found within the anal canal appears to help continence. This pressure results mainly from the activity of two muscles, the internal and external anal sphincters, which form two separate concentric muscle layers encircling the anal canal. The internal anal sphincter (IAS) is composed of circular smooth muscle fibres and is a continuation of the circular muscle layer of the rectum. The boundary between the rectum and IAS is generally accepted as lying at the level of the dentate line. Caudal to this boundary, the thickness of the smooth muscle layer increases (1.5–5 mm) to form the IAS, which varies in length from 2.5 to 3 cm (Stonesifer, Murphy and Lombardo, 1960; Lawson, 1970).

Innervation

The mechanisms responsible for contraction and relaxation of the sphincter muscle, and the influence of extrinsic and intrinsic autonomic nerves, are important when discussing the physiology and pharmacology of the IAS.

IAS function has been investigated in various ways, for example by *in vivo* studies on patients and volunteers and by *in vitro* experiments with isolated muscle strips of sphincter obtained at operation; such *in vitro* work provides additional information about the types of receptors and nerves that might be involved in the motility of the sphincter *in vivo*. Useful information has also arisen from various studies on animals.

Histological examination of IAS muscle has revealed several differences between the sphincter and large intestine in neural organization. E. R. Howard (personal communication) did not find any ganglion cells within the sphincter. Aldridge and Campbell (1968) and Weinberg (1970) found ganglion cells sparsely distributed in the region of the anal canal. Finally, in a comparison of the innervation of the human colon with the IAS, Baumgarten, Holstein and Stelzner (1971, 1973) made the following points:

1. Intrinsic nerve cell perikarya were absent in Auerbach's and Meissner's plexus of the most distal portion of the anal canal.
2. The number of processes of intrinsic neuronal perikarya gradually decreased in the proximal IAS, with virtually none in the distal part of the muscle.
3. More nerve fibres were found innervating the smooth muscle cells of the IAS than the colon. There was twice the concentration of the sympathetic neurotransmitter, noradrenaline, in the IAS than in the colon.

The IAS receives its sympathetic innervation via the hypogastric nerves from the fifth lumbar segment and its parasympathetic supply via the pelvic nerves from the first, second and third sacral segments (Schuster, 1968). According to ideas discussed by Gaskell (1920), the sympathetic nerves would be expected to be excitatory, and the parasympathetic inhibitory to the sphincter. The opposite occurs with non-sphincteric gastrointestinal muscle. Evidence for this theory is incomplete. For instance, when Gaskell first proposed his theory the only evidence for excitatory sympathetic motor nerves to the IAS came from a study using cats, and there was no evidence indicating an inhibitory function for parasympathetic nerves in this or any other sphincter, human or animal.

Since Gaskell proposed his idea, results from both *in vivo* and *in vitro* studies have shown that sympathetic nerve stimulation or the sympathetic neurotransmitter, noradrenaline, contract the IAS. Thus, Rankin and Learmonth (1930) stimulated the peripheral end of cut presacral nerves in a young anaesthetized woman and detected strong contractions of the IAS, indicating that the thoracolumbar outflow provides an excitatory motor supply to this muscle. Shepherd and Wright (1968) were unable to confirm these observations. They reported that stimulation of the presacral nerves in patients caused sphincter relaxation, which was unaffected by atropine 1 mg. These authors were not convinced that adrenergic nerves have an inhibitory function in the IAS, because the presacral outflow might contain functionally mixed nerves rather than just adrenergic fibres, and the concentration of atropine in tissues might have been less than that needed to block a cholinergic effect. Also, it is doubtful that normal responses could be expected from their 11 subjects who were suffering from Hirschsprung's disease.

A study by Frenckner and Ihre (1976) on the influence of autonomic nerves on the IAS confirmed the observation made by Rankin and Learmonth (1930). Eight subjects receiving high spinal anaesthesia (T_6–T_{12}) and five subjects receiving low anaesthesia (S_5–S_1) were investigated; the results were compared with those of an earlier study (Frenckner and Euler, 1975) where 10 healthy subjects had pudendal nerve block, which paralysed the external sphincter without affecting the autonomic nerve supply to the internal sphincter. They concluded that, at rest, there is a tonic excitatory sympathetic discharge to the IAS, and if this is abolished, anal pressure falls by nearly 50 per cent. This excitatory effect is not present when the sphincter is relaxed after rectal distension. There is also pharmacological evidence that IAS tone is partly due to continuous sympathetic nerve activity (Gutierrez and Shah, 1975). Infusions of methoxamine, an α-adrenoceptor agonist, into healthy volunteers consistently increased sphincter pressure. A selective α-adrenoceptor blocker, phentolamine, caused profound inhibition of the IAS tone. Inhibition of basal tone by phentolamine was about 50 per cent, similar to the degree of inhibition found when sympathetic nerve activity was abolished by high spinal anaesthesia.

Low resting anal sphincter pressures have also been found in some individuals suffering from diabetes mellitus (Schiller *et al.*, 1982). Incontinent diabetics had a mean anal sphincter pressure of 37 mmHg, whereas the pressure in the normal subjects was 63 mmHg. External sphincter function appeared to be normal. It was suggested that autonomic neuropathy of the gastrointestinal tract may have also simultaneously affected anal sphincter function in the incontinent diabetics. The nerves affected would probably have been the extrinsic sympathetic adrenergic supply, which contributes towards basal IAS tone. The diarrhoea found in these subjects may also indicate selective impairment of gastrointestinal sympathetic adrenergic nerves. Whether the incontinent diabetics had disturbances in the intrinsic autonomic nerve supply to the IAS is not known, as the potency of the rectosphincteric relaxation reflex was not assessed.

Until 1975, no clear function had been defined for the parasympathetic nerve supply. Then Gutierrez and Shah (1975) established that the infusion of a muscarinic receptor agonist, bethanechol, into volunteers relaxed the IAS, leading to reduced anal pressure. However, other studies have either shown that parasympathetic nerves do not influence tone (Frenckner and Ihre, 1976), or that they are partially responsible for maintaining it (Meunier and Mollard, 1977).

Anal canal pressure

The IAS may be considered to be a typical sphincter of the gastrointestinal tract since it can be differentiated, *in vivo*, from adjacent non-sphincteric areas. It has a higher resting pressure than adjacent non-sphincteric muscle and gives a rapid reflex relaxation in response to an appropriate proximal distant stimulus. Also, relaxation of the sphincter does not depend upon the arrival of a wave of peristalsis from above (Bass *et al.*, 1972).

In situ, the IAS has a high degree of tone; that is, it is normally in a state of permanent contracture, only relaxing in response to rectal distension. The tone is measured as intraluminal pressure within the anal canal and the maximum pressure shows individual variation ranging from 25 to 85 cmH_2O compared with a mean resting rectal pressure of only 2–5 cmH_2O. The high intraluminal pressures recorded from the anal canal are the result of activity of both internal and external sphincters, and perhaps also the puborectalis muscle (Taylor, Beart and Phillips, 1984). The major contribution comes from the IAS, the evidence being the high anal pressures recorded in paraplegics with external sphincter paralysis or in normal subjects with bilateral pudendal nerve block. There was also a marked reduction in anal pressure after total internal sphincterectomy (Schuster, 1968).

When anal continence was assessed dynamically, by rectal infusion of saline, external anal sphincter contractions only occurred with 60 per cent of IAS relaxations and did not prevent the maximum decrease in anal pressure (Haynes and Read, 1982). This suggests that phasic contraction of the external sphincter does not play a major role in maintaining continence; when the IAS relaxes, continence is maintained by a combination of puborectalis muscle and external sphincter tone, residual IAS tone and rapid recovery of maximum IAS tone.

Wheatley, Hardy and Dent (1977) do not think that the IAS is so important in maintaining continence, because they found the IAS contributed much less to anal canal resting pressure. Thus, the pressure was 116 mmHg in normal subjects compared with 63 mmHg in subjects with spinal cord lesions, so the pressure in the latter subjects was halved despite the IAS being intact. The rather high resting pressure recorded in normal subjects may be explained by improved methodology, which utilized perfused sleeve manometry. This technique avoids problems due to mechanical properties of balloons and also of the resistance of sphincters to the presence of balloons. It also avoids inaccuracies of non-perfused water-filled catheters and the displacement of constantly perfused catheters.

Even after sympathetic nerve activity is abolished, the IAS still retains about 50 per cent of its normal basal tone (Gutierrez and Shah, 1975; Frenckner and Ihre, 1976), which is probably myogenic in origin. In the resting state, electrical activity has been recorded from the smooth muscle cells of the IAS. This activity consists of slow sinusoidal waves called basic electrical rhythm (BER). Basic electrical rhythm recorded from the IAS (6–26 c/min) is greater than that of rectal circular smooth muscle (3–6 c/min) and is unaccompanied by spike potentials (Wankling et al., 1968; Ustach et al., 1970; Monges et al., 1980). Despite this lack of spike potential, Gutierrez, Oliai and Chey (1975), using intraluminal pressure recording, found the motility of the IAS was characterized by slow oscillations in pressure with a frequency of 1/min. Superimposed on these manometric ultra-slow oscillations, they recorded small waves with a frequency of 10–20/min. The association of high-frequency BER with high resting pressure and the inhibition of BER with sphincter relaxation suggests that the maintenance of sphincter tone is an active process governed by BER (Bass, Ustach and Schuster, 1972). However, such a myoelectrical control system for IAS could not be demonstrated by Weinbeck and Altaparmacov (1980), who found no relationship between slow-wave frequency or amplitude and absolute sphincter pressure.

Strips of smooth muscle cut from the IAS developed tone (continual state of contraction) that was high compared with circular muscle from the human colon. As tetrodotoxin had no effect on this tone (*Figure 2.1*), it was assumed to be myogenic in origin. Proximal muscle strips usually showed greater spontaneous activity (i.e. rhythmic or irregular contractions and relaxations) than muscle strips from the distal half of the sphincter (Burleigh, D'Mello and Parks, 1979). This spontaneous activity had a frequency of 10–12 contractions/min (Burleigh, unpublished observations), which was in the range of fluctuations in membrane potential.

Rectosphincteric relaxation reflex

This reflex refers to relaxation of the IAS that occurs almost immediately when the rectum or rectosigmoid is distended (Gowers, 1877; Denny-Brown and Robertson, 1935). It is a neurogenic response elicited by stimulation of mechanoreceptors in the rectum; these may also be present to some degree in the sigmoid colon (Schuster, Hendrix and Mendeloff, 1963). Exactly how far up the colon these receptors can be found is obviously important with regard to mechanisms of defaecation. In various animal species, the myenteric plexus of the distal colon shows some unique features, for instance large nerve bundles containing many myelinated nerve fibres. These large nerve bundles or shunt fascicles may be specialized pathways for two-way communication between the distal rectum and sigmoid colon (Christensen et al., 1984). When inflation of a balloon in the distal colon of humans excites relaxation of the IAS, the shunt fascicles could well be the pathways involved. Peristalsis is not involved as, in the few instances where peristalsis is present, the sphincter relaxes at the moment of rectal distension before the peristaltic wave of contraction reaches the sphincter. Rapid intermittent rectal distension causes prolonged relaxation of the IAS, whereas continuous rectal distension initially causes sphincter relaxation, but the muscle gradually returns to its resting tone despite continual rectal distension.

It is generally agreed that the reflex is independent of neural centres higher than the

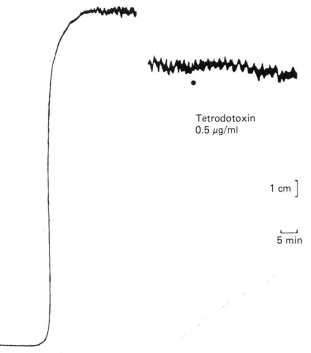

Tetrodotoxin
0.5 µg/ml

1 cm]

⊔
5 min

Figure 2.1. Development of muscle tone by an isolated strip of human internal anal sphincter muscle *in vitro*. The selective blocker of nerve conduction, tetrodotoxin, has no effect on this tone thus indicating its myogenic nature

spinal cord, as it can be obtained in individuals with spinal cord transections. A normal reflex is obtained in patients after hypogastric nerve resections, or after destruction of sacral nerve roots by cauda equina lesions; so Denny-Brown and Robertson (1935) proposed that the reflex is purely intrinsic, that is, located within the bowel wall. Meunier and Mollard (1977) found that, although the reflex depended mainly on the intramural nerve network, its activity could be modulated by the sacral cord. Their evidence for this view is as follows:

1. Shepherd and Wright (1968) stimulated human presacral nerves and obtained IAS relaxation identical to that produced by rectal distension.
2. In subjects with meningocele, the nature of the reflexly induced relaxation became abnormal.
3. No inhibitory reflex was found in individuals suffering from spinal shock.

Histochemical evidence for modulation of the reflex by extrinsic nerve activity comes from an investigation of the myenteric plexus of the distal colon of various species (Christensen *et al.*, 1984). The myenteric nerve fibres in the myenteric plexus could be preganglionic fibres of sacral visceral nerves. These myelinated fibres may be specialized pathways by which central activity can additionally affect certain regions of the colon and thence the sphincter (see above).

Shepherd and Wright (1968) were cautious in interpreting their results because they believed that 'anatomic distinction in the autonomic nervous system has little functional significance beyond certain limits'. Also the relaxation obtained by presacral nerve stimulation was not identical to that produced by rectal distension as it could be obtained in patients with Hirschsprung's disease, whereas rectal distension was ineffective under such circumstances.

The importance of the myenteric nerve plexus for a normal rectosphincteric reflex is shown by studies of bowel function in patients with Hirschsprung's disease (Lawson and Nixon, 1967; Schnaufer et al., 1967; Tobon et al., 1967). In this disorder there are no ganglion cells in variable lengths of the rectum and colon. In such patients, when the rectum was distended recordings of the IAS muscle activity showed that the sphincter did not relax. There is only one report of a normal rectosphincteric relaxation reflex in patients with Hirschsprung's disease (Schuster, Hendrix and Mendeloff, 1963). However, this result might have been due to the cumbersome recording techniques (Schuster, 1968). The rectosphincteric reflex is also abolished if there is an anastomosis of the bowel between the site of distension and the sphincter (Gaston, 1948; Schuster, Hendrix and Mendeloff, 1963), although one report did claim that the reflex could be obtained across an anastomosis and that this was probably due to regeneration of intramural nerves across the anastomosis (Lane and Parks, 1977).

Vesico-anal reflex

As the urethral and anal sphincters receive a common vegetative and somatic innervation by hypogastric (sympathetic), pelvic (parasympathetic) and pudendal (somatic) nerves, it was thought interesting to study anal sphincter function in man during micturition (Salducci, Planche and Naudy, 1982). During micturition, external sphincter electrical activity was totally inhibited, whereas IAS electrical activity was increased. It was concluded, therefore, that IAS activity plays a specific and important functional role in maintaining anal continence during micturition. A similar extrinsic nerve reflex has been described in anaesthetized cats, where strong contractions of the IAS occurred during both urinary bladder compression and spontaneous micturition (Garrett, Howard and Jones, 1974).

Pharmacology of the internal anal sphincter

The high pressure region found in the anal canal is mainly due to contraction of the IAS caused by the high tone of the smooth muscle fibres as well as an excitatory innervation involving sympathetic (thoracolumbar) nerves impinging on α-adrenoceptors. The major reflex response of the muscle is a relaxation thought to be initiated by rectal distension and mediated through intrinsic nerves in the gut wall. However, in vivo studies leave a number of questions unresolved:

1. Do cholinergic nerves or drugs affect IAS motility only indirectly? Gutierrez and Shah (1975) suggested that bethanechol could increase rectal motility, thereby relaxing the IAS by reflex activity.
2. What is the role of β-adrenoceptors? The IAS relaxes when presacral nerves are stimulated (Shepherd and Wright, 1968), and after infusion of isoprenaline (Gutierrez and Shah, 1975).
3. Is the final nerve pathway mediating the rectosphincteric relaxation reflex cholinergic, adrenergic, or is some other type of autonomic fibre involved?

These and other questions relating to drug action on the IAS muscle may be answered by in vitro pharmacological studies using muscle strips, and a complete understanding of normal IAS functions will only be possible through a combination of *in vivo* physiological and *in vitro* pharmacological investigations.

Sympathomimetic amines

The effects of catecholamines on isolated human IAS muscle are well documented (Parks and Fishlock, 1967; Friedmann, 1968; Parks *et al.*, 1969; Ustach and Schuster, 1970; Burleigh, 1978; Burleigh, D'Mello and Parks, 1979; Paskins, Clayden and Lawson, 1982). Muscle strips contract to noradrenaline, give a variable response to adrenaline, and always relax to isoprenaline. Analyses of these responses using the appropriate adrenoceptor antagonists show that sphincter muscle possesses α-adrenoceptors mediating contractions and β-adrenoceptors mediating relaxation. Contractions to noradrenaline can be converted to relaxations by an α-adrenoceptor antagonist such as phenoxybenzamine or phentolamine; these relaxations can be abolished by β-adrenoceptor antagonists such as pronethalol or propranolol. Responses to catecholamines are not affected by the region of sphincter muscle on which they are tested (Friedmann, 1968; Parks *et al.*, 1969). Dopamine contracts sphincter muscle (Burleigh, D'Mello and Parks, 1979), whereas tyramine gives a biphasic response (Burleigh, 1978).

Investigations of the role of adrenoceptors *in vivo* in the human IAS have supported results using isolated muscle strips. Mechanical activity of the IAS was recorded from volunteers and measured as manometric pressure in the anal canal. Infusion of isoprenaline decreased manometric pressure, i.e. it relaxed the sphincter, and this response was abolished by propranolol. Infusion of an α-adrenoceptor agonist, methoxamine, increased sphincter pressure, and this effect was abolished by phentolamine (Gutierrez and Shah, 1975). The different responses to noradrenaline between sphincteric and non-sphincteric muscle appear to be due to a dominant population of excitatory α-adrenoceptors located on the smooth muscle fibres of the IAS. In circular colonic muscle the excitatory α-adrenoceptors are revealed only after blocking β-adrenoceptors (Gagnon, Devroede and Belisle, 1972).

Acetylcholine and bethanechol

Preliminary observations showed that sphincteric muscle was either insensitive to acetylcholine or gave inconsistent responses, including contractions (Parks *et al.*, 1969; Bass, Ustach and Schuster, 1970; Shepherd, 1972). Detailed re-examination of the effects of acetylcholine on sphincter muscle has shown that the drug has a predominantly inhibitory effect (Burleigh, D'Mello and Parks, 1979; Paskins, Clayden and Lawson, 1982) in proximal and distal regions. Bethanechol, a cholinergic agonist that selectively stimulates muscarinic receptors, also relaxed sphincter strips in the majority of cases (Burleigh, D'Mello and Parks, 1979).

Disagreement over the effects of acetylcholine on sphincter muscle may be explained by the different sources of muscle strips. Burleigh, D'Mello and Parks (1979) only obtained muscle strips from operations where the entire anal canal was removed, whereas Parks *et al.* (1969) sometimes obtained distal sphincter muscle from local operative procedures such as haemorrhoidectomy. It is possible that, during the preparation of muscle strips, intrinsic nerves were damaged and resulted in insensitivity and inconsistent responses to electrical field stimulation and acetylcholine. This is particularly relevant because relaxations of sphincter muscle to acetylcholine are mediated partly by nerve stimulation.

The actions of acetylcholine on isolated sphincter muscle are complex. Relaxations to acetylcholine are competitively blocked by hyoscine (Burleigh, D'Mello and Parks, 1979; Paskins, Clayden and Lawson, 1982) and are partly mediated by an effect on intrinsic nerves, because tetrodotoxin could inhibit the response to varying degrees. They are not significantly affected by concentrations of hexamethonium, which antagonized relaxations to nicotine and dimethylphenylpiperazinium, or by concentrations of propranolol that blocked relaxations to isoprenaline (Burleigh, D'Mello and Parks, 1979). They were, however, reduced or abolished by indomethacin (D'Mello, Burleigh and Parks, 1975). There are muscarinic receptors in para-sympathetic and sympathetic ganglia, although in the latter they do not seem essential for normal neurotransmission (Volle and Koelle, 1975). It is doubtful whether the neuronal muscarinic receptors are located on ganglia in the IAS, as there are few if any ganglion cells in the muscle (Aldridge and Campbell, 1968; Weinberg, 1970; Baumgarten, Holstein and Stelzner, 1971, 1973).

A few muscle strips gave a biphasic response (contraction followed by relaxation) to acetylcholine. The contractile phase is small compared with the subsequent relaxation, is not dose related and is due to stimulation of muscarinic receptors on smooth muscle cells, being abolished by hyoscine but unaffected by tetrodotoxin. Direct excitatory effects of acetylcholine are probably best explained by the presence of a small residual population of excitatory muscarinic receptors of the type normally found on the adjacent smooth muscle cells of the circular layer of the rectum (Burleigh, D'Mello and Parks, 1979). A predominantly inhibitory role for sphincter muscarinic receptors has also been demonstrated in an *in vivo* study in which bethanechol decreased sphincter muscle pressure, and this effect was reversed by atropine (Gutierrez and Shah, 1975).

It is difficult to predict the extent to which there is a physiological role for the variety of receptors and mechanisms involved in the action of acetylcholine *in vitro*. For instance, Carpenedo *et al.* (1983) sought a pharmacological treatment for spasm of the IAS, which is frequently associated with anal fissures. They chose caerulein (a CCK-related peptide) as the spasmolytic, because it was known to be very potent in relaxing the sphincter of Oddi. Although caerulein relaxed the IAS *in vitro*, largely by releasing ACh, the compound was inactive *in vivo*. Such inactivity could have been due to fibrosis, caused by the anal fissures, hindering relaxations; or cholinergic neurons may be unimportant in controlling IAS tone. However, in a recent investigation with sphincter muscle removed from children with chronic constipation, cholinergic agonists and electric field stimulation caused contraction rather than relaxation, and the authors concluded that this may explain the poor relaxation of the sphincter after rectal distension (Paskins, Clayden and Lawson, 1982). The muscle strips from the constipated children were obtained by internal anal sphincterotomy, whereas control IAS muscle was obtained from adults undergoing abdominal–perineal resection of the rectum. The sphincterotomy might have caused more trauma to the IAS muscle than the condition of constipation; as a consequence, intrinsic nerves might have been damaged during the operation, resulting in the sphincter muscle strips contracting rather than relaxing to acetylcholine and electrical field stimulation.

To summarize, acetylcholine has a predominantly inhibitory effect on sphincter muscle strips; this response is mediated by muscarinic receptors which seem to be located on both nerve and muscle tissue. Contractions to acetylcholine, when they occur, could be due to stimulation of excitatory muscarinic receptors similar to those found in adjacent rectal circular muscle. The non-adrenergic nerves stimulated by acetylcholine may release prostaglandin E_2; alternatively, the actions of acetylcholine may be enhanced by a prostaglandin (Hedqvist, 1977).

Nicotine and dimethylphenylpiperazinium (DMPP)

These compounds are classified as ganglion stimulants, but sphincter muscle has few, if any, ganglion cells. The effects of both these drugs on sphincter muscle strips are more likely due to actions on nerve axons or terminals. Parks *et al.* (1969) first described the actions on nicotine on the human IAS. Strips from the lower half of the sphincter were insensitive to nicotine, while those from the upper half were relaxed by the drug. The relaxation to nicotine was blocked by hexamethonium, procaine and pronethalol, which suggested that the drug was acting on nerve tissue to release a catecholamine. Friedmann (1968) showed that nicotine usually relaxed proximal sphincter strips, while DMPP usually contracted them; he proposed that, because of a difference in molecular size, the two drugs acted at different sites, one releasing noradrenaline onto inhibitory β-adrenoceptors, the other releasing noradrenaline onto excitatory α-adrenoceptors. Relaxation of sphincter muscle strips by ganglion stimulant drugs was thought either to be due to release of an isoprenaline-like substance (Parks *et al.*, 1969) or to release of noradrenaline in close proximity to inhibitory β-adrenoceptors (Friedmann, 1968). More recent investigations have shown that stimulation of nicotinic receptors relaxes muscle strips from all regions of the sphincter. The idea of noradrenaline release is supported by the observation that when sphincter muscle strips pre-incubated with (^{3}H)-noradrenaline relax to DMPP, there is simultaneous increased release of tritiated (^{3}H) material (Burleigh, 1978).

The actions of acetylcholine, noradrenaline and DMPP on IAS muscle, and for comparison circular muscle strips from the sigmoid colon, are shown in *Figures 2.2* and *2.3*.

Histamine, 5-hydroxytryptamine and prostaglandins

Histamine relaxes sphincter muscle probably by an action on H_1 receptors, as the response is blocked by mepyramine, an H_1 antagonist. 5-Hydroxytryptamine and PG $F_{2\alpha}$ contract sphincter muscle, whereas prostaglandin E_2 relaxes it (Burleigh, D'Mello and Parks, 1979). Continuous release of prostaglandins affects both tone and spontaneous activity of human intestinal muscle strips (Burleigh, 1977). Such an effect on sphincter strips is unlikely because indomethacin, a compound that inhibits prostaglandin synthesis, has no effect on sphincter muscle tone or spontaneous activity. A physiological role for prostaglandins in the IAS cannot be completely discounted, as indomethacin prevented relaxation of sphincter strips to acetylcholine (D'Mello, Burleigh and Parks, 1975).

Morphine and loperamide

The antidiarrhoeal effect of morphine is believed to be caused by an increase in non-propulsive motility of the intestine and contraction of sphincters (Weinstock, 1971). Although it is a typical sphincter, strips from the IAS are not affected by morphine. The drug has no effect on tone and does not prevent the relaxation of muscle strips by nerve stimulation (Burleigh, 1983). Similarly, loperamide, which increases anal canal pressure and the stimulus required to produce the rectosphincteric relaxation reflex (Read, Read and Duthie, 1980), does not increase the tone of muscle strips and only slightly affects relaxation due to field stimulation (McKirdy, 1981). The insensitivity of isolated sphincter muscle to morphine and loperamide indicates that the drugs affect sphincter motility by indirect mechanisms (Stewart, Weisbrodt and Burks, 1978; Burleigh,

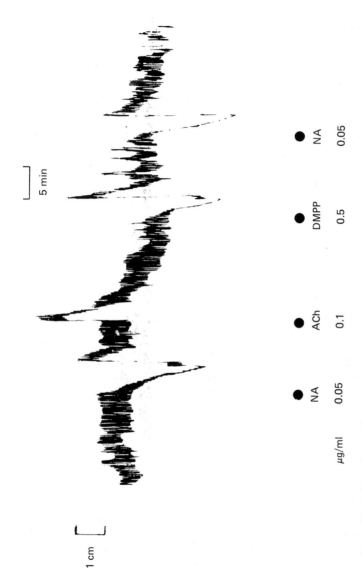

Figure 2.2. Actions of some drugs on isolated circular muscle from the human sigmoid colon. Note relaxations to noradrenaline (NA), contractions to acetylcholine (ACh) and a biphasic response to dimethylphenylpiperazinium (DMPP)

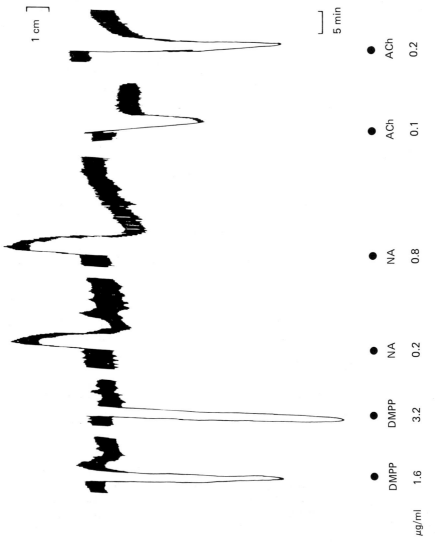

Figure 2.3. Actions of some autonomic drugs on isolated circular muscle from the human internal anal sphincter *in vitro*. Note, in contrast to *Figure 2.2*, contractions to noradrenaline (NA) and relaxations to acetylcholine (ACh). The response to dimethylphenylpiperazinium (DMPP) is changed to relaxation only

Galligan and Burks, 1981) which are absent in *in vitro* preparations. What these might be was further discussed by Read, Read and Duthie (1982) in their investigation on loperamide and anal sphincter function. Loperamide improved continence to rectal infusion of 1500 ml of saline. This effect was accompanied by an increase in maximum basal sphincter pressure and an increase in the degree of rectal distension required to inhibit recovery of IAS tone. Both these actions were attributed to an increase in tone of anorectal smooth muscle which the authors believed was mediated via intrinsic nerves controlling smooth muscle, rather than being an effect on the smooth muscle itself or on the central nervous system. An action on presynaptic terminals to inhibit acetylcholine release was proposed as a possible mechanism. In fact, these nerves would probably have to be preganglionic as the final inhibitory neuron mediating relaxation is non-cholinergic, non-adrenergic.

This is an interesting difference between the mechanism of action of loperamide and a preparation (Lomotil) containing another opiate, diphenoxylate, and atropine. Harford *et al.* (1980) investigated the effects of Lomotil therapy in patients with chronic diarrhoea and incontinence; Lomotil had no effect on continence for saline infused into the rectum, but the average stool frequency and weight were reduced.

Vasoactive intestinal peptide and adenosine triphosphate

Vasoactive intestinal peptide (VIP) has been found in nerves supplying the IAS (Alumets *et al.*, 1978). This peptide is more potent than any other compound tested in causing relaxations of sphincter muscle strips, and has been proposed as a neurotransmitter in the lower oesophageal sphincter (Goyal, Rattan and Said, 1980). Adenosine triphosphate (ATP) also relaxed sphincter muscle strips; the relaxations could be abolished by the ATP antagonist 2′,2′-pyridylisatogen tosylate, or by desensitization using high concentrations of ATP (Burleigh, D'Mello and Parks, 1979).

Hormonal influences

Rab-Choudhury and Lorber (1977) investigated the actions of glucagon and secretin on activity in the distal gut induced by food and morphine. Neither glucagon nor secretin inhibited the elevated pressure of the IAS produced by morphine, although glucagon did inhibit the morphine-induced motor activity in the distal colon and rectum. The inactivity of glucagon on the IAS was surprising, as an earlier study had shown that pulse injections of the hormone relaxed the unstimulated muscle (Gardner, Malloy and Hogan, 1973).

Responses of IAS muscle to intrinsic nerve stimulation

As it is not possible to obtain human sphincter muscle strips with an extrinsic nerve supply, nerve fibres are stimulated by placing the entire muscle strip in an electrical field generated by passing an electric current between two platinum wire electrodes, one on either side of the tissue. Sphincter muscle either relaxed to electrical field stimulation (EFS) (Burleigh, D'Mello and Parks, 1979), or gave small irregular responses (Friedmann, 1968) (relaxations or contractions). In the latter report, similar incon-sistencies were found in the response to acetylcholine, and it is possible that intrinsic nerves were damaged during preparation of the muscle strips, resulting in insensitivity and inconsistent responses to both acetylcholine and EFS. The relaxation to EFS was not due to an action on smooth muscle fibres as only stimuli of short pulse durations

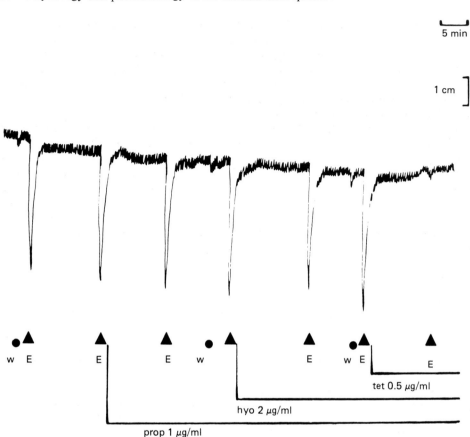

Figure 2.4. Human internal anal sphincter strips relax to electrical field stimulation (E, 14 V, 1 ms, 4 Hz for 15 s). A combination of propranolol and hyoscine had no effect on the relaxation to stimulation, but the response was blocked by tetrodotoxin. w, Additional changes of bath fluid. (From Burleigh, D'Mello and Parks (1979), by permission of the publishers; copyright 1979 by The American Gastroenterological Association)

were used ($\leqslant 1$ ms); furthermore, the relaxation was abolished by tetrodotoxin (*Figure 2.4*) (Burleigh, D'Mello and Parks, 1979), a selective antagonist of nerve function (Kao, 1966). It appears that the majority of intrinsic nerve pathways are inhibitory and that relaxation of the IAS in response to EFS may involve the same nerve pathway that mediates relaxation of the sphincter in the rectosphincteric relaxation reflex, as these nerves are also intrinsic nerves (Howard and Nixon, 1968).

What is the neurotransmitter that causes relaxation of sphincter muscle after EFS? It is not noradrenaline, as this substance contracts sphincter muscle; furthermore, neither guanethidine nor propranolol antagonized the relaxation to EFS. It is unlikely to be acetylcholine, as hyoscine in concentrations blocking relaxations to acetylcholine has no effect on the relaxation to EFS (*Figure 2.4*). Other substances discounted as mediators of the relaxation include prostaglandins E_2 and $F_{2\alpha}$, histamine, 5-HT and dopamine. Prostaglandin $F_{2\alpha}$, 5-HT and dopamine contract sphincter muscle, while prostaglandin E_2 and histamine (H_1 receptors) relax it. Relaxations to EFS are unaffected by mepyramine or indomethacin. It appears that a non-adrenergic, non-cholinergic nerve is involved in relaxing sphincter muscle strips. Such nerves have been postulated to release ATP (Burnstock, 1975) and, indeed, high concentrations of ATP relax sphincter muscle. An inhibitory neurotransmitter role for ATP in the IAS could be confirmed using a selective antagonist; the evidence obtained so far is inconclusive as both ATP desensitization and the ATP agonist 2',2'-pyridylisatogen tosylate only reduced responses of sphincter muscle to ATP in concentrations that also reduced relaxations to isoprenaline (Burleigh, D'Mello and Parks, 1979).

An alternative to ATP as a neurotransmitter of these nerves is VIP (Alumets *et al.*, 1978; Goyal, Rattan and Said, 1980), and selective antisera have been developed for VIP. However, these compounds were only partially effective in reducing relaxations to VIP or non-cholinergic, non-adrenergic stimulation of opossum lower oesophageal sphincter, perhaps because their large molecular structure prevented access to all functional synapses (Goyal, Rattan and Said, 1980). The actions of VIP may also be antagonized by proteolytic enzymes such as α-chymotrypsin (Mackenzie and Burnstock, 1980). While α-chymotrypsin significantly reduced relaxations of IAS to VIP, it had no attenuating effect on relaxations due to electrical field stimulation (Burleigh, 1983).

The *in vitro* pharmacology of this muscle is extremely complex and may be summarized as follows:

1. Electrical stimulation of intrinsic nerves causes relaxation of sphincter muscle strips. The transmitter liberated by these nerves does not appear to be acetylcholine or noradrenaline.
2. Many compounds have been eliminated as neurotransmitter candidates for this non-adrenergic, non-cholinergic inhibitory nerve, but adenosine triphosphate and vasoactive intestinal peptide still remain possibilities. Confirmation of a neurotransmitter role for these substances awaits the synthesis of selective antagonists.
3. As was originally predicted by Gaskell (1920), acetylcholine relaxes the IAS muscle. Detailed analysis of this response, only possible using isolated tissue, has shown that the effect of acetylcholine is partly indirect and may indicate a preganglionic cholinergic nerve synapsing with a non-adrenergic inhibitory neuron.
4. Relaxation of sphincter muscle to ganglion stimulant drugs is almost certainly due to release of noradrenaline. Thus, while electrical field stimulation of intrinsic nerves does not appear to release noradrenaline, chemical stimulation by nicotine or DMPP might do so.

There appear to be at least two types of synapses where inhibitory nerves impinge on sphincter smooth muscle. One involves adrenergic and a second involves non-cholinergic, non-adrenergic nerves. Inhibitory adrenergic nerves may represent the final efferent stage of an extrinsic inhibitory nerve pathway, as demonstrated by Shepherd and Wright (1968). The non-cholinergic, non-adrenergic inhibitory nerves are possibly the final efferent neuron involved in the rectosphincteric relaxation reflex. A schematic representation of excitatory and inhibitory influences acting on human internal anal sphincter is shown in *Figure 2.5* (see also *Table 2.1*).

Comparative studies

Innervation of the IAS has been studied in a number of animal species. Most authors agree that the motor supply to the sphincter is provided by the lumbar sympathetic outflow in the hypogastric nerves (*Table 2.2*), although Learmonth and Markowitz (1929) also found that stimulation of lumbar sympathetic colonic nerves contract dog

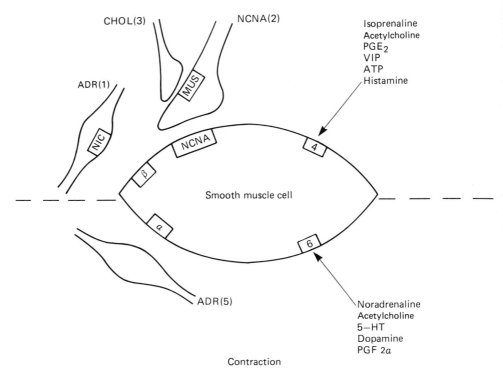

Relaxation

CHOL(3)   NCNA(2)   Isoprenaline
Acetylcholine
PGE$_2$
VIP
ATP
Histamine

ADR(1)

Smooth muscle cell

ADR(5)   Noradrenaline
Acetylcholine
5–HT
Dopamine
PGF 2a

Contraction

Figure 2.5. Diagram showing which nerves and drugs act on the isolated human internal anal sphincter muscle to cause relaxation or contraction (for a comprehensive list of drugs and their effects see *Table 2.1*). Relaxation of sphincter muscle may be caused by activation of nicotinic (NIC) receptors on adrenergic (ADR) nerve varicosities resulting in β-adrenoceptor stimulation (1) or electrical field stimulation of non-cholinergic, non-adrenergic (NCNA) nerves (2). Non-cholinergic, non-adrenergic nerves may have a presynaptic cholinergic (CHOL) input which increases the release of NCNA neurotransmitter through activation of muscarinic (MUS) receptors (3). This cholinergic input appears to be facilitated by a prostaglandin, probably PGE$_2$. A number of substances produce relaxation by acting directly on sphincter muscle cells (4). Contraction of sphincter muscle *in vivo* results from stimulation of adrenergic nerves causing activation of α-adrenoceptors (5). Finally, a variety of substances contract sphincter muscle by a direct action on the smooth muscle cell (6)

IAS. There may be some inhibitory fibres within the hypogastric nerve because contractions could be converted to relaxations by phentolamine (*Table 2.2*). Contractions and relaxations are probably mediated by α- and β-adrenoceptors, respectively.

The nature of the inhibitory nerve supply to the IAS is still not resolved. Stimulation of sacral nerves generally produces relaxation of sphincter muscle, although contraction due to activation of adrenergic nerve fibres has been observed. The response to sacral nerve stimulation was unaffected by atropine, so cholinergic nerves do not appear to form the final inhibitory pathway mediating relaxation of the muscle, despite a very dense innervation of the IAS by cholinergic nerves (Garrett, Howard and Jones, 1974). Animal studies *in vitro* also present a conflicting picture for the role of cholinergic nerves. Stimulation of muscarinic receptors on circular sphincteric muscle caused relaxation (Penninckx, Kerremans and Beckers, 1973), contraction (Rayner,

TABLE 2.1. Response of human internal anal sphincter to drugs

Drug	Response*	
	In vitro	*In vivo*
Acetylcholine	(↑ or ↓)[1], 0 or ↑ or ↓[2], 0[3], ↓(↑, ↑↓)[7], ↓(0 or ↑)[9], ↓[11]	
Bethanechol	↓[7]	↓[5]
Noradrenaline	↑[1], ↑[2], ↑[7], ↑[9]	
Methoxamine		↑[5]
Adrenaline	↓ or ↑[1], ↑ or ↓[2], ↑[3]	
Isoprenaline	↓[1], ↓[2], ↓[7], ↓(0)[9], ↓[11]	↓(0)[5]
Dopamine	↑[7]	
5-Hydroxytryptamine	↑[7]	
Histamine	↓[7]	
Prostaglandin E$_2$	↓[7]	
Prostaglandin F$_{2\alpha}$	↑[7]	
Adenosine triphosphate	↓[7]	
Nicotine	↓ or 0(↑)[1], ↓ or 0[2], ↓[7]	
DMPP	↓[7], ↓[9]	
Morphine	0[10]	↑[6]
Loperamide	↓[8]	↑[9]
Leu-enkephalin	0[10]	
γ-Amino butyric acid	↑[10]	
Substance P	↑[10]	
Bradykinin	↓[10]	
Caerulin	↓[11]	0[11]
Glucagon		0[6], ↓[4]
Secretin		0[6]
Pentagastrin		↑[4]
Hyoscine	0[7]	
Atropine		↑[5]
Phentolamine	0[7]	↓[5]
Propranolol	0[7]	↑[5]
Tetrodotoxin	0(↑)[10]	

* ↑ Contraction; ↓ relaxation; ↑↓ or ↓↑ biphasic response; 0 no effect; ( ) infrequent type of response.

References: [1]Friedmann (1968); [2]Parks *et al.* (1969); [3]Bass, Ustach and Schuster (1970); [4]Gardner, Malloy and Hogan (1973); [5]Gutierrez and Shah (1975); [6]Rab-Choudhury and Lorber (1977); [7]Burleigh, D'Mello and Parks (1979); [8]McKirdy (1981); [9]Read, Read and Duthie (1982); [10]Burleigh (1983); [11]Carpenedo *et al.* (1983).

TABLE 2.2. Response of the internal anal sphincter to extrinsic nerve stimulation

Species	Response*	
	Lumbar nerves (hypogastric)	Sacral nerves (pelvic)
Cat	↑[1] ↑[4] ↑[6] ↓[4]†	↓[3] ↓↑[1] ↑ or ↓[4] ↓[4]† ↓[6]‡
Dog	↑[2] ↑[1] ↓[2]†	↑ or ↑↓[1]†
Rabbit	↑ or ↓[1]	↑↓[1]
Monkey	↑[5]	↑[5]

* ↑ Contraction; ↓ relaxation; ↑↓ or ↓↑ biphasic response.
† Response obtained in the presence of phentolamine.
‡ Relaxation unaffected by atropine and therefore attributed to non-cholinergic inhibitory nerves.

References: [1]Langley and Andersen (1895); [2]Learmonth and Markowitz (1929); [3]Garry (1933); [4]Garrett, Howard and Jones (1974); [5]Rayner (1979); [6]Bouvier and Gonella (1981b).

1979; Adebanjo, Ambache and Verney, 1976), or no response (Bass, Ustach and Schuster, 1970; Bouvier and Gonella, 1981a). These varied responses might have been due to intermingled longitudinal muscle fibres. Since there is a well-defined longitudinal smooth muscle layer in the cat anal sphincter, which contracts to acetylcholine (Penninckx, Kerremans and Beckers, 1973; Bouvier and Gonella, 1981b), changing tone of the muscle strips might have been the cause, as when tone falls contractile response to acetylcholine may appear (Burleigh, D'Mello and Parks, 1979). Bouvier and Gonella (1981b) proposed that cholinergic nerves modulate the actions of extrinsic sympathetic excitatory nerves and intramural inhibitory nerves. In their analysis of the recto-anal reflex in cats *in vitro*, Penninckx and Mebis (1982) demonstrated that ganglion cells, muscarinic receptors on nerve tissue and non-adrenergic, non-cholinergic inhibitory nerves are required for the reflex, but that adrenergic nerves are not involved.

In cats, reflex relaxation of the sphincter by rectal distension was unaffected by atropine, propranolol or pretreatment of animals with 6-hydroxydopamine. The non-cholinergic, non-adrenergic nerves mediating the reflex were located in the bowel wall, as section of the extrinsic nerve supply did not affect the reflex (Garrett and Howard, 1975). Relaxations due to stimulation of non-cholinergic, non-adrenergic nerves have been demonstrated in isolated sphincter muscle from rabbit, pig, dog and cat (Adebanjo, Ambache and Verney, 1976). A single concentration of ATP (18 µm) failed to relax sphincter muscle from any of these species; this concentration was relatively low compared with the range 1–1600 µm of ATP required to relax isolated human IAS (Burleigh, D'Mello and Parks, 1979).

Conclusions

Early investigations into the control of IAS motility were carried out in human volunteers, including patients, and anaesthetized animals. As predicted by Gaskell (1920), the dominant extrinsic autonomic innervation to the IAS is sympathetic, causing sphincter contraction. This may explain why some diabetics, with autonomic neuropathy, had a low resting anal canal pressure and diarrhoea (Schiller *et al.*, 1982). Of greater importance clinically was the location of sensory receptors and neural pathways involved in the rectosphincteric relaxation reflex. Sensory receptors for the reflex are located in the rectum, and only intrinsic nerves are involved in mediating the reflex. Anatomical studies in animals have shown that there are specialized intrinsic nerves, running from the sigmoid colon to the distal rectum, which have unique features suited to rapid conduction of the reflex impulses mediating sphincter relaxation (Christensen *et al.*, 1984). Apart from the rectosphincteric relaxation reflex, there is also a contraction reflex mediated by extrinsic nerves. This contraction reflex is activated when the bladder is being emptied and serves to help maintain anal continence during micturition (Salducci, Planche and Naudy, 1982).

In vitro studies have been used to investigate the actions of drugs and intrinsic nerves in modifying sphincter muscle activity. Relaxation of muscle strips could be produced by electrical field stimulation. Pharmacological analysis of such responses showed that non-cholinergic, non-adrenergic nerves were involved. These nerves are involved in control of gastrointestinal motility such as peristalsis and relaxation of sphincters (Burnstock, 1975), although the transmitter they release remains unidentified. Acetylcholine is not the final neurotransmitter involved in relaxing the IAS, but it is probably involved at some stage in transmission of reflex impulses causing relaxation of the muscle. Penninckx and Mebis (1982) showed the reflex can be abolished, *in vitro*, by atropine or hexamethonium. In children with constipation and a poor relaxation reflex, IAS muscle strips uncharacteristically contracted to both acetylcholine and electrical field stimulation.

Histological studies have shown a dense adrenergic and cholinergic innervation of this muscle compared with adjacent intestinal muscle. So what is their function, since *in vitro* evidence showed that relaxation was induced by non-cholinergic, non-adrenergic nerves? Furthermore, what are these non-cholinergic, non-adrenergic nerves? Perhaps they release a neurotransmitter other than noradrenaline or acetylcholine, or perhaps there are novel cholinoceptors or adrenoceptors unaffected by existing antagonists.

References

ADEBANJO, A. O., AMBACHE, N. and VERNEY, J. (1976). The inhibitory transmission to the internal anal sphincter. *British Journal of Pharmacology*, **56**, 392–393P

ALDRIDGE, R. T. and CAMPBELL, R. E. (1968). Ganglion cell distribution in the normal rectum and anal canal. *Journal of Paediatric Surgery*, **3**, 475–490

ALUMETS, J., HAKANSON, R., SUNDLER, F. and UDDMAN, R. (1978). VIP innervation of sphincters. *Scandinavian Journal of Gastroenterology*, **13** (Suppl. 49), 6

BASS, D. D., USTACH, T. J. and SCHUSTER, M. M. (1970). *In vitro* pharmacologic differentiation of sphincteric and non-sphincteric muscle. *Johns Hopkins Medical Journal*, **127**, 185–191

BASS, D. D., VANASIN, B., USTACH, T. J. and SCHUSTER, M. M. (1972). An *in vitro* model demonstrating specificity of sphincteric smooth muscle. *Johns Hopkins Medical Journal*, **131**, 436–440

BAUMGARTEN, H. C., HOLSTEIN, A. F. and STELZNER, F. (1971). Differences in the innervation of the large intestine and internal anal sphincter in mammals and humans. *Verhandlungen der Anatomischen Gesellschaft*, **66**, 43–47

BAUMGARTEN, H. G., HOLSTEIN, A. F. and STELZNER, F. (1973). Nervous elements in the human colon of Hirschsprung's disease. *Virchows Archives of Pathology and Anatomy*, **358**, 113–136

BOUVIER, M. and GONELLA, J. (1981a). Electrical activity from smooth muscle of the anal sphincter area of the cat. *Journal of Physiology*, **310**, 445–456

BOUVIER, M. and GONELLA, J. (1981b). Nervous control of the internal anal sphincter of cat. *Journal of Physiology*, **310**, 457–459

BURLEIGH, D. E. (1977). The effects of indomethacin on the tone and spontaneous activity of the human small intestine in vitro. *Archives Internationales Pharmacodynamie et Therapie*, **225**, 240–245

BURLEIGH, D. E. (1978). DMPP causes an increase in ^{3}H overflow from superfused strips of human internal anal sphincter, in *Abstracts of the 7th International Congress of Pharmacology*, 773 pp. Oxford; Pergamon Press

BURLEIGH, D. E. (1983). Non-cholinergic, non-adrenergic inhibitory neurones in human internal anal sphincter muscle. *Journal of Pharmacy and Pharmacology*, **35**, 258–260

BURLEIGH, D. E., D'MELLO, A. and PARKS, A. G. (1979). Responses of isolated human internal anal sphincter to drugs and electrical field stimulation. *Gastroenterology*, **77**, 484–490

BURLEIGH, D. E., GALLIGAN, J. and BURKS, T. F. (1981). Subcutaneous morphine reduces intestinal propulsion in rats partly by a central action. *European Journal of Pharmacology*, **75**, 283–287

BURNSTOCK, G. (1975). Purinergic transmission, in *Handbook of Psychopharmacology*, Vol. 5, pp. 131–194 (L. L. Iversen, S. D. Iversen and S. H. Snyder, Eds). New York; Plenum Press

CARPENEDO, F., INFANTINO, A., FLOREANI, M. and DODI, G. (1983). The relaxing effect of caerulein on isolated human internal anal sphincter. *European Journal of Pharmacology*, **87**, 271–276

CHRISTENSEN, J., STILES, M. J., RICK, G. A. and SUTHERLAND, J. (1984). Comparative anatomy of the myenteric plexus of the distal colon in eight mammals. *Gastroenterology*, **86**, 706–713

DENNY-BROWN, D. and ROBERTSON, E. G. (1935). An investigation of the nervous control of defaecation. *Brain*, **58**, 256–310

D'MELLO, A., BURLEIGH, D. E. and PARKS, A. G. (1975). A non-adrenergic inhibitory mechanism in the human internal anal sphincter probably involving the release of prostaglandin, in *Abstracts of the 6th International Congress of Pharmacology*, 158 pp. Helsinki

DUTHIE, H. L. (1971). Progress report: anal incontinence. *Gut*, **12**, 844–852

FRENCKNER, B. (1975). Function of the anal sphincters in spinal man. *Gut*, **16**, 638–644

FRENCKNER, B. and EULER, C. V. (1975). Influence of pudendal block on the function of the anal sphincters. *Gut*, **16**, 482–489

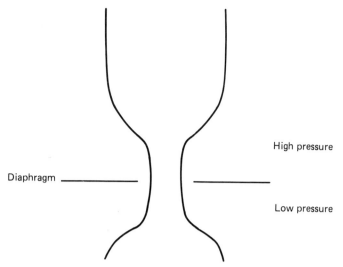

Figure 3.1. Principle of the 'flutter' valve

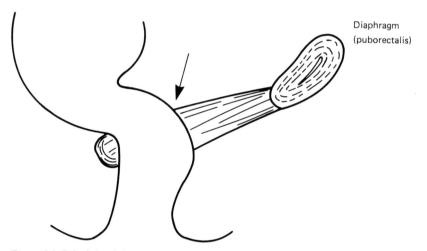

Figure 3.2. Principle of the anorectal 'flap' valve

puborectalis exerts. Such force would permit a valve mechanism similar to a flutter valve to operate.

Parks, Porter and Hardcastle (1966) suggested that contractions of the puborectalis created a 'flap' valve (*Figure 3.2*). A pressure differential must exist between intra-abdominal pressure and that in the anal canal (which is approximately 60–100 cmH$_2$O when measured with a water-filled microballoon). When intra-abdominal pressure is raised by coughing, lifting or sneezing (the pressure may exceed 200 cmH$_2$O), this will compress the anterior rectal wall onto the upper anal canal, so occluding its lumen.

It is doubtful that either theory exclusively accounts for the physical principles involved in continence. Possibly, both principles co-exist, but in practice we believe that the flap-valve mechanism is the dominant factor in continence.

Neuromuscular reflexes in the pelvic floor and external anal sphincter

Where continence is threatened by acts which result in increased intra-abdominal pressure, in addition to the mechanical mechanisms discussed above, a reflex contraction develops within these muscles (Taverner and Smiddy, 1959; Parks, Porter and Melzack, 1962). Taverner and Smiddy (1959) showed that increased motor unit firing occurred in these muscles during coughing, speech and changes in posture. Since this reflex remains intact in patients with complete transection of the cord (Melzack and Porter, 1964), it is presumably mediated within the cord. Melzack and Porter also found that the lower the level of cord section, the greater the amplitude of electrical response induced by a cough effort. They surmised that with lower cord lesions a greater population of trunk musculature remained innervated and higher intra-abdominal pressures were thereby generated.

Sensation and faecal continence

The patient's awareness of rectal distension produced by inflation of a rectal balloon or by the arrival of faecal contents is characterized by a distinct sensation localized to the rectum or sacral area (Goligher and Hughes, 1951). Todd (1959) found that many patients with full-thickness rectal prolapse have a deficient appreciation of rectal distension, as tested by noting the volume of air introduced into a rectal balloon sufficient to cause consciousness of rectal filling. This sensory deficit may partly account for the incontinence many of these patients experience.

The receptors responsible for this sensation probably do not reside in the rectum itself. Hence, patients with rectal carcinoma treated by amputation of the rectum and colo-anal anastomosis preserve a normal sensation of rectal filling (Lane and Parks, 1977). It seems probable that the receptors probably are situated in the nearby pelvic floor muscles. Stretch receptors have been identified in the levator muscles (Winkler, 1958) and in the external anal sphincter muscle spindles, which could carry sensory fibres, have been observed (Walls, 1959).

Goligher and Hughes (1951) considered that the more precise perception of the nature of rectal contents could be a function of intra-rectal pressure. Flatus was responsible for slightly lower intra-rectal pressures than those occurring when faecal matter was introduced into the lumen. Duthie and Bennett (1963) introduced the attractive hypothesis that such discrimination was achieved by means of the sensory receptors situated in the skin of the distal part of the anal canal. A proximal level to which sensation to light touch could be appreciated in the anal canal was determined in a group of normal subjects. In the same subjects, intra-anal and intrarectal pressures were measured. In the resting state, it was found that rectal contents could not reach far enough into the anal canal to make contact with the sensory receptors because of a pressure differential. When the rectum was distended by the arrival of faecal matter or flatus, this caused a reflex fall in intra-anal pressure (caused by internal anal sphincter relaxation) of sufficient degree that it was now possible for rectal contents to make contact with the sensory zone and aid in their recognition.

Goligher (1951) maintains that this function is of considerable importance in the maintenance of continence. He described five patients with carcinoma of the rectum in whom treatment consisted of excision of the rectum at a level just above the anal canal. The colon was subsequently anastomosed by a pull-through technique to the anal canal, the mucosa of which had been denuded. He observed that none of these patients could distinguish between flatus and faeces and were correspondingly incontinent, particularly of flatus and of liquid stool.

Miscellaneous factors

Kerremans (1969) found that the frequency of pressure waves was greater in the distal than the proximal portion of the anal canal. Connell (1964) found that the frequency of pressure waves and the proportion in which motor activity was present were both greater in the rectum than in the sigmoid colon. The suggestion was advanced that, by this mechanism, force vectors acting in a cephalad direction play a part in continence by controlling the entry of faeces into the rectum.

Hill et al. (1960) considered that further resistance to the passage of faeces is offered by the folds of Houston. This conclusion was based on the observation that withdrawal of an open-tipped catheter through the rectum to the anus produced no zones in which a rise in pressure occurred. If, however, this was repeated using a balloon (which resembled a faecal bolus) zones of elevated pressure were recordable. These authors deduced that the balloon encountered resistance as offered by the mucosal folds. No such resistance would be offered to an open tube which merely recorded intra-luminal pressure.

The possibility that an additional contribution to continence is provided by simple surface tension effects created by the close apposition of moist mucosal surfaces in the anal canal has been suggested by Duthie (1975). Harris and Pope (1964) found that lower pressures were generated when a probe was withdrawn from the rectum to the anus than were obtained if the probe was reinserted through the anus. Presumably, this suggests a high resistance to opening in the sphincter, which in turn may be a surface tension effect.

Conclusions

Continence is to a large extent the result of physiological mechanisms which maintain a normal anorectal angle. If the puborectalis is damaged, gross faecal incontinence arises. A sensory deficit and damage to the internal or external anal sphincter, on the other hand, results in only minor degrees of incontinence. The internal sphincter maintains a closed anal canal and probably prevents the inadvertent passage of flatus and liquid stool and can be considered important for fine tuning in continence. The external anal sphincter, by vigorous contraction, may preserve continence in situations in which the normal mechanisms may be severely challenged by profuse liquid stool.

Defaecation

Peristaltic activity in the sigmoid colon may lead to the introduction of flatus or faeces in the rectum. Rectal distension in turn leads to conscious awareness of rectal filling (by stimulating receptors in the surrounding levator muscles). If the situation is not suitable for defaecation, voluntary contraction of the external anal sphincter results in elevation of the pelvic floor, so increasing the anorectal angle and forcing the intruding rectal contents back into the rectal ampulla (Phillips and Edwards, 1965).

Alternatively, if defaecation is to proceed, two distinct events are required to ensure satisfactory voiding of rectal contents. First, intra-abdominal pressure is increased as a result of contraction of the abdominal wall musculature, descent of the diaphragm and closure of the glottis. Secondly, the mechanisms which maintain continence require to be 'unlocked'. Parks, Porter and Melzack (1962) and Porter (1962) demonstrated that a marked inhibition occurred in the pelvic floor muscles and external anal sphincter in subjects who were requested to 'bear down' as if preparing for defaecation. This phenomenon appeared to be the result of a spinal reflex, in that it was preserved in patients with complete transection of the spinal cord. Porter (1962) showed that complete inhibition of electrical activity occurred if an attempt was made to evacuate an intrarectal balloon through the anal canal. Phillips and Edwards demonstrated, by radiographic techniques, that the reflex inhibition in these muscles induced by defaecatory effort caused descent of the pelvic floor and an increased obliquity of the anorectal angle. The mechanisms of the flap/flutter valves are unlocked, the internal sphincter relaxes, presumably as a result of the locally mediated recto-anal visceral reflex, and the external sphincter is inhibited *pari passu* with the puborectalis. The faecal bolus can now be voided.

At the completion of defaecation there is a rapid burst of activity in the external anal sphincter and pelvic floor; this is the so-called closing reflex (Porter, 1962). Cine-radiography reveals a rapid rise of the pelvic floor with reconstitution of the anorectal angle (Phillips and Edwards, 1965).

The central mechanisms in the nervous system controlling defaecatory activity are not understood. Urge incontinence of faeces, like that of urine, can occur as an idiopathic phenomenon, particularly in the presence of diarrhoea or faecal impaction, but it is also a characteristic feature of spinal and cerebral disorders such as multiple sclerosis and stroke. Recent experiments on the cortical localization of the motor cells controlling the anal sphincter suggest that there is a fast-conducting, direct pyramidal pathway to the sacral anterior horn cells supplying the pelvic floor and external sphincter, illustrating the importance of the brain in the normal function of these muscles (see Chapter 7).

B. Colorectal motility

D. Kumar and D. L. Wingate

Introduction

Motility is a descriptive term which is commonly used to describe both the movements of the wall of a viscus and the transit of material through the viscus; in this sense, motility cannot be quantified, since there is no measurement which can simultaneously describe both these variables. Measurements of motility, therefore, usually describe *either* wall movement *or* the transit of material. Terms such as 'increased motility' or 'decreased motility' are imprecise and best avoided. Increased contractile activity at a single site does not necessarily imply increased transit of material; likewise, patterns of transit cannot be deduced from changes in intraluminal pressure or the occurrence of local contractions.

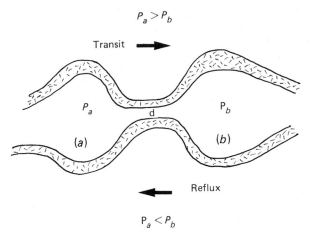

Figure 3.3. Conditions governing transit between adjacent segments of bowel. Two segments, (*a*) and (*b*), with respective intraluminal pressures P_a and P_b, are shown. The direction of flow is determined by the difference between P_a and P_b (ΔP_{ab}), as well as the magnitude of flow. Conventionally, flow in the physiological direction is termed 'transit', while flow in the opposite direction is termed 'reflux', although in the colon (in contrast to, for example, the oesophagus), movement in either direction probably occurs physiologically. The magnitude, but not the direction, of flow is determined by the diameter (*d*) of the aperture through which the segments communicate, and by the viscosity of the contents

Material in a viscus is moved along a pressure gradient, as shown in *Figure 3.3*. The rate and volume of material moved is related to the pressure differential, the diameter of the tube and the viscosity of the material. With this number of variables, observation of transit alone does not allow accurate characterization of the contractile activity responsible for transit. Because of the segmentation of the tube and the partial or complete obstruction of the lumen by its contents, measurements of intraluminal pressure at a single point, or even a series of points, is not always a useful guide to transit; the same applies to the measurement of contraction (or relaxation) of the muscular wall.

The above considerations complicate the description of motility throughout the gastrointestinal tract, but three additional problems bedevil the investigation of colonic motility. First, the luminal content varies between fluid at one end and solid at the other, although the physical characteristics of the content at different levels of the colon have not been characterized and are, indeed, unlikely to be constant even within a single subject. Secondly, the colon is long, wide and inaccessible, allowing only isolated sampling of motor activity; for this reason, most information has been gained from the sigmoid colon which is relatively accessible, but it would be unwise to assume that the motor activity of the sigmoid is representative of the rest of the colon. Thirdly, the considerable variation in colonic morphology and function between different species has meant that the validity of animal models as representative of another species, including man, is doubtful.

Most of the features of colorectal motility now known to us were, in fact, observed and recorded at the beginning of this century. Bayliss and Starling (1900) recorded the motility of isolated canine colon and postulated that, just as at the beginning of the alimentary canal there is a gradual transit from the cerebrospinal reflex of swallowing to the local intestinal reflex of peristalsis so, at the lower end of the gut, there is a change in the reverse direction from the automatic reflexes of the upper part of the colon to the spinal reflex which, in defaecation, affects the lower segment of the large intestine. Cannon (1902) used X-rays to study the colon of cats. He observed segmental and peristaltic movements and also suggested the presence of antiperistaltic waves. Although the use of more sophisticated techniques has provided us with a better understanding of colonic motor activity, the relationship between electrical and mechanical activity and its significance in the transit of luminal contents in health and disease still remains controversial (Misiewicz, 1975).

Colonic musculature

The smooth muscle of the colon has an outer longitudinal layer and an inner circular layer. In the sacculated segments of the colon, the longitudinal layer is present as three thick bundles, the taeniae coli and the circular layer which constitutes most of the muscle wall. The latter causes slight bulges, giving rise to the sacculated appearance. The circular muscle layer also forms the haustra, which can be detected as early as 11 weeks of gestation (Pace, 1971). In the distal sigmoid colon and rectum, the two layers of muscle are similar in thickness.

In the anal canal, the circular muscle layer is thickened to form the internal anal sphincter. The external anal sphincter is formed by a ring of striated muscle which is part of the pelvic floor musculature.

Innervation of the large bowel

The intrinsic nerves

The intrinsic nerve supply to the colon is via the myenteric plexus and the submucosal plexuses. The distribution density of ganglion cells appears uniform along the colon. In recent studies (Christensen, 1983), a sharp difference in the plexus between the proximal colon and the rectosigmoid colon of monkey has been detected. In the proximal colon, the plexus appears to have large ganglia joined by thick nerve bundles. In the rectum, the ganglia are small and few and the nerve bundles are thin. The intrinsic nerves of the colon have been shown to contain various regulatory peptides; immunofluorescence has demonstrated the presence of substance-P, VIP, neurotensin and CCK, among others. The role of these peptides in this location has not been elucidated, although it is likely that they act either as neuromodulators, or even as neurotransmitters. Infusion of exogenous peptides has been shown to alter rectosigmoid motility (Snape, Matarazzo and Cohen, 1978), but it would be naive to assume, from this type of evidence, that the peptides are acting as 'gut hormones'. The consequences of neuropathy will be discussed below; suffice it to state, at this point, that impaired nerves result in impaired function even when the distribution and release of peptides is apparently unimpaired.

The extrinsic nerves

The extrinsic nerve supply to the colon is via the craniosacral and thoracolumbar nerves. The thoracolumbar supply is through splanchnic nerves originating from retroperitoneal ganglia. These ganglia receive the preganglionic fibres of the sympathetic system. The superior mesenteric ganglion supplies the part of the colon which receives its blood supply from the superior mesenteric artery. The rest of the colon is supplied by the inferior mesenteric ganglion. The craniosacral nerve supply to the colon is through the sacral outflow.

The efferent sympathetic supply to the distal rectum comes from the hypogastric plexus, and to the proximal rectum from the inferior mesenteric plexus. The parasympathetic innervation to the rectum is via nervi erigentes. The parasympathetic motor supply is excitatory for the rectum and inhibitory for the internal anal sphincter. It has been suggested (Devroede and Lamarche, 1974) that the nervi erigentes have ramifications to the left colon and left half of transverse colon in man and that these are important in the maintenance of normal defaecation.

Receptors

Storage in and voiding from the rectum are complex phenomena. The rectal wall accommodates well to distension and seems to have properties similar to the urinary bladder. Not only filling of the rectum but also both the rate of filling and the level of accommodation are important in prompting the urge to defaecate. While the receptors of the rectum and of the distal colon are poorly understood, the existence of several types of receptor can be inferred. Not only can rectal distension be perceived by normal individuals, but the nature of the distension can also be discriminated. Since individuals can distinguish between fluid, solid and gaseous distension, it seems clear that several types of mucosal receptor must exist and, in addition, it is probable that there are stretch receptors within the muscle layers. The difficulty of characterizing the receptors lies in the problem of applying stimuli which will only affect one population of receptors. A number of clinical tests that depend upon rectal and sigmoid sensation have been used in the assessment of colorectal functions; such tests include rectal distension with fluid, or with balloons inflated with air or water, but the results of such tests are difficult to interpret in terms of neurophysiology and neuroanatomy. What is clear is that a healthy human can distinguish between gaseous and solid or fluid distension with sufficient confidence to allow the passage of flatus in social circumstances where the passage of faeces would be unacceptable.

The motor activity of the colon and rectum

The problems of studying colonic and rectal motor activity have already been mentioned. The studies that have been carried out fall into two categories. Pressure sensors have been used to study pressure changes at selected points within the rectum and colon, usually by the retrograde introduction of probes fitted with pressure sensors; such studies have usually been carried out in human subjects. Alternatively, the electrical activity of the smooth muscle has been recorded from electrodes which are placed, in man, adjacent to the mucosa and, in animals, usually sutured directly to the serosal surface of the bowel. Before summarizing the phenomena described from these two modes of study, some general comments may be helpful:

1. The correlation between the mechanical and electrical phenomena that have been recorded is not clear. Even though it seems obvious that the electrical activity that is recorded must, in some way, correspond to muscle movement, the fact remains that it is difficult to correlate the patterns of electrical discharge with the organized movements familiar to the radiologist.
2. Further confusion in this field has been generated by the extrapolation of results

obtained in one species to other species, even though there is considerable evidence of morphological and functional differences between mammalian species.
3. Information of the functional motor activity of the rectum itself is very limited. The motor events which occur in the rectum during defaecation can only be studied during defaecation, but the available methods of study either inhibit normal defaecation or are invalidated during defaecation.

Organized movements of the colon

Three types of colonic movement have been identified from radiographic observation:

1. *Retrograde propulsion.* These are contractions originating in the transverse colon and travelling towards the caecum (Cannon, 1902; Elliott and Barclay-Smith, 1904). These contractions are believed to retard the forward flow of colonic luminal contents, allowing greater exposure of luminal contents to the colonic mucosa, resulting in complete absorption of salt and water (Cohen and Snape, 1983).
2. *Segmental non-propulsive movements.* These movements are demonstrated on radiographic studies (Ritchie, 1968). They comprise retrograde and anterograde movement of contents in a segment. The luminal contents are carried forwards by a propulsive contraction. The transit of contents in the right colon is slower in comparison with the transverse and descending colon.
3. *Mass movement.* This was first described by Hertz (1907). It is the movement of a long faecal bolus over a long colonic segment. It occurs only a few times during the day and lasts for a few seconds.

Contractile activity of the colorectal muscle

Although radiology has demonstrated what appear to be the common types of organized movement of the colon, it is not helpful for the detailed examination of patterns of local contraction in man. Radiology can only demonstrate changes in contour, which may be either active or passive. The slow rate of contraction in the colon would require an impermissible amount of radiation exposure for accurate recording.

Contractile activity has been recorded in man from the colonic lumen, usually in the rectum or rectosigmoid (*Figure 3.4*). Pressure recording systems have consisted of tubes with attached water- or air-filled balloons, or strain gauges; some workers have also employed multilumen perfused tubes attached to strain gauge transducers. Since there is a limit to the tolerance of subjects for lying still with tubes *in situ*, such studies are usually of relatively short duration (45–90 min).

Little useful information has emerged from such studies. It has been shown that propagated contractions may be recorded, but no characteristic pattern of contraction has been observed. It is generally agreed that contractile activity, as represented by an arbitrary 'motility index', is decreased by anticholinergic drugs, and increased by cholinergic drugs, and also by food. The limited value of such studies has been shown recently by Dinoso *et al.* (1983), who found variations in contractile activity between different subjects which were no greater than the variations in the same subject studied on different occasions. Such pressure studies have so far contributed little to physiology, diagnosis, or therapeutics. Most data available on colonic motility refer to the distal 30 cm of the colon, because sigmoid and rectosigmoid are the only easily accessible areas (Connell, 1968).

Radiotelemetry capsules have been used in the study of the colon, but the difficulty of

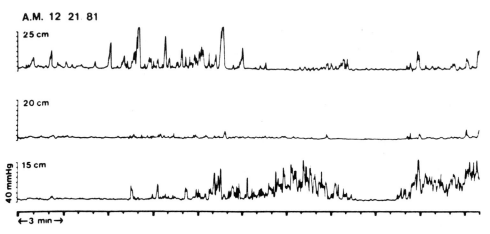

Figure 3.4. An example of activity of the distal colon in a normal subject. Intraluminal pressure changes 25, 20 and 15 cm from the anal verge over 30 min are shown (Reprinted by permission of Elsevier Science Publishing Co., Inc. from Dinoso *et al.* (1983). Copyright 1983 by The American Gastroenterological Association)

maintaining them at a constant site without intermittent loss of signal has not, so far, encouraged their use in the study of the colon and rectum.

Colorectal myoelectric activity

Since the study of the electroenterogram by Alvarez and Mahoney, in 1921, enteric electromyography has been an important method of experimental study; in recent years, electromyography of the stomach and small intestine has led to the recognition of the interdigestive migrating myoelectric—or motor—complex (MMC) of the stomach and small bowel, and its modulation by peptides and nutrients. In the proximal digestive tract, the main components of the electrical signal are the *rhythmic slow waves*, or basic electrical rhythm, regulated by pacemaker sites and, phase-locked to these slow waves, the *spike bursts* which are known correlates of muscle contraction. Slow waves are generated as a result of cyclic depolarizations in the cell membranes of adjacent smooth muscle cells in the syncytial mass, which are electrically coupled. These cyclic depolarizations are co-ordinated in such a manner that the signal appears to migrate.

Colonic electromyography has been carried out in various species, including the human. In experimental animals, recordings are made from implanted monopolar or bipolar serosal electrodes. In man, recordings are made from a series of bipolar electrodes in the form of rings of wire arrayed along a tube introduced per rectum (*Figure 3.5*); there is no method available by which such electrodes can be made to adhere continuously to the mucosa, and the recordings obtained in this way are therefore distorted by changes in signal strength due to alterations in the contact between electrode and tissue.

Colonic slow waves differ from slow waves of other parts of the gastrointestinal tract in that (a) slow waves in the colon originate from the circular muscle layer, whereas slow waves in the rest of the gastrointestinal tract originate in the longitudinal layer; (b) colonic slow waves are less frequent than gastric slow waves; (c) slow waves in the colon seem to be capable of producing a contraction since contractions may occur without

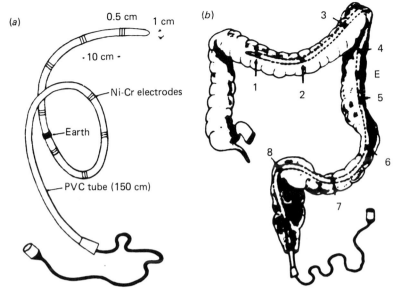

Figure 3.5. A colonic EMG recording probe with multiple bipolar electrodes (*a*) and its location during a recording session (*b*) (From Bueno *et al.* (1980), by permission of the Editor and publishers of *Gut*)

the appearance of spike bursts. Furthermore, although gastric and small bowel slow wave activity is regular and omnipresent, similar regular slow wave activity has only been observed in colonic muscle *in vitro*. In the mammalian colon *in vivo*, there is evidence of rhythmic slow wave activity for only about 30–70 per cent of a period of continuous recording, depending upon the region, species and the experimental conditions (*Figure 3.6*). Moreover, when slow wave activity is present, the signal is often distorted and consisting of activity at multiple frequencies. The difficulties of identifying regular slow waves from real-time analysis of colonic electromyograms has led to the use of averaging techniques of frequency analysis (*Figure 3.7*), usually involving the use of Fast Fourier Transforms (Sarna *et al.*, 1982).

The consensus of evidence allows some broad conclusions to be drawn about colonic slow wave activity. The frequency of slow waves in the cat colon averages between 4.5 c/min in the proximal colon to about 6 c/min in the distal colon (Christensen, Anuras and Hauser, 1974). Slow waves in the lower rectum are more constant and regular (Provenzale and Pisano, 1971; Taylor *et al.*, 1974). In humans, the slow wave frequency between ascending and descending colon is 11 c/min (Taylor *et al.*, 1975). The frequency decreases in the sigmoid colon. The slow wave frequency in the human sigmoid colon and rectosigmoid appears to be about 6 c/min (Snape, Carlson and Cohen, 1977). In the small intestine, the frequency of the slow waves seems to be determined by temperature and metabolic rate (Christensen, Schedl and Clifton, 1964, 1966). It is not clear whether this is also the case in the colon, although similar modulation of myoelectric activity at this site is likely. The normal internal sphincter has slow waves with a mean frequency of 20 c/min (Kerremans, 1968). The same slow wave frequency is present in the external sphincter, which suggests an autonomous mechanism that is independent of the electrical activity of the rectum.

In the *in vitro* cat preparation, which exhibits regular slow wave activity, the proximal colon has a slower and irregular slow wave frequency, while distal segments

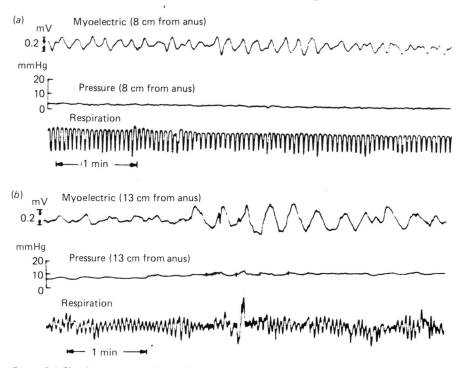

Figure 3.6. Simultaneous recordings of myoelectric activity, intraluminal pressure and respiration: (*a*) Record obtained in a normal subject; the slow wave frequency is 6.2 c/min; (*b*) record obtained in a patient with 'irritable bowel' syndrome; the slow wave frequency is 3.1 c/min (From Snape *et al.* (1977), by permission of The Williams and Wilkins Co., Baltimore, USA)

of the colon have a faster slow wave frequency. This has been interpreted as evidence of a pacemaker for the generation of slow waves in the transverse colon, which would allow for the bidirectional propagation of slow waves, and hence of colonic contents (Christensen, Anuras and Hauser, 1974). Evidence of this type of electrical activity in man is lacking.

The second type of electrical activity in colonic muscle is the spike burst. Spike bursts reflect the summated action potentials which accompany contraction occurring in individual (but synchronized) muscle cells. In theory, spike potentials always occur during a fixed portion of slow wave cycle, and the frequency of intestinal contractions or the frequency of spike bursts is thus dependent on the slow wave frequency. Since every slow wave cycle does not carry a spike burst, the contractions may be irregular, but cannot occur more frequently than the slow waves. This relationship between spikes and slow waves, which holds good for the distal stomach and the entire small bowel, is not necessarily true in the colon. In the isolated cat colon, which exhibits regular slow activity, two patterns of spike burst are seen (Christensen, Anuras and Hauser, 1974): (a) spike bursts superimposed on the slow waves and (b) migrating spike bursts. Migrating spike bursts are not related to slow wave activity and result in strong contractions of the circular muscle layer.

A third type of spike potential, the oscillatory spike potential, has also been described. It occurs in the proximal colon and is associated with powerful contractions of the intestine (Christensen, 1975); an increase in spike activity in the colon is

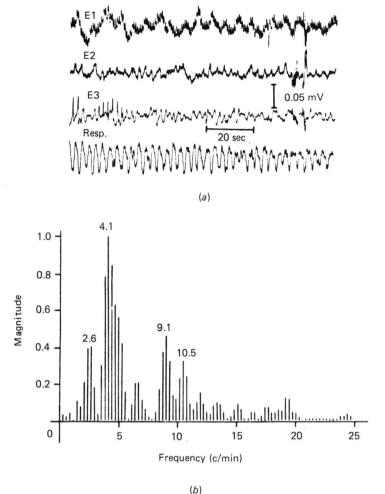

(a)

(b)

Figure 3.7. (a) Electrical activity from three electrodes placed on the human ascending colon; (b) power spectrum of 1 min of electrical activity at electrode 1 above. Peaks at 2.6, 4.1, 9.1 and 10.5 c/min indicate dominant frequencies identifiable by computer analysis, but not by visual inspection of the record (From *Gastrointestinal Motility*, by Sarna *et al.* (1980), with permission of Raven Press, New York)

accompanied by an increase in the intraluminal pressure. The oscillatory potential complex migrates distally at a rate of 4 cm/s (Sarna *et al.*, 1981) and is more rapid than the mass propulsion seen radiographically (Ritchie, 1968).

Detailed correlation of electrical spike bursts and mechanical events in conscious animal or human subjects is fraught with difficulty, but recordings have been made from the canine and human colon over periods of several hours to determine the overall pattern of spike bursts. In the dog, spike activity appears to be phasic, with periods of activity every 20–30 min, separated by periods of relative quiescence (Fioramonti and Bueno, 1983). In these studies (Sarna, London and Cowels, 1984), groups of spike bursts detected sequentially at three or more recording sites were considered to be colonic migrating complexes; these complexes do not appear to have discrete phases, as in the

CNS neuropathy

Glick *et al.* (1982) showed absence of postprandial stimulation of sigmoid motility in patients suffering from multiple sclerosis and demonstrated the same phenomenon (Glick *et al.*, 1984) in patients following traumatic thoracic spinal cord injury. Menardo *et al.* (1984) studied paraplegic patients and found that the major delay in transit occurred in the left colon and rectum. They concluded that transection of the spine between C4 and L5 causes alteration of large bowel motor activity mainly at the level of the segments innervated by the parasympathetic sacral outflow. Constipation also complicates a number of other CNS disorders, such as Parkinson's disease, but specific studies on colonic motility in neurological patients are lacking; moreover, in these diseases, drugs and inanition, rather than the actual nerve lesions, may be important.

Autonomic neuropathy

Autonomic neuropathy may also lead to constipation. This is a feature of the Shy–Drager syndrome and also, in some patients, of diabetic neuropathy. As in cord transection, diabetic patients have an impaired postprandial colonic motor response (Battle *et al.*, 1980).

Enteric neuropathy

Damage to the myenteric plexuses, which probably predominantly affects non-adrenergic, non-cholinergic neurons, results in delayed transit and constipation, leading to the syndrome of chronic intestinal pseudo-obstruction. The causes of this syndrome are numerous (Faulk, Anuras and Christensen, 1978), being both systemic and local and affecting either nerve or muscle or both. In terms of the number of patients affected, the most important cause is Chagas' disease, caused by infection with *T. cruzii*, leading to megacolon (Earlam, 1972), but the estimated 10 million sufferers from this disease are to be found only in South America. Hirschsprung's disease is due to a defined short segment of aganglionosis, but other types of primary neuropathy of the myenteric plexus, categorized as chronic idiopathic intestinal pseudo-obstruction (CIIP), apparently less common, involve a more generalized loss of ganglia (Dyer *et al.*, 1969). The interest in these conditions is two-fold. First, while florid cases of CIIP are rare, it is likely that some of the cases of chronic refractory constipation are due to milder forms of CIIP, in which laxative abuse with consequent enteric neuropathy may well play a part. Secondly, such cases emphasize the importance of intact innervation in normal colonic function, and it is in the understanding of neural control that further progress in this field depends.

Conclusions

The motor physiology of the rectum and colon remains largely obscure. The inaccessibility of the organ, and the technical difficulties of obtaining reliable and prolonged recordings of contractile or electrical activity in subjects under physiological conditions, have prevented us from obtaining a clear and coherent picture of the physiology of the organ. Fragmentary or corrupt data has often been over-interpreted, while techniques which are essentially invalidated have often been used. There is a relatively clear understanding of the morphology of the organ, of its innervation and of the structure and function of the contractile elements. What we do not yet understand is how these elements are combined to produce organized and functional movements, nor how these relationships are disturbed in disease. Abnormalities of colonic motility undoubtedly exist; these may be secondary to disease processes as in diarrhoea (Connell, 1968), or may be primary as in the pathogenesis of diverticula (Arfwidsson, 1964). Neuropathy, as in Hirschsprung's disease, and myopathy, as in pseudo-obstruction (Christensen, 1983), are expressed as motility disorders. It is widely believed that disordered motility underlies the 'irritable colon' syndrome. The fact remains that, at the present time, both the normal range of colorectal motor activity and its variation in disease have yet to be clearly defined.

References

ARFWIDSSON, S. (1964). Pathogenesis of multiple diverticula of the sigmoid colon in diverticular disease. *Acta Chirurgica Scandinavica*, Supplement 342

BATTLE, W. M., SNAPE, W. J., ALAVI, A., COHEN, S. and BRAUNSTEIN, S. (1980). Colonic dysfunction in diabetes mellitus. *Gastroenterology*, **79**, 1217–1221

BAYLISS, W. N. and STARLING, E. H. (1900). The movements and innervations of the large intestine. *Journal of Physiology*, London, **26**, 107–118

BENNETT, R. C. and DUTHIE, H. L. (1964). The functional importance of the internal sphincter. *British Journal of Surgery*, **51**, 355–357

BISHOP, B. (1959). Reflex activity of the external anal sphincter of the cat. *Journal of Neurophysiology*, **22**, 679–692

BUENO, L., FIORAMONTI, J., RUCKEBUSCH, Y., FREXINOS, J. and COULOM, P. (1980). Evaluation of colonic myoelectrical activity in health and functional disorders. *Gut*, **21**, 480–485

CANNON, W. B. (1902). The movements of the intestine studied by means of roentgen rays. *American Journal of Physiology*, **6**, 251–277

CHRISTENSEN, J. (1975). Myoelectric control of cat colon. *Gastroenterology*, **68**, 601–609

CHRISTENSEN, J. (1983). In *A Guide to Gastrointestinal Motility*, pp. 199–213 (J. Christensen and D. L. Wingate, Eds). Bristol; Wright

CHRISTENSEN, J., ANURAS, S. and HAUSER, R. L. (1974). Migrating spike bursts and electrical slow waves in the cat colon: effect of sectioning. *Gastroenterology*, **66**, 240–247

CHRISTENSEN, J., SCHEDL, H. P. and CLIFTON, J. A. (1964). The basic electrical rhythm of the duodenum in normal human subjects and in patients with thyroid disease. *Journal of Clinical Investigations*, **43**, 1659–1667

CHRISTENSEN, J., SCHEDL, P. and CLIFTON, J. A. (1966). The small intestine basic electrical rhythm frequency gradient in normal men and in patients with a variety of diseases. *Gastroenterology*, **5**, 309–315

COHEN, S. and SNAPE, W. J. (1983). Movement of the small and large intestine, in *Gastrointestinal Disease*, 3rd edn, pp. 859–873 (J. Fordtran and M. Sleisenger, Eds.). New York; McGraw-Hill

COLLINS, C. D., DUTHIE, H. L., SHELLEY, T. and WHITTAKER, G E. (1967). Force in the anal canal and anal continence. *Gut*, **8**, 354–360

CONNELL, A. M. (1964). The clinical physiology of colonic muscle. *Proceedings of the Royal Society of Medicine*, **57**, 283–286

CONNELL, M. L. (1968). Motor action of the large bowel, in *Handbook of Physiology, Alimentary Canal*, Section 6, Vol. 4, pp. 2075–2091 (C. F. Code, Ed.). Washington, D.C.; American Physiological Society

DEVROEDE, G. and LAMARCHE, J. (1974). Functional importance of extrinsic parasympathetic innervation to the distal colon and rectum in man. *Gastroenterology*, **66**, 273–280

DINOSO, V. P. JR, MURPHY, S. N. S., GOLDSTEIN, J. and ROSNER, B. (1983). Basal motor activity of the distal colon: a reappraisal. *Gastroenterology*, **85**, 637–642

DUTHIE, H. L. (1975). In *Surgery of the Anus, Rectum and Colon*, p. 47 (J. C. Goligher, Ed.). London; Baillière, Tindall and Cox

DUTHIE, H. L. and BENNETT, R. C. (1963). The relation of sensation in the anal canal to the functional anal sphincter; a possible factor in anal incontinence. *Gut*, **4**, 179–182

DUTHIE, H. L. and WATTS, J. M. (1965). Contribution of the external anal sphincter to the pressure zone in the anal canal. *Gut*, **6**, 64–68

DYER, N. H., DAWSON, A. M., SMITH, B. F. and TODD, I. P. (1969). Obstruction of bowel due to lesion in the myenteric plexus. *British Medical Journal*, **i**, 686–689

EARLAM, R. J. (1972). Gastrointestinal aspects of Chagas disease. *American Journal of Digestive Diseases*, **17**, 559–571

ELLIOTT, T. R. and BARCLAY-SMITH, E. (1904). Antiperistalsis and other muscular activities of the colon. *Journal of Physiology*, London, **31**, 272–304

FAULK, D. L., ANURAS, S. and CHRISTENSEN, J. (1978). Chronic intestinal pseudo-obstruction. *Gastroenterology*, **74**, 922–931

FIORAMONTI, J. and BUENO, L. (1983). Diurnal changes in colonic motor profile in conscious dogs. *Digestive Diseases and Sciences*, **28**(3), 257–264

FLOYD, W. F. and WALLS, E. W. (1953). Electromyography of the sphincter ani externus in Man. *Journal of Physiology*, London, **122**, 599–609

GLICK, M. E., MESHKIPOUR, H., HALDEMAN, S., BHATIA, N. N. and BRADLEY, W. E. (1982). Colonic dysfunction in multiple sclerosis. *Gastroenterology*, **83**, 1002–1007

GLICK, M. E., MESHKIPOUR, H., HALDEMAN, S., HOEHLER, F., DOWNEY, N. and BRADLEY, W. E. (1984). Colonic dysfunction in patients with thoracic spinal cord injury. *Gastroenterology*, **86**, 287–294

GOLIGHER, J. C. (1951). The functional results after sphincter saving resections of the rectum. *Annals of the Royal College of Surgeons of England*, **8**, 421–439

GOLIGHER, J. C. and HUGHES, E. S. R. (1951). Sensibility of the rectum and colon: its role in the mechanism of anal continence. *Lancet*, **1**, 543–548

HARDCASTLE, J. D. and PARKS, A. G. (1970). A study of anal incontinence and some principles of surgical treatment. *Proceedings of the Royal Society of Medicine*, **63**, Suppl., 116–118

HARRIS, L. D. and POPE, C. E. (1964). Squeeze vs resistance: an evaluation of the mechanism of sphincter competence. *Journal of Clinical Investigation*, **43**, 2272–2278

HERTZ, A. F. (1907). The passage of food along the human alimentary canal. *Guy's Hospital Reports*, **61**, 389–427

HILL, J. R., KELLEY, M. L., SCHLEGEL, J. F. and CODE, C. F. (1960). Pressure profile of rectum and anus of healthy persons. *Diseases of Colon and Rectum*, **3**, 203–209

HOLDSTOCK, D. J., MISIEWICZ, J. J., SMITH, T. and ROWLANDS, E. N. (1970). Propulsion in the human colon and its relationship to meals and somatic activity. *Gut*, **11**, 91–99

KERREMANS, R. (1968). Electrical activity and motility of the internal anal sphincter. *Acta Gastroenterologia Belgica*, **31**, 465–482

KERREMANS, R. (1969). In *Morphological and Physiological Aspects of Anal Continence and Defaecation*. Brussels; Editions Arscia

LANE, R. H. S. and PARKS, A. G. (1977). Function of the anal sphincters following colo-anal anastomosis. *British Journal of Surgery*, **64**, 596–599

MELZACK, J. and PORTER, N. H. (1964). Studies of the reflex activity of the external sphincter ani in spinal man. *Paraplegia*, **1**, 277–296

MENARDO, G., FAZIO, A., MARANGI, A., GENTA, V., MARENCO, G., BAUSANO, G. and CORAZZIARI, E. (1984). Large bowel transit in patients with paraplegia. *Gut* (Abstract in press)

MILLIGAN, E. T. C. and MORGAN, C. N. (1934). Surgical anatomy of the anal canal with special reference to anorectal fistulae. *Lancet*, **2**, 1150–1156

MISIEWICZ, J. J. (1975). Colonic motility. *Gut*, **16**, 311–314

PACE, J. L. (1971). The age of appearance of the haustra of the human colon. *Journal of Anatomy*, **109**, 75–80

PAINTER, N. S., ALMEIDA, A. Z. and COLEBOURNE, K. W. L. (1972). Unprocessed bran in treatment of diverticular disease of the colon. *British Medical Journal*, **ii**, 137–140

PARKS, A. G., PORTER, N. H. and HARDCASTLE, J. D. (1966). The syndrome of the descending perineum. *Proceedings of the Royal Society of Medicine*, **59**, 477–482

PARKS, A. G., PORTER, N. H. and MELZACK, J. (1962). Experimental study of the reflex mechanism controlling the muscles of the pelvic floor. *Diseases of the Colon and Rectum*, **5**, 407–414

PHILLIPS, S. F. and EDWARDS, D. A. W. (1965). Some aspects of anal continence and defaecation. *Gut*, **6**, 396–405

PORTER, N. H. (1962). A physiological study of the pelvic floor in rectal prolapse. *Annals of the Royal College of Surgeons of England*, **31**, 379–404

PROVENZALE, L. and PISANO, M. (1971). Methods for recording electrical activity of the human colon *in vivo*. *American Journal of Digestive Diseases*, **16**, 712–722

RITCHIE, J. A. (1968). Colonic motor activity and bowel function. Normal movement of contents. *Gut*, **9**, 442–456

SARNA, S. K., BARDAKJIAN, B. L., WATERFALL, W. E., LIND, J. F. and DANIEL, E. E. (1980). The organisation of human colonic control activity, in *Gastrointestinal Motility*, pp. 403–410 (J. Christensen, Ed.). New York; Raven Press

SARNA, S., LATIMER, P., CAMPBELL, D. and WATERFALL, W. E. (1982). Effect of stress, meal and neostigmine on rectosigmoid electrical control activity (ECA) in normals and in irritable bowel syndrome patients. *Digestive Diseases and Sciences*, **27**(7), 582–591

SARNA, S., LONDON, R. and COWELS, V. (1984). Colonic migrating and non-migrating motor complexes in dogs. *American Journal of Physiology*, **246**, 355–360

SARNA, S. K., WATERFALL, W. R., BARDAKJIAN, B. L. and LIND, J. F. (1981). Type of human colonic electrical activities recorded postoperatively. *Gastroenterology*, **81**, 61–70

SNAPE, W. J. JR., CARLSON, G. M. and COHEN, S. (1976). Colonic myoelectric activity in the irritable bowel syndrome. *Gastroenterology*, **70**, 326–330

SNAPE, W. J. JR., CARLSON, G. M. and COHEN, S. (1977). Human colonic myoelectrical activity in response to prostigmine and the gastrointestinal hormones. *American Journal of Digestive Diseases*, **22**, 881–887

SNAPE, W. J. JR, CARLSON, G. M., MATARAZZO, S. A. and COHEN, S. (1977). Evidence that abnormal myoelectric activity produces colonic motor dysfunctions in the irritable bowel syndrome. *Gastroenterology*, **72**, 382–387

SNAPE, W. J. JR, MATARAZZO, S. A. and COHEN, S. (1978). The effect of eating and gastrointestinal hormones on human colonic myoelectric and motor activity. *Gastroenterology*, **75**, 373–378

SNAPE, W. J., WRIGHT, S. H., COHEN, S. and BATTLE, W. M. (1979). The gastrocolonic response: evidence for a neural mechanism. *Gastroenterology*, **7**, 12–35

SULLIVAN, M. A., COHEN, S. and SNAPE, W. J. JR (1978). Colonic myoelectrical activity in the irritable bowel syndrome: effect of eating and anticholinergics. *New England Journal of Medicine*, **298**, 878–883

TAVERNER, D. and SMIDDY, F. G. (1959). An electromyographic study of the normal function of the external anal sphincter and pelvic diaphragm. *Diseases of the Colon and Rectum*, **2**, 153–160

TAYLOR, I., DARBY, C. and HAMMOND, P. (1978). Comparison of recto-sigmoid myoelectric activity in the irritable colon during relapses and remissions. *Gut*, **19**, A457

TAYLOR, I., DUTHIE, H. L., SMALLWOOD, R., BROWN, B. H. and LINKENS, D. (1974). The effect of stimulation on the myoelectrical activity of the rectosigmoid in man. *Gut*, **15**, 599–607

TAYLOR, I., DUTHIE, H. L., SMALLWOOD, R. and LINKENS, D. (1975). Large bowel myoelectrical activity in man. *Gut*, **16**, 808–814

TODD, I. P. (1959). Etiological factors in the production of complete rectal prolapse. *Postgraduate Medical Journal*, **35**, 97–100

WALLS, E. W. (1959). Recent observations of the anatomy of the anal canal. *Proceedings of the Royal Society of Medicine*, **52**, Suppl., 85–87

WINKLER, G. (1958). Remarques sur la morphologie et l'innervation du muscle releveur de l'anus. *Archives Anatomie et Histologie et Embryologie*, Strasbourg, **41**, 77–95

WRIGHT, S. H., SNAPE, W. J. JR, BATTLE, W. M., COHEN, S. and LONDON, R. L. (1980). Effect of dietary components on the gastrocolonic response. *American Journal of Physiology*, **238**, G228–G232

Part II

Investigation of the pelvic floor

Chapter 4

Anorectal manometry: techniques in health and anorectal disease

N. W. Read and J. J. Bannister

Anatomy

The anal canal is a narrow muscular channel, which is 2.5–5 cm long and passes downwards and posteriorly through the pelvic floor. It is surrounded by two muscular sleeves, the internal anal sphincter (IAS), composed of visceral smooth muscle, and the external anal sphincter (EAS), consisting of striated muscle. It is normally closed due to the tonic activity of both of these muscles and forms an anteroposterior slit for most of its length. The junction between the rectum and anal canal occurs at an angle of about 80–100°. The anorectal angle is maintained by the tonic contraction of the puborectalis sling of muscle, looping behind the anorectum and attached to the posterior surface of the pubis.

Internal anal sphincter

The IAS is the caudal extension of the circular muscle of the rectum. Its intrinsic nerve supply comes from the myenteric plexus, but it is also supplied by extrinsic sympathetic nerves from the hypogastric plexus and parasympathetic nerves from the sacral outflow.

The tone of the IAS is maintained by the inherent contractility of the circular smooth muscle, but is enhanced by activity in the sympathetic and probably parasympathetic (cholinergic) nerves (Garrett, Howard and Jones, 1974; Frenckner and Ihre, 1976). Rectal distension causes a reduction in IAS tone mediated by inhibitory intramural non-adrenergic, non-cholinergic neurons (Rayner, 1971; Garrett and Howard, 1972) and possibly also by a reduction in the sympathetic tone (Frenckner and Ihre, 1976; Bouvier and Gonella, 1981).

External anal sphincter

The EAS is continuous with the puborectalis muscle of the pelvic floor. It surrounds the IAS, overlapping it caudally by about 1 cm, and is thickest in the lower two-thirds of the anal canal. Shafik (1975) studied the anatomy of the anal sphincter in 18 cadavers and suggested that the EAS is composed of three distinct loops. The top loop is indistinguishable from the puborectalis muscle and lies around the posterior aspect of the upper anal canal, pulling it forward. The middle loop is attached to the coccyx posteriorly and loops around the anterior aspect of the middle third of the anal canal, pulling it backwards. The base loop is attached to the perianal skin anteriorly and loops around the posterior aspect of the lowest part of the anal canal, pulling it forwards. This triple-loop system may kink the anal canal, allowing the most efficient use of the easily fatigued striated fibres of the EAS to prevent incontinence (Shafik, 1975).

The EAS consists of Type 1 fibres, adapted for tonic contraction, and Type 2 fibres, adapted for rapid contraction (Beersiek, Parks and Swash, 1979). The EAS can be controlled voluntarily. According to Shafik (1975), the top and base loops of the EAS are supplied by the inferior haemorrhoidal branch of the pudendal nerve, while the intermediate loop is supplied by the perineal branch of S4. Recent studies involving nerve stimulation at operation suggests that the puborectalis is not innervated by the pudendal nerve, but is supplied by branches of the sacral nerves (Percy et al., 1981).

Physiology of defaecation

Defaecation is probably initiated by propagated contractions in the sigmoid or more proximal colon. Arrival of faecal matter or gas in the rectum may then stimulate rectal contractions (Scharli and Kiesewetter, 1970) which are associated with relaxations of the IAS. Some, but not all, of the rectal contractions may propagate through the rectum. Rectal contractions and IAS relaxations can be elicited by inflation of a balloon in the rectum, and the integrated responses to rectal distension have been termed the 'defaecation reflex', and as such is analogous to the micturition reflex in the urinary bladder. The desire to defaecate appears to be induced by stretch receptors in the puborectalis (Scharli and Kiesewetter, 1970), probably stimulated by the arrival of a mass in the lower rectum. If conditions are appropriate for defaecation the subject squats, the puborectalis and the external anal sphincter are inhibited, straightening the anorectal angle and converting the anorectum into a funnel shape. The bolus is then expelled by contractions of both the abdominal muscles and the smooth muscle of the rectum. The latter may be mediated by stimulation of stretch receptors in the puborectalis, since they may be produced by traction on the puborectalis (Scharli and Kiesewetter, 1970). Although defaecation can occur automatically in spinal patients, it has to be facilitated in normal subjects by the central nervous system in much the same way as micturition (Bradley et al., 1976).

Methods of recording anal manometry

Pressures in the anal canal can be measured by water-filled catheters, water- or air-filled balloons, diaphragm or sleeve catheters and force transducers. Each technique measures a somewhat different aspect of contractile activity and each has particular advantages and disadvantages.

Open-tip perfused catheters

Modern perfusion systems employ pressurized bottles containing boiled (degassed) water, connected via capillary tubing to pressure transducers and the anal probe. The latter is constructed from low compliance tubing, fitted with side-opening ports. Such systems respond rapidly to changes in pressure and use low flow rates which do not distort organ function by increasing intraluminal volume.

The pressure in the catheter is an index of the resistance to flow of fluid out of the catheter. In the anal sphincter, where the wall is closely apposed to the side opening of the catheter, fluid is initially trapped in a relatively small space, and pressures may increase to a point when the fluid escapes either inwards or outwards. The point at which this occurs is known as the yield pressure (Harris and Pope, 1964; Harris, Winnans and Pope, 1966; Katz, Kaufman and Spiro, 1967) and is influenced by the surface tension between adjacent walls of the canal as well as by the muscular tone. For comparative results, it is important that fluid is perfused into the canal until the yield pressure is attained. In modern systems, this point is reached rapidly.

The pressures measured by open-tip perfused catheters depend on the compliance of the catheter system and the rate of perfusion. Systems employing low compliance catheters and large side openings provide a more sensitive index of anal contractility. Thus, data from different laboratories using open-tip perfused catheters must be interpreted with caution.

Open-tip perfused catheters are of particular value in recording pressures in sphincters, where they may localize a contraction. A side-opening port localizes a contraction better than an end-opening where the wall is not apposed to the outflow from the catheter. Open-tip perfused catheters are less useful for recording pressures in large hollow organs where a contraction anywhere within the space will cause a rise in pressure. An important source of error with these pressure systems is that fluid infused into the anal canal may irritate the mucosa and cause a contraction.

Sleeve catheters

A sleeve catheter is often used in conjunction with an open-tipped perfused catheter. Fluid is perfused through a sleeve or tunnel formed by a flexible silastic membrane which is glued over a smooth silastic base (Dent, 1976) (*Figure 4.1*). When the probe is in the anus, the sleeve spans the sphincter so that a contraction anywhere along its length will cause an increased resistance to the flow of fluid and is measured as an increase in pressure in the catheter. Thus, the sleeve catheter provides a convenient means of

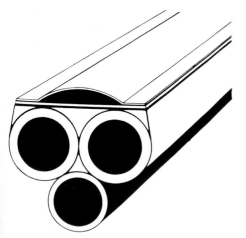

Figure 4.1. Diagram of the distal end of the sleeve catheter developed for sphincter recording by Dent (1976)

determining the net resistance of the whole sphincter to the flow of fluid, although it does not localize the site of resistance and it cannot distinguish between IAS and EAS activities.

Balloons

Fluid- or air-filled balloons are connected by a catheter to pressure transducers. Balloons distend the anal canal and the pressure measured may provide a more sensitive index of the resistance to distension than open-tipped catheters. Duthie and Watts (1965) were unable to demonstrate any effect of anaesthesia and muscle relaxants on anal tone when they used open-tipped catheters, but recorded a 40 per cent decrease in pressure using a balloon.

The pressures that are recorded depend on the size of the balloon that has been used: resistance to distension will increase as the diameter of the balloon is increased, depending upon the viscoelastic properties of the balloon as well as the anus. The effect of the wall of the balloon can be determined by inflation outside the body. The pressures obtained can then be subtracted from the measurements recorded when the balloon is *in situ*. The balloon may also directly influence sphincter tone, since distension of the anus has been shown to cause anal contraction followed by relaxation (Gowers, 1877; Denny-Brown and Robertson, 1935), whereupon the balloon may be expelled.

The 'Schuster' probe (Schuster *et al.*, 1965) (*Figure 4.2*) consists of a rigid metal cylinder, which is clamped in the anal canal by inflating two balloons in such a manner that the external balloon appears to record the EAS contractions, while the internal balloon records predominantly the activity of the IAS. This ingenious device provides a simple and convenient means of recording external and internal sphincter components independently, although the overlap of the two sphincters limits the interpretation of the data. Another possible drawback is that large balloons that stretch the sphincter may alter anorectal contractility to a greater extent than small balloons or perfused catheters.

Rectal tone and compliance are measured using large, floppy, thin-walled balloons inflated with increasing volumes of air or water; a condom is ideal, although smaller balloons have been used to measure the contractility of the rectal ampulla (Bubrick, Godec and Cass, 1980). Clearly, large rectal balloons only measure the integrated pressure inside the rectal cavity; smaller balloons are preferable if one wants to localize rectal contractions.

Results from rectal distension may differ according to whether the balloon is filled with air or water. Fluid-filled balloons are heavy, and if studies are carried out in patients in the upright position their weight on the pelvic floor may stretch the puborectalis and induce rectal contractions and IAS relaxations (Scharli and Kiesewetter, 1970).

Other devices

Gaston (1948) measured anal pressures with an obturator, one inch (25 mm) in diameter, covered in thin rubber, which enclosed a chamber connected by means of a tube to a pressure transducer. In a modification of this method, a metal septum was fixed in the middle of the obturator, separating it into proximal and distal compartments, so that events occurring in the upper and lower anal canal could be

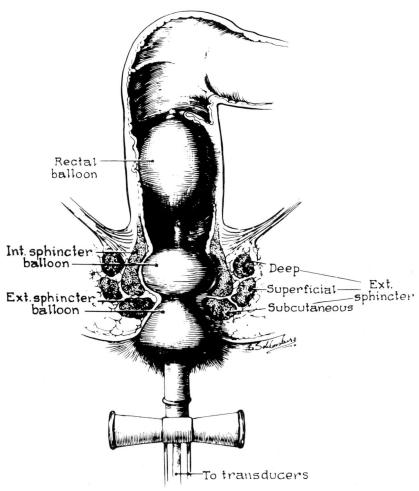

Rectal balloon

Int. sphincter balloon

Ext. sphincter balloon

Deep
Superficial
Subcutaneous

Ext. sphincter

To transducers

Figure 4.2. 'Schuster' probe *in situ* in the anorectum (From Schuster *et al.* (1965), by permission of the publishers)

recorded independently. Similar devices have been used by other workers (Lawson and Nixon, 1967; Molnar *et al.*, 1983).

Several attempts have been made to measure the radial force of anal contraction. One device consisted of 16 steel cantilevers in groups of four, each cantilever being bonded to a semiconductor strain gauge. This allowed simultaneous measurements of pressure at four longitudinal positions and four radial positions in the anal canal (Collins *et al.*, 1969).

Sphincter pressures have also been measured with radiotelemetering capsules (Scharli and Keisewetter, 1970) and more recently strain gauge transducers have been made small enough to fit in the anal canal (Loening-Baucke, 1983; Rosenberg and Vela, 1983). Microtransducers do not distend the anus and avoid many of the problems associated with balloons or perfused catheters.

Problems of interpreting anal pressures

Use of pressures as an index of resistance

The anal pressure is often used as an index of the resistance of the sphincter to the passage of faecal material from the rectum. This seems reasonable, since balloons and perfused catheters actually measure the force required to distend the sphincter, and there are significant correlations between sphincter pressure and the force required to pull a spherical ball through the anal canal (Diamant and Harris, 1969; Read *et al.*, 1979). Other factors, however, contribute to the resistance of the anal canal. They include the anorectal angulation; if the anorectal angle is sufficiently acute, only very low anal pressures are needed to keep the mass in the rectum (Kerremans, 1969).

Whether pressures can be used to provide a useful index of the resistance of the anal canal also depends upon the size of the probe. Narrow probes may give an erroneous index of the resistance that the anal canal may have to the passage of a solid stool. Normally, the anal canal is fairly elastic and can relax to accommodate quite large probes (Duthie, Kwong and Brown, 1970), but when the canal is scarred or when it contains engorged anal cushions, higher pressures than normal may be recorded with large-diameter probes, but not necessarily small-diameter probes.

Radial and longitudinal differences

Variations in pressures exist at different sites within the anal canal. The highest pressures are recorded in the lower canal, corresponding with the anatomical position of the bulk of the EAS. Radial pressures in the upper canal, measured by a rigid probe, are lower anteriorly than posteriorly both at rest and during voluntary contraction (Collins *et al.*, 1969; Taylor, Beart and Phillips, 1984). This would correspond with the anatomy of the puborectalis which loops around the back of the canal and is deficient anteriorly. These pressures are particularly low in women who have had a vaginal delivery and may explain the occurrence of rectocele. Radial pressures are approximately equal in the mid-canal, but Taylor, Beart and Phillips (1984) found that both resting and squeeze pressures in the lower canal were lower posteriorly. Thus, the manometric recordings are consistent with the existence of a forwardly directed top loop and a backwardly directed loop below it (Shafik, 1975), but they do not confirm Shafik's forwardly directed base loop. It is possible, however, that the radial differences recorded by Taylor and his colleagues are caused by the unavoidable leverage applied to the sphincter in order to get the tip of their rigid probe into the rectum.

Manipulation of the probe

Movement of the probe within the anal canal may reflexly increase anorectal pressure (*Figure 4.3*). Thus, higher pressures may be recorded if the probe is continuously pulled through the canal, than if the probe is left at one site for at least 30 s to allow the pressure to fall to steady levels before being moved (station pull-through).

Normal records

Anal canal

Resting pressures

The resting pressure in the anal canal undergoes regular fluctuations. These consist of slow waves (amplitude 5–25 cmH$_2$O; frequency between 10/min and 20/min) and much

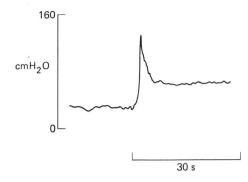

160 — cmH₂O

0 —

|————————————|
30 s

Figure 4.3. Movement of probe within the anal canal showing a reflex rise in anal pressure returning in a few seconds to new baseline

larger amplitude, ultra-slow waves (amplitude 30–100 cmH₂O; frequency <3/min) (Kerremans, 1969; Hancock and Smith, 1975; Haynes and Read, 1982). Slow and ultra-slow waves are generated by the IAS, since electrical recordings from the IAS show fluctuations occurring at the same frequencies (Bouvier and Gonella, 1981), and rectal distension reduces the tone of the IAS and abolishes both electrical and pressure fluctuations.

The frequency of the slow wave is higher in the lower canal than in the upper canal (Kerremans, 1969; Penninckx, Kerremans and Beckers, 1973; Hancock, 1976). This suggests that an inwardly directed contraction gradient may propel small amounts of material in the anal canal back into the rectum.

Ultra-slow waves are associated with particularly high resting pressures. In our studies we found them in about 40 per cent of normal subjects, but only when the resting pressure was above 140 cmH₂O (Haynes and Read, 1982). Other workers have reported ultra-slow waves in only 5 per cent of normal subjects, but in 45 per cent of patients with haemorrhoids and 80 per cent of patients with anal fissures (Hancock, 1976, 1977). Resting sphincter pressures are often very high in both of these conditions.

Tonic contractions of both the internal and the external sphincters contribute to the resting pressure. Studies in which the EAS component was blocked by anaesthesia of the pudendal nerve showed that about 15 per cent of the resting pressure, measured by a 7 mm anal balloon, came from the EAS (Frenckner and von Euler, 1975). On the other hand, IAS myotomy for fissures produces a 50 per cent drop in sphincter pressure measured with narrow open-ended polythene tubes (Bennett and Duthie, 1964).

Resting anal pressure is reduced in patients with meningocele, spinal shock (Meunier and Mollard, 1977), spinal anaesthesia (Frenckner and Ihre, 1976) and in patients who have had a sacral resection with ablation of sacral nerves on one or both sides (Gunterberg *et al.*, 1976). It is not, however, lowered in chronic paraplegics (Denny-Brown and Robertson, 1935; Frenckner, 1975; Meunier and Mollard, 1977). These data suggest that the anal tone is enhanced by a spinal mechanism which can operate independently of any cerebral control, although it is not certain whether this mechanism influences anal tone by altering activity in the EAS, IAS or both. Anal pressure is increased in the upright posture (*Figure 4.4*) and is associated with an increased electrical activity in the external sphincter (Kerremans, 1969). Coughing or increases in intra-abdominal pressure also increases the external sphincter activity (Floyd and Walls, 1953; Parks, Porter and Melzack, 1962; Kerremans, 1969), possibly by stimulation of stretch receptors in the pelvic floor.

Resting pressures in women, particularly those who have had several children, are

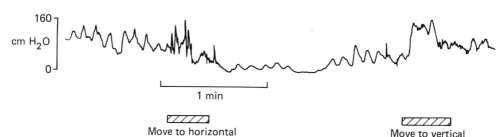

Move to horizontal   Move to vertical

Figure 4.4. Influence of posture on the anal pressure. The subject is tilted to the vertical plane keeping the transducers level with the anal canal. After approximately 2 min, the subject is tilted back to the horizontal plane

lower compared with men, and in elderly subjects compared with younger subjects (Read *et al.*, 1979; Matheson and Keighley, 1981; Taylor, Beart and Phillips, 1984).

Pressures recorded during voluntary contraction

Phasic contraction of the EAS is under voluntary control and is associated with contraction of the puborectalis sling. Voluntary contraction elevates the pressure throughout the anal canal, but is maximal in the lower canal where the bulk of the EAS is situated. Pressures induced by voluntary contraction are higher in male compared with female subjects and are reduced as subjects get older (Read *et al.*, 1979; Matheson and Keighley, 1981). If subjects are asked to sustain a voluntary contraction, the pressure declines to basal values over a period of up to 3 min (Parks, Porter and Melzack, 1962; Read and Read, 1982). Both the amplitude and duration of the voluntary squeeze pressure are reduced by anaesthesia of the anal mucosa (Read and Read, 1982).

Length of the canal

The length of the anal canal, determined by the pull-through technique, is 2.5–5 cm, and is longer in males compared with females (Nivatvongs, Stern and Fryd, 1981).

Rectal pressures

The rectum is often quiescent under normal resting conditions and exerts a basal pressure of about 5 cmH$_2$O. Rectal contractions may be induced by infusion of air and water in the upper rectum, distension with a balloon or traction on the puborectalis (Connell, 1961; Scharli and Kiesewetter, 1970). Scharli and Kiesewetter described three major types of rectal contractile activity: runs of simple contractions, occurring at a frequency of 5–10 c/min, slower contractions, occurring at a frequency of about 3 c/min and attaining amplitudes of up to 100 cmH$_2$O, and slow contractions of similar characteristics that appear to propagate through the rectum. Propagated contractions were observed in approximately 15 per cent of studies. Similar findings have been reported by other workers (Whitehead, Engel and Schuster, 1980).

The inflation of a balloon with increasing volumes of air or liquid is associated with an initial increase in pressure as the material is introduced. This is often followed by a secondary increase in pressure, probably caused by rectal contraction (see below). The pressure then gradually subsides to a steady baseline as the rectum accommodates to the new volume (*Figure 4.5*). Eventually, however, a volume is attained at which the

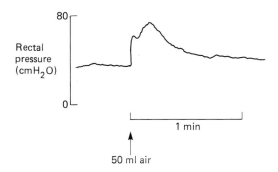

Figure 4.5. Effect of inflation of a rectal balloon upon rectal pressure. A sharp rise in pressure as the air is introduced is followed by a further increase, due possibly to a rectal contraction and by a relaxation

rectum fails to accommodate and a large increase in steady-state pressure is observed when the balloon is distended (Ahran *et al.*, 1976). This increase in pressure is often associated with pain. The slope of the pressure–volume relationship is often used to calculate values for rectal compliance (V/P), although such values depend upon the size and elasticity of the rectal balloon and differ in different laboratories. Values for the tension of the rectal wall have also been calculated from the pressure data by the Laplace law (Ahran *et al.*, 1976). This calculation relies on the assumption that the radius of a rectal balloon *in situ* will be the same as it is outside the body. Changes in gas volume caused by the body warmth and the distortion of the balloon from the spherical by surrounding structures may introduce errors.

Reflex responses to rectal distension

Distension of the rectum with a balloon induces rectal contraction, IAS relaxation and EAS contraction. These recto-anal reflexes may permit the sensitive anal epithelium to sample rectal contents without fear of incontinence (Duthie and Bennett, 1963). Relaxation of the IAS allows the rectal contents to enter the anal canal and stimulate the sensory anal mucosa, which is not exposed to rectal contents under resting conditions. This sensory epithelium can discriminate between solid, liquid and gaseous contents.

If solids and liquids enter the anal canal and conditions are inappropriate for defaecation, strong voluntary contractions of the EAS and puborectalis force the mass back into the rectum, but if the anal contents are gaseous, the contents can be released without fear of soiling.

Rectal response

The rectal contractile response to rectal distension is reduced or absent in patients with lesions involving the spinal cord (Denny-Brown and Robertson, 1935; White, Verlot and Ehrentheil, 1940), suggesting that it is mediated by a spinal reflex.

IAS response

At low distending volumes, a transient reduction in anal pressure is often observed (Meunier and Mollard, 1977). At higher volumes, an initial increase in pressure, caused by contraction of the EAS, is followed by a reduction in pressure, caused by relaxation of the IAS (*Figure 4.6*). As the rectal balloon is distended with larger volumes, the

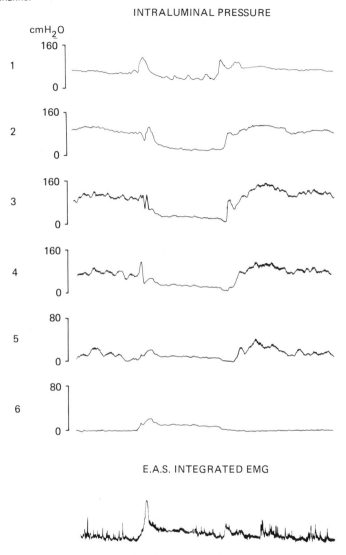

Channel

INTRALUMINAL PRESSURE

E.A.S. INTEGRATED EMG

1 min

Figure 4.6. Pressure recorded at 0.5 cm intervals in the anal canal and rectum and the external anal sphincter electromyogram activity during distension of the rectum with a rectal balloon. The inflation was maintained for 1 min and then the balloon was rapidly deflated. Channel 1 was 0.5 cm and channel 6 was 3 cm from the anal verge

amplitude and duration of the relaxation increases (Schuster *et al.*, 1965; Ahran, Faverdin and Thouvenot, 1972; Meunier and Mollard, 1977) (*Figure 4.7*).

Multi-sensor recordings show that relaxation of the lower canal in response to rectal distension is less than the relaxation of the upper canal, but increases as the rectum is distended with larger volumes (*Figure 4.8*). In some patients, pressures in the lowermost

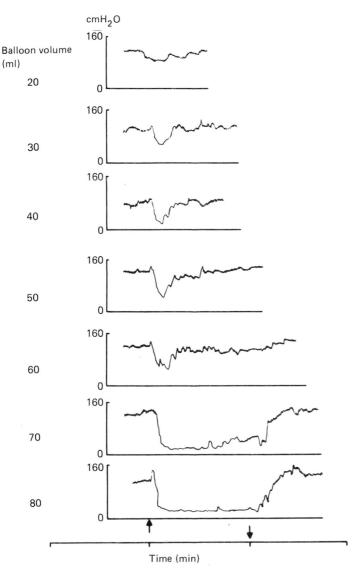

Figure 4.7. Pressure recorded in the anal canal on distension of the rectum with increasing volumes of air in a rectal balloon. The inflation at each volume was maintained for 1 min and then the balloon was deflated

0.5 cm of the anal canal may not fall until the distending volumes become uncomfortable. This is presumably because the IAS does not extend to the lowermost part of the anal canal and the pressures at this site reflect the tonic activity of the EAS.

The relaxation of the IAS in response to rectal distension is probably mediated by an intramural reflex; it is not necessarily abolished by spinal anaesthesia in man (Frenckner and Ihre, 1976), but disappears in experimental animals after rectal application of cocaine and after transection of the low rectum (Gary, 1933). IAS relaxation is, however, modulated by activity in the spinal cord since no reflex is found

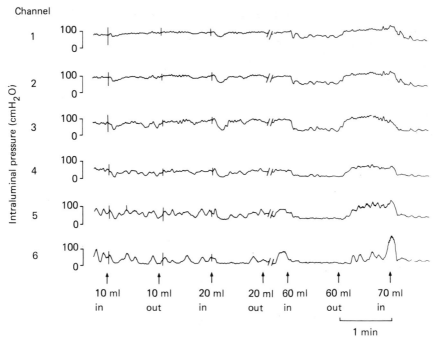

Figure 4.8. Pressure recorded at 0.5 cm intervals in the anal canal during distension of the rectum with progressively large volumes of air in a rectal balloon. The inflation at each volume was maintained for 1 min and then the balloon was deflated. Channel 1 is situated 0.5 cm and channel 6 is 3 cm from the anal verge

during spinal shock, and there is no relationship between the degree of distension and the amplitude of relaxation in patients with meningocele (Meunier and Mollard, 1977). Recent studies have shown that distension of the more proximal regions of the colon (Naudy *et al.*, 1984) may cause IAS relaxation.

Relaxation of the IAS is associated with rectal contraction (Kerremans, 1969; Haynes and Read, 1982), suggesting that it is triggered by stimulation of in-series tension receptors in the rectal wall.

EAS response—the inflation reflex

Balloon distension of the rectum causes an increase in EAS activity at low distending volumes, although this gives way to a relaxation at higher distending volumes (Porter, 1962). Both responses are produced by spinal reflexes. The receptors are thought to lie in the pelvic floor, since the responses can only be produced by distension of the rectum in normal subjects (Parks, Porter and Melzack, 1962) but can be elicited by colonic distension in patients with colo-anal anastomoses (Lane and Parks, 1977).

Dynamic studies of anorectal function

More information on the relationship between anorectal responses and continence may be gained by recording anorectal pressures when the rectum is distended with fluid (Haynes and Read, 1982; Read *et al.*, 1983b). This mimics the situation that occurs when the sphincter is trying to retain a large volume of liquid faeces in the rectum. In our studies, saline was infused into the rectum at a rate of 60 ml/min for 25 min. A few minutes after the start of the infusion, a regular series of anal relaxations developed (*Figure 4.9*). After a few more minutes these were accompanied by contractions of the rectum and the EAS. The frequency of these oscillations was approximately 1/min (similar to that of the ultra-slow wave) and increased as more fluid was infused.

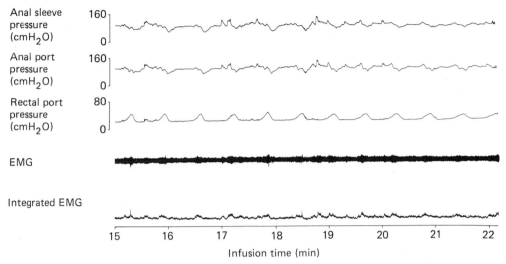

Figure 4.9. Typical record of anal and rectal pressure fluctuations and external sphincter electromyogram (EMG) during rectal infusion of saline in a normal subject. Note that regular increases in rectal pressure occur at the same time as anal relaxations and external sphincter contractions (seen on the anal pressure and EMG channels). (From Read *et al.* (1983b), by permission of the publishers)

In most normal subjects, continence appeared to be maintained during rectal infusion by the residual tone of the sphincter. Inhibition of sphincter tone was less than that which could be elicited by balloon distension of the rectum, and the peak rectal pressures were always lower than the lowest anal sphincter pressures. Phasic contraction of the EAS appeared to play little part in the maintenance of continence in normal subjects, since contraction was only transient and occurred before the deepest relaxation of the IAS (Haynes and Read, 1982). In no subject did we observe sustained forcible contraction of the EAS in an attempt to retain fluid in the rectum (Haynes and Read, 1982; Read *et al.*, 1983b).

Manometry in patients with anorectal disorders

Faecal incontinence

Several factors are thought to maintain continence to faeces. They include the contraction of the IAS and EAS, the acute angulation of the anorectum, reflex contraction of the EAS upon distension of the rectum, the ability of the anal canal to distinguish between solids, liquids and gases, the sensibility of the rectum and the mucosal plug formed by the anal cushions.

Patients with idiopathic faecal incontinence have low basal and squeeze sphincter pressures and obtuse anorectal angulation (Read *et al.*, 1979; Read, Bartolo and Read, 1984). These findings are usually associated with electromyographic evidence of neuropathic damage to the EAS and the puborectalis (Bartolo *et al.*, 1983a, 1983b). Studies in which anorectal pressures have been recorded by a multilumen probe suggest the existence of two different abnormalities of sphincter function in patients with idiopathic faecal incontinence. In some patients, basal sphincter pressures are very low, and rectal distension induces EAS contraction but no IAS relaxation. These patients presumably have severe weakness of the IAS. Other patients have normal sphincter relaxation to rectal distension, although the EAS response is very small. These patients presumably have marked weakness of the EAS. Similar findings were observed during rectal infusion of saline (Read *et al.*, 1983b). Fifty-nine per cent of incontinent patients showed an early and sustained relaxation in sphincter tone (Read *et al.*, 1983b). Thereafter the record consisted of regular contractions visible throughout the rectum and anal canal (*Figure 4.10*) and associated with increases in the electrical activity of the EAS, so that the whole anorectum was behaving as a single fluid-filled compartment and the EAS and possibly puborectalis were contracting in an attempt to prevent leakage induced by increases in rectal pressure. The remaining 41 per cent of incontinent patients demonstrated a normal pattern of regular anal relaxations, rectal contractions and EAS activity. Rectal pressures were, however, abnormally high and incontinence occurred when rectal pressure was higher than the pressure in the anal canal. The EAS response to distension with fluid was often reduced compared with normal subjects (*Figure 4.10*).

The strength of the EAS seems particularly important for maintaining continence to solids, since patients who are incontinent to both solids and liquids have significantly

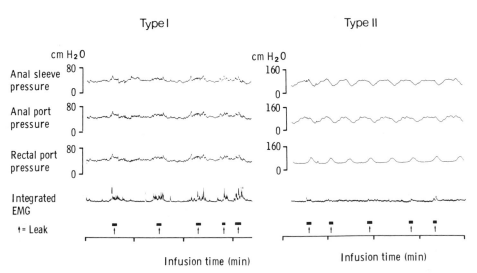

Figure 4.10. Record of anal and rectal pressure fluctuation and external sphincter electromyogram (EMG) during rectal infusion of saline in 2 incontinent patients. In one patient (type I), identical pressure profiles are seen throughout the anorectum. These are associated with a similar profile in the integrated EMG. In the other patient (type II), increases in rectal pressure are associated with anal relaxation and low amplitude increases in external sphincter EMG. In this patient, external sphincter contractions are only just apparent on the anal sleeve channel

lower squeeze pressures than those who are incontinent only to liquids (Read, Bartolo and Read, 1984).

The combination of a weak sphincter and an obtuse anorectal angle seems to be necessary before incontinence will occur. Patients with perineal descent and obtuse anorectal angulation are incontinent only if they also have low sphincter pressures (Bartolo *et al.*, 1983b), while patients who have no IAS or EAS may remain continent as long as the puborectalis can maintain a normal anorectal angle (Varma and Stephens, 1972). Treatment of incontinence by reconstruction of the anorectal angle by postanal repair renders over 80 per cent of patients continent (Parks, 1975), although basal pressures and the maximum squeeze pressures are also increased after this operation (Browning and Parks, 1983; Keighley and Fielding, 1983). The anorectal angle is thought to act as a flap valve; as the intra-abdominal pressure increases, the anterior rectal wall is forced down on top of the anal canal, preventing rectal contents from entering the anus. If the angle is obtuse, rectal contents have a direct passage to the anus, and continence can only be maintained by the resistance of the sphincter.

Incontinence is a complication of diabetes mellitus. Both maximum basal and maximum squeeze pressures are reduced in incontinent diabetics compared with continent diabetics (Schiller *et al.*, 1982; Erkenbrecht *et al.*, 1984). Perhaps more important is the observation that the rectal volume, which induces anal relaxation in incontinent diabetics, is often less than that which can be perceived by the patient (Wald, 1983; Wald and Tunuguntla, 1984). This phenomenon has also been observed in children with meningomyelocele (Wald, 1983), and in children with encopresis (Molnar *et al.*, 1983). It may well be an important factor in causing incontinence, because it means that the stimulus for voluntary protective contraction of the EAS and puborectalis may not occur prior to soiling. In support of this hypothesis, patients with incontinence, particularly those with diabetes and meningocele, often do not demonstrate adequate EAS responses when anal relaxation is induced by rectal distension (Cerulli, Nikoomanesh and Schuster, 1979; Wald, 1981; Wald and Tunuguntla, 1984). Biofeedback training has been used to enhance the EAS response to rectal distension in such patients (Cerulli, Nikoomanesh and Schuster, 1979; Wald, 1981).

Perineal descent

Abnormal descent of the perineum, both at rest and on straining, is found in about 75 per cent of patients with faecal incontinence, as well as in patients who habitually strain at stool but have little or no incontinence. In the latter, the anterior mucosal wall of the rectum may prolapse into the anus, plugging it and producing pain, tenesmus and bleeding (the descending perineum syndrome) (Parks, Porter and Hardcastle, 1966; Hardcastle, 1969; Parks, 1975). Both groups of patients have similar degrees of neuropathic damage to the EAS (Bartolo *et al.*, 1983b).

The manometric findings in patients with perineal descent correlate with the presence or absence of incontinence. We recently examined 53 patients with perineal descent, 32 of whom were incontinent (Bartolo *et al.*, 1983b). Only the group of patients who were incontinent of faeces or rectally infused saline had abnormally low sphincter pressures; the group of patients who were continent had sphincter pressures which were not significantly different from normal. Low sphincter pressures are not the only factor responsible for incontinence in patients with perineal descent. The anorectal angle is often obtuse, and damage to the pudendal nerve will also cause anaesthesia of the anal canal.

Rectal prolapse

Studies carried out in patients with rectal prolapse are difficult to interpret because many of these patients are incontinent; thus the manometric findings may reflect the incontinence rather than the prolapse. In studies carried out in continent patients with prolapse, Neill, Parks and Swash (1981) found reductions in mean sphincter length and resting sphincter pressures, while Matheson and Keighley (1981) found no reductions in sphincter pressures. The majority of continent patients with prolapse show no evidence of external sphincter neuropathy (Neill *et al.*, 1981), unlike patients with perineal descent and anterior mucosal prolapse (Henry, Parks and Swash, 1982; Bartolo *et al.*, 1983b). This observation suggests that the descending perineum syndrome (with anterior mucosal prolapse) and full thickness rectal prolapse in continent patients are not caused by the same mechanism. It seems likely that rectal prolapse may commence as a rectal intussusception, which the patient perceives as a stool and attempts to pass. If this is the case, the patient does not require any abnormality in anal sphincter function to prolapse the rectum.

In incontinent patients with prolapse, sphincter pressures are low, the minimum rectal volume required to cause constant relaxation of the IAS (Ihre, 1974) is less than that which can be perceived and the EAS response to rectal distension is often reduced (Porter, 1962). These abnormalities are found in patients with faecal incontinence associated with other conditions and may have little relevance to rectal prolapse *per se.*

Irritable bowel syndrome

In a recent study of 81 patients with irritable bowel syndrome (IBS) (Cann, Read and Holdsworth, 1983; Cann *et al.*, 1984), we found that 68 per cent complained of urgency and 27 per cent admitted episodes of incontinence when this was enquired about. Other common symptoms included frequent passage of stool, passage of small stools, feeling of wanting to defaecate but an inability to pass anything from the rectum, and feeling of incomplete evacuation after defaecation. All of these symptoms suggest a disturbance of the motor activity of the distal colon and anus.

Patients with IBS generate higher pressures than controls during balloon distension of the rectum, and pain is experienced at lower distending volumes (Ritchie, 1973; Whitehead, Engel and Schuster, 1980). Rectal distension is also more likely to give rise to runs of rectal contractions and associated anal relaxations in patients with IBS (*Figure 4.11*). Thus, the rectum in IBS is hypertonic, hypersensitive and shows increases in contractility.

Proctalgia fugax

Proctalgia fugax is thought to be caused by the spasmodic contraction of the striated muscle of the puborectalis and EAS (Douthwaite, 1962), although to our knowledge anal manometry has not been recorded during a typical episode of pain. Harvey (1979) studied two patients who had lower abdominal pain and 20–60 episodes of perianal pain in 1 h. In each case, perianal pain was associated with sharp increases in pressure in the rectosigmoid, but not in the rectum. Unfortunately, anal sphincter pressures and EMG were not recorded during this study.

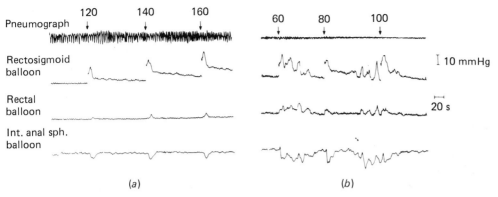

Figure 4.11. Rectal contraction associated with balloon distension of the rectum in a normal control (*a*) and a patient with irritable bowel syndrome (*b*)

Pruritus ani

The majority of patients with this condition have slight soiling. Eyers and Thomson (1979) found that 28 out of 43 patients had minor anorectal conditions, such as fissures, haemorrhoids, skin tags and anal canal polyps. The remaining 15 had normal resting sphincter pressures, but a greater reduction in anal pressure upon rectal distension than either controls or the group with detectable anorectal abnormalities.

Haemorrhoids

Patients with haemorrhoids have very high resting sphincter pressures, often associated with ultra-slow waves (Hancock and Smith, 1975). Maximum squeeze pressures and the recto-anal inhibitory reflex are normal (Read *et al.*, 1983a). It is not entirely certain whether the increased anal pressure is the primary event or whether it occurs secondary to the haemorrhoids. Thomson (1975) has suggested that increased smooth muscle activity may reduce venous drainage, increasing the size of the anal cushions and causing them to prolapse, although it is equally possible that the increased size of the anal cushions may contribute to the anal pressure by directly pressing on the anal probe or by stimulating sphincter contraction.

During continuous infusion of saline into the rectum, patients with haemorrhoids exhibited a regular pattern of EAS contractions, IAS relaxations and rectal contractions (Read *et al.*, 1983a), although rectal peaks were significantly higher in haemorrhoid patients than in normal subjects.

Anal fissure

The resting anal pressure, recorded with a narrow catheter, is normal in patients with anal fissures (Duthie and Bennett, 1964), but if the anal canal is dilated with a wider probe, the pressure is abnormally elevated (Nothmann and Schuster, 1974; Hancock, 1977). Moreover, Hancock (1977) observed ultra-slow waves in 80 per cent of patients with fissures compared with 5 per cent of controls. The IAS can be inhibited by rectal distension, although there is often an overshoot in anal canal pressures above the original values when the rectal balloon is deflated (Nothmann and Schuster, 1974).

Treatment of anal fissure by forcible anal stretch or lateral sphincterotomy lowers anal pressure and reduces the incidence of ultra-slow waves (Duthie and Bennett, 1964).

Constipation

In children with Hirschsprung's disease, the anal pressure does not relax upon rectal distension (Callaghan and Nixon, 1964; Lawson and Nixon, 1967; Meunier, Marechal and Mollard, 1978). However, in order to make this diagnosis, it is important to record pressures from the mid anal canal since the lowermost anal canal in normal subjects may show no relaxation (see above). It is also important to ensure that the recording port does not move into the rectum during rectal distension (Meunier, Marechal and Mollard, 1978). If the rectum is also involved with the condition, it is spastic and resistant to distension.

Most constipated children do not have Hirschsprung's disease (Molnar et al., 1983), although many of them show manometric abnormalities. Meunier, Marechal and de Beaujeu (1979) showed that 46 per cent of such children had elevated resting sphincter pressures and 68 per cent had blunted rectal sensitivity. Encopresis was commoner when the rectal volume, which caused anal relaxation, could not be perceived by the patient (Meunier, Mollard and Marechal, 1976).

Idiopathic constipation in young adults is much more common in women than men. Martelli et al. (1978) carried out anal manometry in 13 constipated patients, who subsequently underwent anal myectomy. Of these, five had an absent recto-anal inhibitory reflex, while in four it was reduced in amplitude. Four patients showed spontaneous variations in pressure in the rectum and anal canal under resting conditions. Recent studies (Behar and Biancani, 1984; Meunier, 1984) have also reported that anorectal manometry is abnormal in a subgroup of adults with idiopathic constipation. The major abnormal findings included high resting sphincter pressures, reduced rectal compliance and reduced anal relaxation upon rectal distension. Perception of a rectal balloon was also significantly reduced in patients with constipation compared with controls (Behar and Biancani, 1984). Lanfranchi et al. (1984) found that the recto-anal manometry and sensation differed according to colonic transit time; patients with slow colonic transit times had lower resting anal pressures, decreased rectal sensitivity and less abdominal pain than patients with normal colonic transit times.

We have recently carried out manometry on 31 women with severe constipation, who have very slow transit times. Basal and squeeze pressures were normal. The anal response to rectal distension, recorded by a multilumen probe, was also normal in the majority of patients. Upon serial distension of the rectum with a balloon, the volume which induced a desire to defaecate was above the normal range in 25 per cent of constipated patients, although the rectal pressures in the whole group were not significantly different from normal. The most striking finding was that constipated patients also had considerable difficulty in passing simulated stools from the rectum. Our data suggest that constipation in this group may be due to an inability to relax the EAS to allow passage of the stool.

Tests carried out in 55 elderly patients with faecal impaction showed that all modalities of rectal sensation were considerably impaired (Abouzekry and Read, unpublished data). Distension of a balloon in the rectum never gave any desire to defaecate in 50 per cent of patients, even at volumes of 500 ml or over. Rectal compliance was markedly increased compared with age and sex-matched normal controls and larger rectal volumes were required to elicit rectal contractions. The anal sphincter relaxed normally upon rectal distension in most patients, although the threshold volume required to induce relaxation was higher than in age and sex-matched controls. Soiling was common in these patients, and may be explained by the observation that constant relaxation of the sphincter often occurred at rectal volumes that cannot be perceived, while anal sensation was absent in the majority of subjects (Abouzekry and Read, unpublished data). These findings resemble those described in patients with damage to the sacral cord and may suggest a common mechanism.

Studies carried out in four patients who became severely constipated following injury to the low spinal cord showed low rectal pressures, high anal pressures and absence of the normal linear relationship between the degree of rectal distension and anal relaxation (Devroede *et al.*, 1979).

Ischaemic rectum

Devroede *et al.* (1982) studied 36 patients who had evidence of rectal ischaemia on mucosal biopsy and who presented with either faecal incontinence or rectal pain. These patients could not tolerate rectal distension with large volumes, and rectal compliance was reduced compared with normal subjects. Although resting sphincter pressures were normal in most patients, the amplitude of relaxation upon rectal distension was less than controls. In addition, a few patients showed an abnormally prolonged anal relaxation.

Spinal cord lesions

Resting sphincter pressures are lower than normal in patients with meningocele or lesions involving cauda equina (Meunier and Mollard, 1977). Similar reduction in resting anal pressure is also seen in patients who have undergone low spinal anaesthesia or bilateral pudendal nerve block (Frenckner and von Euler, 1975; Frenckner and Ihre, 1976). The rectum in patients with low spinal and cauda equina lesions is large and compliant and shows little contractile activity (White, Verlot and Ehrentheil, 1940). Rectal sensation to balloon distension is blunted and felt as abdominal discomfort rather than a perineal sensation (Frenckner and Ihre, 1976). The recto-anal inhibitory reflex is present in patients with low spinal or cauda equina lesions, but the degree of relaxation does not necessarily bear a direct relationship to the distending volume (Meunier and Mollard, 1977). Reflex contraction of the EAS is absent.

Patients with damage to the high spinal cord also have impaired rectal sensation (Frenckner, 1975); although the compliance of the rectum is often normal, it may be increased in some patients (White, Verlot and Ehrentheil, 1940; Frenckner and von Euler, 1975). The recto-anal inhibitory reflex is present, although the relaxation is deeper and lasts longer than in controls (Frenckner, 1975). Reflex contraction of the EAS is usually present, although at higher volumes than normal (Frenckner, 1975). Sphincter pressures are often normal (Denny-Brown and Robertson, 1935; Varma and Stephens, 1972; Frenckner, 1975).

Thus, patients with low spinal cord lesions are most likely to suffer from faecal impaction with overflow incontinence, whereas patients with high spinal lesions, who have intact rectal and IAS reflexes but can exert no control over EAS function, are more likely to suffer from incontinence caused by automatic defaecation.

Is anal manometry of any clinical use?

At present, functional tests of sphincter competence are probably of more clinical value than anorectal manometry. For example, testing the ability of the sphincter to retain a given volume of rectally infused saline provides an index of continence, which may be used to assess the efficacy of treatment and to identify those patients who are likely to become incontinent of faeces after operations which may lead to the passage of liquid motions, such as vagotomy, cholecystectomy or bowel resection (Read *et al.*, 1979). In constipation, assessment of the ability of the patient to pass a simulated stool may separate those patients with a disorder of defaecation from those with colonic inertia and may prove a useful means of assessing the response to biofeedback conditioning or drug therapy.

The most useful piece of information for the surgeon contemplating surgery for faecal incontinence is the measurement of the anorectal angle, since surgery is aimed at correcting the anatomical defect. Anal pressures may, however, have predictive value inasmuch as those patients with low voluntary squeeze pressures have a greater incidence of postoperative incontinence (Keighley and Fielding, 1983).

Manometry is, however, very important in the clinical diagnosis of Hirschsprung's disease, where the demonstration of an anal canal that does not relax on rectal distension is the most reliable simple screening test. In a study of 229 constipated children, manometry had an overall accuracy of 92 per cent, although this accuracy fell to 75 per cent in the neonatal group (Meunier, Marechal and Mollard, 1978).

The importance of anorectal manometry is that when used in combination with radiological and electrophysiological techniques it provides the important basic information for understanding of the physiology of the pelvic floor and the mechanisms of anorectal disorders. Urodynamic investigations are now regarded as an essential part of the assessment of urinary retention and incontinence. Combined manometric radiological and functional studies of anorectal physiology must eventually achieve equivalent importance in the diagnosis and treatment of anorectal disorders.

References

ARHAN, P., FAVERDIN, C., PERSOZ, B., DEVROEDE, G., DUBOIS, F., DORNIC, C. and PELLERIN, D. (1976). Relationship between viscoelastic properties of the rectum and anal pressure in man. *Journal of Applied Physiology*, **41**, 677–682

ARHAN, P., FAVERDIN, C. and THOUVENOT, J. (1972). Anorectal motility in sick children. *Scandinavian Journal of Gastroenterology*, **7**, 309–314

BARTOLO, D. C. C., JARRATT, J. A., READ, M. G., DONNELLY, T. C. and READ, N. W. (1983a). The role of partial denervation of the puborectalis in idiopathic faecal incontinence. *British Journal of Surgery*, **70**, 664–667

BARTOLO, D. C. C., READ, N. W., JARRATT, J. A., READ, M. G., DONNELLY, T. C. and JOHNSON, A. G. (1983b). Differences in anal sphincter function and clinical presentation in patients with pelvic floor descent. *Gastroenterology*, **85**, 68–75

BEERSIEK, F., PARKS, A. G. and SWASH, M. (1979). Pathogenesis of anorectal incontinence: a histometric study of the anal sphincter musculature. *Journal of the Neurological Sciences*, **42**, 111–127

BEHAR, J. and BIANCANI, P. (1984). Rectal function in patients with idiopathic chronic constipation, in *Gastrointestinal Motility*, pp. 459–466 (C. Roman, Ed.). London; MTP Press

BENNETT, R. C. and DUTHIE, H. L. (1964). The functional importance of the internal sphincter. *British Journal of Surgery*, **51**, 355–357

BOUVIER, M. and GONELLA, J. (1981). Nervous control of the internal anal sphincter of the cat. *Journal of Physiology*, **310**, 457–469

BRADLEY, W. E., ROCKSWOLD, G. L., TIMM, G. W. and SCOTT, F. B. (1976). Neurology of micturition. *Journal of Urology*, **115**, 481–486

BROWNING, G. G. P. and PARKS, A. G. (1983). Post anal repair for neuropathic incontinence: correlation of clinical results and anal canal pressures. *British Journal of Surgery*, **70**, 101–104

BUBRICK, M. P., GODEC, C. J. and CASS, A. J. (1980). Functional evaluation of the rectal ampulla with ampullometrogram. *Journal of the Royal Society of Medicine*, **73**, 234–237

CALLAGHAN, R. P. and NIXON, H. H. (1964). Megarectum: physiological observation. *Archives of Diseases in Childhood*, **39**, 153–157

CANN, P. A., READ, N. W. and HOLDSWORTH, C. D. (1983). The irritable bowel syndrome. Relationship of disorders in the transit of a single solid meal to symptom patterns. *Gut*, **24**, 405–411

CANN, P. A., READ, N. W., HOLDSWORTH, C. D. and BARENDS, D. (1984). Role of loperamide and placebo in the management of irritable bowel syndrome. *Digestive Diseases and Sciences*, **29**, 239–247

CERULLI, M. A., NIKOOMANESH, P. and SCHUSTER, M. M. (1979). Progress in biofeedback conditioning for faecal incontinence. *Gastroenterology*, **76**, 742–746

COLLINS, C. D., BROWN, B. H., WHITTAKER, G. E. and DUTHIE, H. L. (1969). New method of measuring forces in the anal canal. *Gut*, **10**, 160–163

CONNELL, A. M. (1961). The motility of the pelvic colon. *Gut*, **2**, 175–186

DENNY-BROWN, D. and ROBERTSON, E. G. (1935). An investigation of the nervous control of defaecation. *Brain*, **58**, 256–310

DENT, J. A. (1976). A new technique for continuous sphincter pressure measurement. *Gastroenterology*, **71**, 263–267

DEVROEDE, G., ARHAN, P., DUGUAY, C., TETREAULT, L., AKOURY, H. and PEREY, B. (1979). Traumatic constipation. *Gastroenterology*, **77**, 1258–1267

DEVROEDE, G., VOBECHY, S., MASSE, S., AHRAN, P., LEGER, C., DUGUAY, C. and HEMOND, M. (1982). Ischaemic fecal incontinence and rectal angina. *Gastroenterology*, **83**, 970–980

DIAMANT, N. E. and HARRIS, L. D. (1969). Comparison of objective measurement of anal sphincter strength with anal sphincter pressures and levator ani function. *Gastroenterology*, **56**, 110–116

DOUTHWAITE, A. H. (1962). Proctalgia fugax. *British Medical Journal*, **ii**, 164–165

DUTHIE, H. L. and BENNETT, R. C. (1963). The relation of sensation in the anal canal to the functional anal sphincter: a possible factor in anal continence. *Gut*, **4**, 179–182

DUTHIE, H. L. and BENNETT, R. C. (1964). Anal sphincter pressure in fissure in ano. *Surgery, Gynecology and Obstetrics*, **119**, 19–21

DUTHIE, H. L., KWONG, N. K. and BROWN, B. (1970). Adaptability of the anal canal to distension. *British Journal of Surgery*, **57**, 388

DUTHIE, H. L. and WATTS, J. M. (1965). Contribution of the external anal sphincter to the pressure zone in the anal canal. *Gut*, **6**, 64–68

ERCKENBRECHT, J. F., WINTER, H. J., CICMIR, I., BERGER, H., BERGES, W. and WIENBECK, M. (1984). Is incontinence in diabetes mellitus due to diabetic autonomous neuropathy?, in *Gastrointestinal Motility*, pp. 483–484 (C. Roman, Ed.). London; MTP Press

EYERS, A. A. and THOMSON, J. P. S. (1979). Pruritus ani: is anal sphincter dysfunction important in aetiology? *British Medical Journal*, **ii**, 1549–1551

FLOYD, W. F. and WALLS, E. W. (1953). Electromyography of the sphincter ani externus in man. *Journal of Physiology*, **122**, 599–609

FRENCKNER, B. (1975). Function of the anal sphincters in spinal man. *Gut*, **16**, 638–644

FRENCKNER, B. and VON EULER, C. (1975). Influence of pudendal block of the function of the anal sphincters. *Gut*, **16**, 482–489

FRENCKNER, B. and IHRE, T. (1976). Influence of autonomic nerves on the internal anal sphincter in man. *Gut*, **17**, 306–312

GARRETT, J. R. and HOWARD, E. R. (1972). Effects of rectal distension on the internal anal sphincter of cats. *Journal of Physiology*, **222**, 85–86P

GARRETT, J. R., HOWARD, E. R. and JONES, W. (1974). The internal anal sphincter of the cat: a study of nervous mechanisms affecting tone and reflex activity. *Journal of Physiology*, **243**, 153–166

GARRY, R. C. (1933). The responses to stimulation of the caudal end of the large bowel in the cat. *Journal of Physiology*, **78**, 208–224

GASTON, E. A. (1948). The physiology of faecal continence. *Surgery, Gynecology and Obstetrics*, **87**, 280–293

GOWERS, W. R. (1877). The automatic action of the sphincter ani. *Proceedings of the Royal Society of Medicine, London*, **26**, 77

GUNTERBERG, B., KEWENTER, J., PETERSEN, I. and STENER, B. (1976). Anorectal function after major resection of the sacrum with bilateral or unilateral sacrifice of sacral nerves. *British Journal of Surgery*, **63**, 546–554

HANCOCK, B. D. (1976). Measurement of anal pressure and motility. *Gut*, **17**, 645–651

HANCOCK, B. D. (1977). The internal sphincter and anal fissure. *British Journal of Surgery*, **64**, 92–95

HANCOCK, B. D. and SMITH, K. (1975). The internal sphincter and Lord's procedure for haemorrhoids. *British Journal of Surgery*, **62**, 833–866

HARDCASTLE, J. D. (1969). The descending perineum syndrome. *The Practitioner*, **203**, 612–619

HARRIS, L. D. and POPE, C. E. (1964). 'Squeeze' vs. resistance: an evaluation of the mechanism of sphincter competence. *Journal of Clinical Investigation*, **43**, 2272–2278

HARRIS, L. D., WINNANS, C. S. and POPE, C. E. (1966). Determination of yield pressures: a method for measuring anal sphincter competence. *Gastroenterology*, **50**, 754–760

HARVEY, R. F. (1979). Colonic motility in proctalgia fugax. *Lancet*, **2**, 713–714

HAYNES, W. G. and READ, N. W. (1982). Anorectal activity in man during rectal infusion of saline: a dynamic assessment of the anal continence mechanism. *Journal of Physiology*, **330**, 45–56

HENRY, M. M., PARKS, A. G. and SWASH, M. (1982). The pelvic floor musculature in the descending perineum syndrome. *British Journal of Surgery*, **69**, 470–472

IHRE, T. (1974). Studies on anal function in continent and incontinent patients. *Scandinavian Journal of Gastroenterology*, **9**, Suppl. 25

KATZ, L. A., KAUFMAN, H. J. and SPIRO, H. M. (1967). Anal sphincter pressure characteristics. *Gastroenterology*, **52**, 513–518

KEIGHLEY, M. R. B. and FIELDING, J. W. L. (1983). Management of faecal incontinence and results of surgical treatment. *British Journal of Surgery*, **70**, 463–468

KERREMANS, R. (1969). *Morphological and Physiological Aspects of Anal Continence and Defaecation*. Brussels; Editions Arscia

LANE, R. H. S. and PARKS, A. G. (1977). Function of the anal sphincter following colo-anal anastomosis. *British Journal of Surgery*, **64**, 596–599

LANFRANCHI, G. A., BAZZOCHI, G., CAMPIERI, M., BRIGNOLA, C., FOIS, F., MARZIO, L. and LABO, G. (1984). Intestinal transit time is related with different anorectal motility patterns in chronic non-organic constipation, in *Gastrointestinal Motility*, pp. 477–481 (C. Roman, Ed.). London; MTP Press

LAWSON, J. O. N. and NIXON, H. H. (1967). Anal canal pressures in the diagnosis of Hirschsprung's disease. *Journal of Paediatric Surgery*, **2**, 544–552

LOENING-BAUCKE, V. A. (1983). Anorectal manometry: experience with strain gauge pressure transducers for the diagnosis of Hirschsprung's disease. *Journal of Paediatric Surgery*, **18**, 595–600

MARTELLI, H., DEVROEDE, G., NARHAN, P. and DUGUAY, C. (1978). Mechanism of idiopathic constipation: outlet obstruction. *Gastroenterology*, **75**, 623–631

MATHESON, D. M. and KEIGHLEY, M. (1981). Manometric evaluation of rectal prolapse and faecal incontinence. *Gut*, **22**, 126–129

MEUNIER, P. (1984). Physiological study of the lower digestive tract in primary constipation, in *Gastrointestinal Motility*, pp. 469–475 (C. Roman, Ed.). London; MTP Press

MEUNIER, P., MARECHAL, J. M. and DE BEAUJEU, M. J. (1979). Rectoanal pressures and rectal sensitivity studies in chronic childhood constipation. *Gastroenterology*, **77**, 330–336

MEUNIER, P., MARECHAL, J. M. and MOLLARD, P. (1978). Accuracy of the manometric diagnosis of Hirschsprung's disease. *Journal of Paediatric Surgery*, **13**, 411–415

MEUNIER, P. and MOLLARD, P. (1977). Control of the internal anal sphincter (manometric study with human subjects). *Pflügers Archiv für die gesamte Physiologie des Menschen und der Tierre*, **370**, 233–239

MEUNIER, P., MOLLARD, P. and MARECHAL, J. M. (1976). Physiopathology of megarectum: the association of megarectum with encopresis. *Gut*, **17**, 224–227

MOLNAR, D., TAITZ, L. S., UNWIN, O. M. and WALES, J. K. H. (1983). Anorectal manometry results in defaecation disorders. *Archives of Diseases in Childhood*, **58**, 257–261

NAUDY, B., PLANCHE, D., MONGES, B. and SALDUCCI, J. (1984). Relaxations of the internal anal sphincter, elicited by rectal and extra-rectal distensions in man, in *Gastrointestinal Motility*, pp. 451–458 (C. Roman, Ed.). London; MTP Press

NEILL, M. E., PARKS, A. G. and SWASH, M. (1981). Physiological studies of the anal sphincter musculature in faecal incontinence and rectal prolapse. *British Journal of Surgery*, **68**, 531–536

NIVATVONGS, S., STERN, H. S. and FRYD, D. S. (1981). The length of the anal canal. *Diseases of the Colon and Rectum*, **24**, 600–601

NOTHMANN, M. E. and SCHUSTER, M. M. (1974). Internal sphincter derangement with anal fissure. *Gastroenterology*, **67**, 216–220

PARKS, A. G. (1975). Anorectal incontinence. *Proceedings of the Royal Society of Medicine*, **68**, 681–690

PARKS, A. G., PORTER, N. H. and HARDCASTLE, J. D. (1966). The syndrome of the descending perineum. *Proceedings of the Royal Society of Medicine*, **59**, 477–482

PARKS, A. G., PORTER, N. H. and MELZACK, J. (1962). Experimental study of the reflex mechanism controlling the muscles of the pelvic floor. *Diseases of the Colon and Rectum*, **5**, 407–414

PENNINCKX, F., KERREMANS, R. and BECKERS, J. (1973). Pharmacological characteristics of the non-striated anorectal musculature in cats. *Gut*, **14**, 393–398

PERCY, J. P., NEILL, M. E., SWASH, M. and PARKS, A. G. (1981). Electrophysiological study of motor nerve supply of the pelvic floor. *Lancet*, **1**, 16–17

PORTER, N. H. (1962). Physiological study of the pelvic floor in rectal prolapse. *Annals of the Royal College of Surgeons of England*, **31**, 379–404

RAYNER, V. (1971). Observations on the internal anal sphincter and the rectum in the vervet monkey. *Journal of Physiology*, **286**, 383–389

READ, N. W., BARTOLO, D. C. C. and READ, M. G. (1984). Differences in anal function in patients with incontinence to solids and in patients with incontinence to liquids. *British Journal of Surgery*, **71**, 39–42

READ, N. W., BARTOLO, D. C. C., READ, M. G., HALL, J., HAYNES, W. G. and JOHNSON, A. G. (1983a). Differences in anorectal manometry between patients with haemorrhoids and patients with descending perineum syndrome: implications for management. *British Journal of Surgery*, **70**, 656–659

READ, N. W., HARFORD, W. V., SCHMULEN, A. C., READ, M. G., SANTA ANA, C. and FORDTRAN, J. S. (1979). A clinical study of patients with faecal incontinence and diarrhoea. *Gastroenterology*, **76**, 747–756

READ, N. W., HAYNES, W. G., BARTOLO, D. C. C., HALL, J., READ, M. G., DONNELLY, T. C. and JOHNSON, A. G. (1983b). Use of anorectal manometry during rectal infusion of saline to investigate sphincter function in incontinent patients. *Gastroenterology*, **85**, 105–113

READ, M. G. and READ, N. W. (1982). Role of anorectal sensation in preserving continence. *Gut*, **23**, 345–347

RITCHIE, J. (1973). Pain from distension of the pelvic colon by inflating a balloon in the irritable colon syndrome. *Gut*, **14**, 125–132

ROSENBERG, A. J. and VELA, A. R. (1983). A new simplified technique for pediatric anorectal manometry. *Paediatrics*, **71**, 240–245

SCHARLI, A. F. and KEISEWETTER, W. B. (1970). Defaecation and continence: some new concepts. *Diseases of the Colon and Rectum*, **13**, 81–107

SCHILLER, L. R., SANTA ANA, C. A., SCHMULEN, A. C., HENDLER, R. S., HARFORD, M. V. and FORDTRAN, J. S. (1982). Pathogenesis of fecal incontinence in diabetes mellitus. Evidence for internal anal sphincter dysfunction. *New England Journal of Medicine*, **307**, 1666–1671

SCHUSTER, M. M., HENDRIX, T. R. and MENDELOFF, A. I. (1963). The internal anal sphincter response: manometric studies on its normal physiology, neural pathways and alteration in bowel diseases. *Journal of Clinical Investigation*, **42**, 196–207

SCHUSTER, M. M., HOOKMAN, P., HENDRIX, T. R. and MENDELOFF, A. I. (1965). Simultaneous manometric recording of internal and external anal sphincter reflexes. *Bulletin of the Johns Hopkins Hospital*, **116**, 79–88

SHAFIK, A. (1975). A new concept of the anatomy of the anal sphincter mechanism and the physiology of defaecation. The external anal sphincter: a triple-loop system. *Investigations in Urology*, **12**, 412–419

TAYLOR, B. M., BEART, R. W. and PHILLIPS, S. F. (1984). Longitudinal and radial variations of pressure in the human anal sphincter. *Gastroenterology*, **86**, 693–697

THOMSON, W. H. F. (1975). The nature of haemorrhoids. *British Journal of Surgery*, **62**, 542–552

VARMA, K. K. and STEPHENS, D. (1972). Neuromuscular reflexes of anal continence. *Australian and New Zealand Journal of Surgery*, **41**, 263–272

WALD, A. (1981). Biofeedback therapy for faecal incontinence. *Annals of Internal Medicine*, **95**, 146–149

WALD, A. (1983). Biofeedback for neurogenic faecal incontinence: rectal sensation is a determinant of outcome. *Journal of Paediatric Gastroenterology and Nutrition*, **2**, 302–306

WALD, A. and TUNUGUNTLA, A. K. (1984). Anorectal sensation dysfunction in fecal incontinence and diabetes mellitus. *New England Journal of Medicine*, **310**, 1282–1287

WHITE, J. C., VERLOT, M. G. and EHRENTHEIL, O. (1940). Neurogenic disturbances of the colon and their investigation by the colonmetrogram. *Annals of Surgery*, **112**, 1042–1057

WHITEHEAD, W. E., ENGEL, B. T. and SCHUSTER, M. M. (1980). Irritable bowel syndrome: physiological and psychological differences between diarrhoea predominant and constipation predominant patients. *Digestive Diseases and Sciences*, **25**, 404–413

Chapter 5

Electromyography in pelvic floor disorders

M. Swash and S. J. Snooks

Introduction

Electromyography (EMG) is a powerful investigative technique which is much used in neurological and orthopaedic practice in the investigation of patients with neuro-muscular diseases, particularly in the evaluation of disorders in which the nerve supply of muscles is damaged, whether from diseases of the spinal cord, spinal nerve roots or peripheral nerves (Swash and Schwartz, 1981). The technique depends on the recording of electrical activity arising in muscle fibres during voluntary contraction and at rest. A number of different methods for quantification of this electrical activity are available, but these are not all applicable to the EMG analysis of the pelvic floor musculature and, as with most measurement techniques in medicine, it is important to recognize the advantages and limitations of the different methods. The related technique of nerve conduction studies is discussed in Chapter 7.

In pelvic floor disorders, EMG can provide useful clinical information about the function of the pelvic floor musculature, particularly the external anal sphincter and puborectalis muscles (Kerremans, 1969; Jesel, Isch-Treussard and Isch, 1973; Neill and Swash, 1980; Neill, Parks and Swash, 1981; Bartolo et al., 1983). The levator ani is not readily accessible for EMG exploration. The more anteriorly situated perineal muscles, particularly the peri-urethral striated musculature, are also accessible to EMG evaluation (Chantraine, 1973).

EMG can be used as a functional test of muscle activity. For example, quantitative measurements of electrical activity in the external anal sphincter or puborectalis muscles during rest and straining have been applied to the investigation of patients with incontinence, rectal prolapse and solitary rectal ulcer syndrome (*Figures 5.1* and *5.2*). Measurements of the amplitude, duration and number of phases of motor unit action potentials, on the other hand, provide information about the innervation and functional state of individual motor units within the muscle. The electrical activity in muscles can be recorded using surface electrodes, monopolar electrodes, concentric needle electrodes or single fibre EMG electrodes. These techniques will be discussed separately in this chapter.

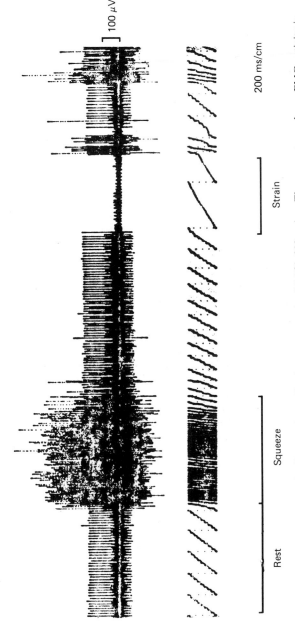

Figure 5.1. Puborectalis muscle. Concentric needle electromyography (EMG), 200 ms/cm. The upper trace shows EMG activity in this muscle. The lower trace shows the summated rectified EMG activity expressed in volt-seconds. The trace rises with the acquisition of potentials until 1 V has been stored, so that the quantitative activity in the muscle is represented by counting the number of accessions during a period of 1 s (or less). At rest there is some ongoing basal activity. The amount of EMG activity, and of muscle contraction, increases during voluntary squeezing of the anal sphincter muscle. This gradually relaxes after cessation of voluntary activity. During an attempted strain, as if in defaecation, the puborectalis muscle relaxes and EMG activity in this muscle decreases. Basal activity is resumed at the end of the voluntary strain, and increases during a cough, seen at the end of the recording

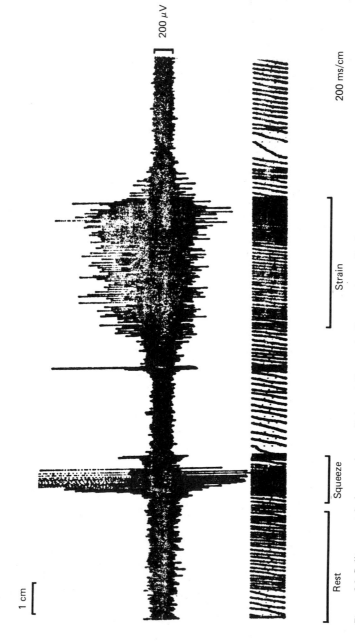

1 cm

200 µV

Rest

Squeeze

Strain

200 ms/cm

Figure 5.2. Solitary rectal ulcer syndrome. Puborectalis muscle. Concentric needle electromyography, 200 ms/cm. The recording resembles *Figure 5.1.* Basal activity is rather more evident. During straining, there is a paradoxical increase in activity in the puborectalis muscles (see Chapter 13)

Basic concepts of EMG

All electromyographic techniques depend on the recording of electrical activity generated in muscle fibres during voluntary contraction, or occurring in abnormally innervated muscle fibres at rest. The electrical activity of contracting muscle was first recorded with a string galvanometer from the human forearm flexor muscles by Piper (1908), but the technique did not come into clinical use until the advent of the coaxial (concentric) needle electrode devised by Adrian and Bronck (1929). In normal muscle, depolarization of the muscle fibre membrane, leading to the generation of the muscle action potential which is propagated along the length of the muscle fibre at a velocity of about 3 m/s, is initiated by depolarization at the specialized motor end-plate zone. This is caused by the arrival of quanta of acetylcholine released from the presynaptic motor nerve terminal by the nerve impulse. When the muscle fibre membrane becomes depolarized, the process of excitation contraction coupling is initiated, resulting in shortening of the actin myosin bands by sliding of one filament inside the other in each sarcomere. This is an energy-dependent process. Individual muscle fibres show specialization into fibres adapted for continuous contraction (tonic fibres) and those adapted for brief forceful contractions (phasic fibres). These physiological characteristics can be correlated with the Type I and Type II enzyme histochemical types determined by light microscopy (see Swash and Schwartz, 1981, 1984; and Chapter 8 of this volume).

The motor unit

Our concept of the organization of the innervation of muscle fibres within individual muscles derives from the work of Sherrington, who recognized that individual muscles contained more muscle fibres than the large heavily myelinated motor nerve fibres innervating these muscles. The term 'motor unit', which he introduced, refers to the anterior horn cell, its axon, and the axonal branches, motor end-plates and muscle fibres innervated by this cell. In some muscles, for example the intrinsic muscles of the hand, there are relatively small numbers of muscle fibres innervated by individual axons, perhaps only 6–10 muscle fibres, whereas in other muscles, for example the hip flexor muscles, much larger numbers of muscle fibres (for example 100–200) are innervated by an individual axon. The motor unit is thus smaller in the intrinsic hand muscles than in the hip flexor muscles. The former are specialized for fine and carefully controlled movements, and the latter for movements requiring considerable force.

Electromyography allows the recording of action potentials derived from motor units within a contracting muscle. The muscle fibres making up individual motor units are scattered quasi-randomly through the cross-sectional area of individual muscles in such a way that a mosaic pattern of muscle fibres representing interlocking motor units can be demonstrated in experimental studies. In pathological studies of human skeletal muscles, it is possible only to recognize the mosaic pattern of Type I, Type IIa and Type IIb fibres within the cross-section of muscles—an appearance resembling a chequer-board. During voluntary contraction of individual units, the individual muscle fibre action potentials derived from the contracting unit summate to form the motor unit action potential, a potential of larger amplitude and longer duration than that derived from single muscle fibres. Because of the small size and brief duration of individual muscle fibre action potentials, such potentials can only be recorded when the recording electrode is in close proximity to the fibre undergoing contraction, but motor unit action potentials, representing the activity of several fibres within a motor unit, can be recorded at a greater distance.

Changes in disease

There are two broad classes of neuromuscular disease—the myopathies and the neurogenic disorders. These can usually be distinguished with EMG techniques by the different patterns of electrical activity recorded in the two groups of disorders. However, EMG of the pelvic floor musculature is not usually applied to this kind of investigative problem, which is better approached by EMG of limb muscles. In pelvic floor disorders, the major indications for EMG are to assess the functional activity of the pelvic floor muscles during voluntary contraction, e.g. straining at stool or in reflexly controlled contractions, as in the cough reflex or the recto-anal sphincteric reflex, or, as in recent work from St. Mark's Hospital, in order to assess the presence of damage to the innervation of these muscles. The latter application has become of increasing importance in clinical practice.

Changes in EMG activity related to neurogenic disturbances

When the nerve supply of a muscle is damaged, some or all of the muscle fibres become denervated. This loss of functional innervation of muscle fibres leads to loss of responsiveness of those muscle fibres to nerve fibre activity, and to atrophy of the affected fibres. This can be recognized pathologically by the presence of scattered atrophic muscle fibres (see Chapter 8). If the process is incomplete, and reinnervation occurs either by regrowth of the damaged axons from the site of damage in the nerve itself, or by sprouting of nearby unaffected axons within the muscle so as to take on the innervation of neighbouring denervated fibres, effective reinnervation may occur. This process begins within a few days of nerve injury and may result in effective recovery during a period of a few days to several weeks, depending on the site of the injury. Sprouting of axons within the damaged muscle leads to a change in the distribution of muscle fibres within motor units, so that there is a tendency for these fibres not to retain their random distribution within the muscle, but to be clustered together in small groups of fibres innervated by branches of a single axon. This process is called fibre-type grouping. This change in the spatial distribution of muscle fibres within motor units results in a change in the amplitude and duration of motor unit action potentials recorded by EMG.

It is important to recognize that denervated muscle fibres cannot contract in response to voluntary activity and that the EMG changes during slight voluntary activity thus reflect the process of reinnervation rather than the process of denervation. Denervated muscle fibres may show spontaneous activity at rest—fibrillations, fasciculations and positive sharp waves (see Swash and Schwartz, 1981, for descriptive details)—but, while these are relatively easy to recognize in limb muscles, they are difficult to find in sphincter muscles.

Special characteristics of pelvic floor and anal sphincter muscles

The muscles of the pelvic floor differ from most striated muscles both anatomically and physiologically. The pelvic floor muscle fibres are generally smaller than striated muscle fibres (see Chapter 8) and contain a higher proportion of Type I, tonic muscle fibres than do the limb muscles. The external anal sphincter muscle, puborectalis muscle and periurethral striated musculature particularly show these differences. The external anal sphincter muscle is further unusual in that it consists of two deep parts and a superficial part. The latter inserts into skin and the former portions insert not into tendons or fascia, but into the endomysium of the muscle itself, since it occupies a circular position around the anal orifice. However, the muscle fibres in these muscles, like all other striated muscles in the body with the exception of the external ocular muscles, are each innervated by a single motor end-plate. Muscle spindles, the stretch sensitive receptors of striated muscles, have been identified in the levator ani, puborectalis and external anal sphincter muscles (Swash, 1982) and they presumably also exist in the periurethral striated sphincter muscle. These muscles might therefore be expected to respond to stretch by reflex contraction generated by a reflex arc dependent on the anterior horn cells in the spinal cord.

Because the muscle fibres in the external anal sphincter and puborectalis muscles are smaller than those in other striated human muscles, the amplitude of action potentials derived from individual fibres, and therefore of the motor unit action potentials themselves, might be expected to be somewhat smaller than in other striated muscles. This point is of particular importance in single fibre electromyography and in quantitative concentric needle EMG techniques.

Recording of spontaneous activity, that is, activity not generated by voluntary contraction, in these muscles is difficult to evaluate, since the external anal sphincter muscle, and probably the puborectalis muscle, shows a continuous tonic contraction (Floyd and Walls, 1953). The periurethral sphincter muscle also exhibits slow continuous electrical activity. This activity varies from moment to moment, but has been shown to be present even during sleep. This observation illustrates the importance of these muscles in the maintenance of continence. During defaecation or micturition, the activity of the sphincters ceases.

EMG recording techniques

EMG apparatus is readily available commercially. The apparatus consists of a recording electrode, a pre-amplifier, amplifier and loudspeaker, and an oscilloscope for display of electrical activity. Most modern EMG equipment provides variable amplitude and time-base duration controls within a range suitable for electromyography, together with low pass and high pass filter options suitable for the various recording techniques in common use. A number of computer-assisted methods for data analysis are available, but these have not yet been applied, in practical terms, to sphincter EMG.

Surface electrodes

Electrical activity recorded with surface electrodes is difficult to assess because each electrode is at some distance from the muscular activity, and particularly because it is not always possible to be sure that the activity recorded is actually generated within the muscle close to the electrode. Adjacent muscles, which might also be in contraction, will also contribute to the activity recorded by the surface electrodes. Surface electrodes are usually mounted in pairs on a muscle to be assessed, with a ground electrode at a distance. Surface electrode recording techniques are particularly applicable to motor nerve conduction velocity and terminal motor latency measurements in which muscle

electrode within the individual insertions during the process of the recording. In normal subjects, the fibre density in most muscles is less than two (Stalberg and Trontelj, 1979), although after the age of 60 years this value increases slightly. In the external anal sphincter muscle, the normal fibre density is 1.5 ± 0.16 (Neill and Swash, 1980). The calculation of fibre density is dependent on the acquisition of recordings of sufficient clarity to allow the measurement. By convention, in limb muscles, components used for triggering must be greater than 150 μV in amplitude but, because of the smaller size of the muscle fibres in the pelvic sphincter muscles, potentials of greater than 100 μV are accepted. During the process of reinnervation and fibre-type grouping, with increasing compaction of the muscle fibres within individual motor units, the fibre density will increase because there are more fibres within the uptake area of the electrode innervated by an individual axon or its branches and measurement of the fibre density is thus a useful parameter for assessing reinnervation (*Figure 5.4*). Further, it lends itself to sequential studies during the natural history of a disease. It is important to recognize that the observer must be scrupulous in technique. *All potentials in which a component is greater than 100 μV must be included in the calculation of the mean derived from the 20 recordings.* Thus, single recordings must all be included. It is tempting during the recording to discard single recordings in favour of the more visually exciting multiple-phase action potentials and so to obtain a higher value for the fibre density artificially. It is our practice to record all the potentials recorded during the EMG analysis on the paper printout of the EMG machine and to calculate the fibre density sequentially from the first recording that fulfils the technical criteria for the technique. This method enables the fibre density to be checked by several observers from the paper printouts.

Neuromuscular jitter

The variability in the time interval between the triggering potential and the other potential or potentials belonging to the same motor unit recorded in the uptake area of the single fibre EMG electrode is called the neuromuscular jitter (Ekstedt, 1964; Stalberg and Trontelj, 1979). This jitter is mainly due to variation in the time of onset of the action potential generated by the end-plate potential and thus reflects variabilities in the onset of threshold for depolarization of the muscle fibres with respect to each other. It is thus mainly a measure of end-plate function. It has been much used in the study of neuromuscular diseases, particularly in neurogenic disorders, in limb muscles, but has not hitherto been much studied in pelvic floor disorders. In neurogenic disorders affecting limb muscles, the neuromuscular jitter is characteristically increased and there may be blocking of transmission at high rates of motor unit firing at individual motor end-plates. These two aspects of single fibre EMG, i.e. fibre density and jitter measurements, lend themselves to computer-based quantification (Davis *et al.*, 1983) and may prove useful in pelvic floor disorders in the future.

Practical applications of pelvic floor EMG

EMG recordings of pelvic floor muscles, particularly of the striated anal and urinary sphincter musculature, can provide information relevant to the diagnosis and management of patients with faecal incontinence, urinary incontinence or double incontinence. It is also useful in the investigation of patients with other disorders of the pelvic floor, particularly rectal prolapse, solitary rectal ulcer syndrome (Rutter and

Riddell, 1975; Snooks *et al.*, 1985) and anal pain in adults. In infancy, EMG of the anal sphincter has a particular value in mapping the position of the anal sphincter in congenital atresia of the anorectum prior to reparative surgery. Similarly, in adults, sphincter mapping procedures are used when surgical attempts to reconstruct the anal canal are planned after trauma or, in some patients, after cancer surgery. EMG techniques have also been used in the assessment of retention of urine in women.

Normal EMG of the external anal sphincter muscle

The EMG activity of the striated anal sphincter was recorded by Beck (1930), Floyd and Walls (1953), Kawakami (1954), Taverner and Smiddy (1959), Ruskin and Davis (1969), Chantraine (1966) and Jesel, Isch-Treussard and Isch (1973), using conventional concentric needle EMG techniques. These studies have revealed that the external anal sphincter shows continuous low frequency activity at rest, and even during sleep (Floyd and Walls, 1953). This activity consists of contraction of individual motor unit potentials at low firing rates, and of low amplitude (<500 μV). Distension of the rectum, or of the bladder, increases this basal activity in the anal sphincter muscle. Resting activity is also increased by changes in position, and by coughing (the cough reflex). During attempts at defaecation, electrical silence occurs in the anal sphincter muscle and similar switching off of EMG activity occurs in the external urinary sphincter during the several seconds prior to detrusor contraction during micturition (Hutch and Elliott, 1968). There is thus a degree of co-contraction, or reciprocal innervation, between the voluntary vesical and anorectal sphincter musculature.

Voluntary activity of the external anal sphincter muscle, as when asking the patient to squeeze the sphincter tight, produces an interference pattern comparable with that found during maximal voluntary contraction of a limb muscle. Summation of individual motor unit action potentials occurs so that the oscilloscope screen is filled with activity (*Figure 5.1*). The motor unit potentials reach 2 or 3 mV in amplitude, although the mean amplitude is somewhat lower (200–600 μV) (Jesel, Isch-Treussard and Isch, 1973). The mean duration of motor unit potentials during voluntary activity in the striated urinary and anal sphincter muscles is 5–7.5 ms (Petersen and Franksson, 1955; Chantraine, 1966). Bartolo, Jarratt and Read (1983) found that in normal subjects there was a wide variation in motor unit potential duration, and that this increased slightly with age, from a mean value of 5 ms at age 20 years to a mean of 6.5 ms at age 80 years (*Figure 5.3*). This observation, together with the finding in several of the studies discussed above that polyphasic units are more common in elderly subjects than in young adults, is consistent with our findings using single fibre EMG (Neill and Swash, 1980; Neill, Parks and Swash, 1981; Percy *et al.*, 1982) that the fibre density in single fibre EMG recordings increases after the age of about 60 years. In 34 subjects less than 30 years old, the fibre density in the external anal sphincter was 1.37 ± 0.09 (Snooks, Barnes and Swash, 1984), but in people aged up to about 65 years it is 1.5 ± 0.16 (Percy *et al.*, 1982). At the age of 75 years, the upper limit of normal is 1.75 (Percy *et al.*, 1982).

Reflex activity

EMG activity increases in the anal sphincter muscle during coughing (the cough reflex), in response to scratching the anal skin (the anal reflex) or by eliciting the bulbo-cavernosus reflex. Further, stretching the anal sphincter by digital examination would itself result in activity in the external anal sphincter muscle. The latter method is used to increase anal sphincter activity during the acquisition of motor unit potentials for analysis during both conventional needle EMG and single fibre EMG in our laboratory (Neill and Swash, 1980).

Clinical methods

The patient lies on an electrically insulated mat in the left lateral position on a couch in a warm room. The ground electrode is strapped to the right thigh. Where possible, the sphincter ring is palpated, the perianal skin cleaned and dried and, having warned the patient, the electrode is inserted 12 cm posterior to the anal verge at an angle of 45° to the skin. By inserting the needle nearly to its hilt, its tip enters the puborectalis, a position that can be ascertained by controlling the position of the tip of the needle with a finger in the rectum. More superficial needle placement records activity in the external anal sphincter muscle. A few minutes' rest must be allowed to elapse after needle or patient movement, for the muscle activity to settle to a steady resting state. The patient is asked to squeeze the anus as hard as possible in order to record maximal voluntary contraction. Activity during straining can also be recorded, the patient being asked to strain as though having his bowels open. Activity gradually increases during this manoeuvre during a period of 5–10 s.

For single fibre EMG recordings, activity in the external anal sphincter and puborectalis muscles is induced by the insertion of a balloon into the rectum, a 150 g weight tension being applied to this by allowing a string ending in the weight to dangle over the edge of the couch. This is sufficient to induce continuous low-grade activity suitable for recording individual motor unit potentials for single fibre EMG and quantitative concentric EMG analysis (Neill and Swash, 1980; Neill, Parks and Swash, 1981).

Anal mapping

This is performed by inserting a concentric needle electrode into the external anal sphincter muscle in the four quadrants of the muscle. Posterior insertion usually produces copious EMG activity, but anterior insertion in women is painful and the muscle very thin at this site even in normal subjects. Using this technique, by repeated adjustments in needle placement without the necessity of further skin insertions, the distribution of muscle fibres within the external anal sphincter can be accurately mapped and, in the case of patients with sphincter division (Kiff, 1983), and in infants with imperforate anus (Archibald and Goldsmith, 1967; Chantraine, 1973), the position of the muscle, or the remaining fibres of the muscle, can be accurately mapped so that appropriate surgery can be planned (see Kiff, Barnes and Swash, 1984).

We have used a simple quantitative method in concentric needle EMG recording in carrying out sphincter mapping analysis by measuring the amount of EMG activity (voltage) occurring during 1 s periods. This requires the use of rectified EMG activity during successive 1 s activation periods.

Incontinence

In patients with idiopathic anorectal (neurogenic) incontinence, characteristic EMG abnormalities are found in the external anal sphincter and puborectalis muscles. In the most severely affected patients, EMG activity is decreased and zones of the sphincter muscles may be electrically silent. The potentials recorded are of larger amplitude and longer duration than normal and show multiple phases when examined with a trigger delay line, both in concentric needle and single fibre EMG recordings. The fibre density, therefore, is increased (Neill and Swash, 1980; Neill, Parks and Swash, 1981; Snooks, Barnes and Swash, 1984; Snooks et al., 1985). In less severely affected patients, the maximal amplitude during voluntary contraction is increased and the major abnormality consists of the polyphasic motor unit potentials and the increased fibre density. There may be an increased neuromuscular jitter between components of these polyphasic potentials, indicating an instability of innervation. Similar abnormalities are found in the puborectalis as in the external sphincter muscle (Bartolo et al., 1983; Snooks, Henry and Swash, 1985). In patients with rectal prolapse, the EMG activity in these two muscles is abnormal only if there is associated incontinence (Neill, Parks and Swash, 1981).

Recordings of the external anal sphincter have been used to monitor activity in the external urinary sphincter in patients with urinary incontinence, and an increase in fibre density has been described in the external anal sphincter muscle in such patients (Anderson, 1983). The use of the external anal sphincter muscle in such patients implies that a similar abnormality has occurred in both muscles in the presence of urinary incontinence without faecal incontinence. This implication has not been thoroughly investigated and the use of the external anal sphincter EMG in this way seems insecurely based. Nevertheless, in patients with double incontinence similar abnormalities are found in the external anal and external urinary sphincter muscles (Snooks, Barnes and Swash, 1984).

These findings, particularly the single fibre EMG feature of an increased fibre density, the increased motor unit potential duration, presence of polyphasic potentials, and increased amplitude in concentric needle electrode recordings, with increased jitter between individual components, are consistent with a neurogenic abnormality, that is with denervation and reinnervation of muscle fibres, in patients with incontinence. This EMG abnormality is consistent also with the histological features found in biopsies of the external anal sphincter and puborectalis muscles in patients with incontinence (see Chapter 8) and it is this combination of histological and EMG abnormalities that has led to electrophysiological investigation of the innervation of the pelvic floor muscles using the new techniques of pudendal nerve terminal motor latency measurement, and latency measurements from spinal stimulation in the cauda equina (see Chapter 7).

Monitoring during neurosurgery

EMG of the anal sphincter has been used as a monitoring technique during neurosurgical procedures in which the conus medullaris and sacral nerve roots are vulnerable (James et al., 1979).

Practical applications

These EMG methods provide useful clinical information in the investigation of patients with pelvic floor disorders, particularly incontinence. The finding of an increased fibre density, or of abnormalities in quantitive concentric needle EMG studies, suggests that there has been damage to the innervation of the pelvic floor muscles. Taken together with the clinical data, this information can be used in planning treatment and management. Since pelvic floor weakness, as is found in patients with perineal descent, is likely to be a progressive disorder, these investigations carry the practical advantage that they may be repeated during the natural history of the disorder without harm to the patient.

References

ADRIAN, E. D. and BRONCK, D. W. (1929). The discharge of impulses in motor nerve fibres. *Journal of Physiology*, London, **67**, 119–151

ANDERSON, R. S. (1983). Increased motor unit fibre density in the external anal sphincter in genuine stress incontinence: a single fibre EMG study. *Neurology and Urodynamics*, **2**, 45–50

ARCHIBALD, K. C. and GOLDSMITH, E. J. (1967). Sphincteric electromyography. *Archives of Physical Medicine and Rehabilitation*, **48**, 2349–2352

BARTOLO, D. C. C., JARRATT, J. A. and READ, N. W. (1983). The use of conventional electromyography to assess external sphincter neuropathy in man. *Journal of Neurology, Neurosurgery and Psychiatry*, **46**, 1115–1118

BARTOLO, D. C. C., JARRATT, J. A., READ, M. G., DONNELLY, T. C. and REED, N. W. (1983). The role of partial denervation of the puborectalis in idiopathic faecal incontinence. *British Journal of Surgery*, **70**, 664–667

BECK, A. (1930). Electromyographische Untersuchungen am Sphinkter ani. *Archiv. Physiologie*, **224**, 278–292

BUCHTHAL, F. (1977). Diagnostic significance of the myopathic EMG, in *Pathogenesis of Human Muscular Dystrophies*, pp. 205–218 (E. P. Rowland, Ed.). Amsterdam; Excerpta Medica International Congress Series 404

CARUSO, C. and BUCHTHAL, F. (1965). Refractory period of muscle and EMG findings in relatives of patients with muscular dystrophy. *Brain*, **88**, 29–50

CHANTRAINE, A. (1966). Electromyographie des sphincters striés urétral, cerebral et anal humains: etude descriptive et analytique. *Revue Neurologique*, **115**, 396–403

CHANTRAINE, A. (1973). EMG examination of the anal and urethral sphincters, in *New Developments in Electromyography and Clinical Neurophysiology*, vol. 2, pp. 421–432 (J. E. Desmedt, Ed.). Basle; Karger

DAVIS, G. R., BROWN, I. T., SCHWARTZ, M. S. and SWASH, M. (1983). A dedicated microcomputer-based instrument for internal analysis of multi-component waveforms in single fibre EMG. *Electroencephalography and Clinical Neurophysiology*, **56**, 110–113

EKSTEDT, J. (1964). Human single muscle fiber action potentials. *Acta Physiologica Scandinavica*, **61**, Suppl. 226, 1–98

FLOYD, W. F. and WALLS, E. W. (1953). Electromyography of the sphincter ani externus in man. *Journal of Physiology*, London, **122**, 500–609

HUTCH, J. A. and ELLIOTT, H. W. (1968). Electromyographic study of electrical activity in the paraurethral muscles prior to and during voiding. *Journal of Urology*, **99**, 759–765

JAMES, H. E., MULCAHY, J. J., WALSH, J. W. and PALPAN, G. W. (1979). Use of anal sphincter EMG during operations on the conus medullaris and sacral nerve roots. *Neurosurgery*, **4**, 821–823

JESEL, M., ISCH-TREUSSARD, C. and ISCH, F. (1973). Electromyography of striated muscles of anal and urethral sphincters, in *New Developments in Electromyography and Clinical Neurophysiology*, vol. 2, pp. 406–420 (J. E. Desmedt, Ed.). Basel; Karger

KAWAKAMI, M. (1954). Electromyographic investigation of the human external sphincter muscle of anus. *Japanese Journal of Physiology*, **4**, 1961

KERREMANS, R. (1969). *Morphological and Physiological Aspects of Anal Continence and Defaecation*. Brussels; Editions Arscia

KIFF, E. S. (1983). The clinical use of anorectal physiology studies. *Annals of the Royal College of Surgeons of England*, Sir Alan Parks Symposium, pp. 27–29

KIFF, E. S., BARNES, M. and SWASH, M. (1984). Evidence of pudendal neuropathy in patients with perineal descent and chronic straining at stool. *Gut*, **25**, 1279–1282

NEILL, M. E., PARKS, A. G. and SWASH, M. (1981). Physiological studies of the anal sphincter musculature in faecal incontinence and rectal prolapse. *British Journal of Surgery*, **68**, 531–536

NEILL, M. E. and SWASH, M. (1980). Increased motor unit fibre density in the external sphincter muscle in ano-rectal incontinence: a single fibre EMG study. *Journal of Neurology, Neurosurgery and Psychiatry*, **43**, 343–347

PERCY, J. P., NEILL, M. E., KANDIAH, T. K. and SWASH, M. (1982). A neurogenic factor in faecal incontinence in the elderly. *Age and Ageing*, **11**, 175–179

PETERSEN, I. and FRANKSSON, E. E. (1955). Electromyographic study of the striated muscles of the male urethra. *British Journal of Urology*, **27**, 148–153

PIPER, H. (1908). Über die Leitungsgeschwindigkeit in den markhaltigen, menslichen Nerven. *Pflüger's Archiv für die gesamte Physiologie des Menschen und der Tiere*, **124**, 591–600

ROSENFALCK, P. (1969). Intra and extra cellular potential fields of active nerve and muscle fibres. *Acta Physiological Scandinavica*, Suppl., **321**, 1–168

ROSENFALCK, P. (1975). *Electromyography: Sensory and Motor Conductions. Findings in Normal Subjects.* Copenhagen; Rikshospitalet Laboratory of Clinical Neurophysiology

RUSKIN, A. P. and DAVIS, J. E. (1969). Anal sphincter electromyography. *Electroencephalography and Clinical Neurophysiology*, **27**, 713

RUTTER, K. R. P. and RIDDELL, R. H. (1975). The solitary rectal ulcer syndrome. *Clinical Gastroenterology*, **4**, 505–530

SNOOKS, S. J., BARNES, P. R. H. and SWASH, M. (1984). Abnormalities of the innervation of the voluntary anal and vertebral sphincters in incontinence: an electrophysiological study. *Journal of Neurology, Neurosurgery and Psychiatry*, **47**, 1269–1273

SNOOKS, S. J., HENRY, M. M. and SWASH, M. (1985). Anorectal incontinence and rectal prolapse: differential assessment of the innervation of the puborectalis and external anal sphincter muscle. *Gut* (in press)

SNOOKS, S. J., NICHOLLS, R. J., HENRY, M. M. and SWASH, M. (1985). Electrophysiological and manometric assessment of the pelvic floor in the solitary rectal ulcer syndrome. *British Journal of Surgery* (in press)

SNOOKS, S. J. S., SWASH, M., SETCHELL, M. and HENRY, M. M. (1984). Injury to the innervation of pelvic floor sphincter musculature in childbirth. *Lancet*, **ii**, 546–550

STALBERG, E. and THIELE, B. (1975). Motor unit fibre density in the extensor digitorum communis muscle. *Journal of Neurology, Neurosurgery and Psychiatry*, **38**, 874–880

STALBERG, E. S. and TRONTELJ, V. (1979). *Single Fibre Electromyography.* Old Woking, U.K.; Mirvalle Press

SWASH, M. (1982). Idiopathic faecal incontinence, in *Recent Advances in Neuropathology*, vol. 2, pp. 243–271 (J. B. Cavanagh and W. Thomas Smith, Eds). Edinburgh; Churchill-Livingstone

SWASH, M. and SCHWARTZ, M. S. (1981). *Neuromuscular Disorders: A Practical Approach to Diagnosis and Management.* Berlin; Springer-Verlag

SWASH, M. and SCHWARTZ, M. S. (1984). *Biopsy Pathology of Muscle.* London; Chapman and Hall

TAVERNER, D. and SMIDDY, F. G. (1959). An electromyographic study of the normal function of the external anal sphincter and pelvic diaphragm. *Diseases of Colon and Rectum*, **2**, 153–160

Chapter 6

The anal reflex

E. Pedersen

Introduction

The classical anal reflex is elicited by pricking the anal mucosa or the perianal skin; the response is observed as dimpling of the perianal skin caused by the contraction of the external anal sphincter. The original description of the reflex was given by Rossolimo (1891), who reported the anal reflex present in all normal subjects. By transections of the spinal cord and the sacral nerve roots in dogs, he was able to localize the anatomical centre for the reflex in the sacral part of the cord; the reflex persisted until the fourth posterior sacral nerve roots were cut.

The original description thus recognizes a spinal reflex connection between the skin around the anus and the external anal sphincter. Stimulation of the perianal skin, however, also gives rise to simultaneous reflex reactions elsewhere, particularly in the external urethral sphincter and in the bulbocavernosus muscle (Allert and Jelasic, 1974; Pedersen, 1978; Vodušek, Janko and Lokar, 1983). This parallelism between the external anal sphincter, external urethral sphincter and the bulbocavernosus muscle allows some conclusions about the activity in one of the muscles to be applied to the others. Such conclusions are, of course, invalid in the case of peripheral neuromuscular lesions, since in such cases differences in responses in these muscles can be informative about the site of the lesion.

Reflex reactions can also be found in the ischiocavernosus, puborectalis and part of the levator ani muscles, but systematic investigations of these muscles in humans are not available.

Reflex reactions in the external anal sphincter can also be provoked by stimulating the glans penis, the clitoris, the mucosa of the rectum, urethra and bladder, and the skin of the distal parts of the leg as used for elicitation of the flexor reflex, e.g. the plantar response. Reflex reactions from the rectum, colon and the bladder can, however, also inhibit activity in the anal sphincters, e.g. distension or contraction of visceral smooth muscle may initiate evacuation of the rectum.

Elicitation by electrical stimulation and electromyography (EMG) of the anal reflex is a useful supplement to its mechanical stimulation and visual observation, and such a technique is necessary for accurate measurements of threshold and latency. Recording of sphincter reactions by pressure measurement can also be useful and can sometimes be used instead of EMG when the latter technique is difficult to apply or not accepted by the patient.

Technique

The routine elicitation of the anal reflex can be performed by single or repetitive pin-pricks or scratching of the perianal skin. In normal subjects, a contraction of the stimulated side is usually accompanied by a reaction on the opposite side, but often to a lesser degree. Stimulation of both sides of the anus is therefore recommended.

Electrical stimulation can be achieved by surface electrodes fixed to the perianal skin, for example by using EEG electrodes or by an electrode montage. We prefer a specially constructed pencil with two metal-tipped electrodes of 3 mm diameter arranged 10 mm apart. The skin impedance of the stimulating electrode should preferably be below 5 kΩ.

Single electrical shocks or a train of stimuli can be used. A train of pulses is the most effective for eliciting polysynaptic reflexes, like the anal reflex. Such stimulation is often necessary for obtaining minimal latencies and maximal reactions in polysynaptic reflexes, as exemplified by studies of the flexor reflex (Tørring, Pedersen and Klemar, 1981). Due to the short distance between stimulating and recording electrodes in anal reflex studies, the time covered by the stimulus train will exclude observation of the reaction and, in addition, the amplifier will often be saturated for even longer periods. Single shocks are therefore the most appropriate in studies of early reactions, and pulses of 0.1–0.2 ms duration are usually used.

External anal sphincter EMG recording

EMG of the anal sphincter can be obtained by surface electrodes placed on the perianal skin, by anal plug electrodes or by intramuscular electrodes. Surface and anal plug electrodes are able to collect electrical signals from a larger area of the anal sphincter than the intramuscular electrodes, but they are often disturbed by movement artefacts. We generally use bipolar needle electrodes inserted just outside the anocutaneous junction on one or both sides of the anus or sometimes in the midline position posterior to the anal verge. The intramuscular electrodes are thus inserted into the superficial part of the external sphincter. The procedure can be facilitated if the examiner inserts a finger into the rectum and requests the patient to contract around it. The patient may be placed in the dorsal or the left lateral position, but investigation in the sitting or standing position is also possible.

External urethral sphincter EMG recordings

In men, EMG of the external urethral sphincter is carried out in the left lateral position with flexion of the hip and knee joints. A 50–90 mm needle is introduced through the perineum 2 cm in front of the anus and approximately 0.5 cm above the midline and, guided by the examiner's left finger, is inserted into the rectum and placed on the middle lobe of the prostate. A slight resistance is usually felt when the needle penetrates the muscle. This coincides with the appearance of EMG activity on the oscilloscope and in the loudspeaker of the EMG equipment.

In women, the dorsal position is the most convenient for this investigation. A 42 mm needle electrode is introduced through the vaginal mucosa next to the outer urethral orifice. The urethral sphincter is located at a depth of approximately 1.5 cm. The introduction of the electrode can be facilitated by an intra-urethral catheter. In both sexes, EMG can be obtained by ring electrodes in contact with mucosa at the relevant urethral site. This non-traumatic method can, however, activate mucosal reflexes.

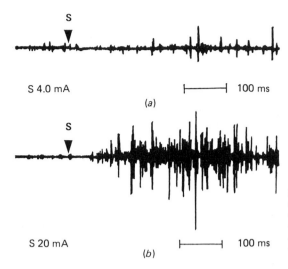

S 4.0 mA   ⊢————⊣ 100 ms

(a)

S 20 mA   ⊢————⊣ 100 ms

(b)

Figure 6.1. Anal reflex elicited by electrical stimulation perianally and recording by electromyography with needle electrode from the anal sphincter. The reflex in the upper trace is elicited by a stimulus intensity near the threshold; the reflex in the lower trace by higher stimulation. S, stimulation

Bulbocavernosus EMG recordings

The classical way of testing the bulbocavernosus reflex is with the patient in the supine position. By palpating the bulbocavernosus and ischiocavernosus muscles, a response can be felt on stimulation of glans penis or clitoris. This contraction in the muscle can facilitate the placing of surface electrodes or the introduction of a needle into the muscle.

Recording of the signals from the electrode can be fed through a conventional amplifier to an oscilloscope and recording equipment, e.g. an ink writer or a videotape. Movement of the needle electrode alters EMG activity as electrical activity from neighbouring muscles may then be picked up. This can disturb quantitative measurements of the activity of the striated muscles. In such cases, a special amplifier recording a number of units firing over a certain threshold can be of value (Klemar, Pedersen and Tørring, 1981).

The classical anal reflex

The visible contraction of the anus on mechanical stimulation of the perianal skin can be analysed by EMG from the anal sphincter. The analysis can be improved by replacing the mechanical stimulation by electrical stimulation and such an analysis will generally reveal a complex response, including early responses of short duration and later responses of longer duration. These latter responses are the background for the visible response and for the mechanically elicited reflex.

The latency of the late response is, within certain limits, dependent on the intensity of stimulation (*Figure 6.1*). On stimulation by a train of five square pulses of 1 ms duration and separated by 1 ms, the average threshold in normal subjects is 3.6 mA (s.d. 1.82) and the latency at threshold 200 ms (s.d. 80). By increasing the stimulation intensity, the latency is reduced on average to 50 ms (s.d. 10.5) (Pedersen *et al.*, 1978). This relation between stimulation intensity and latency was confirmed by Vodušek, Janko and Lokar (1983), who found, however, a wider spread of minimal latencies, namely from 38 to 83 ms. These workers used a technique based on the application of single electrical stimuli which does not, in all cases, result in a minimal latency. In addition, such high-voltage single stimuli can be more painful. With increasing stimulation intensity, the duration and voltage of the reflex response is increased, often with a tendency to rhythmicity, and it can have a duration of up to several hundred milliseconds.

The constancy of this reflex was originally described by Rossolimo (1891), but was later questioned (Allert and Jelasic, 1974). Other studies have confirmed the original observation that the reflex is present in normal subjects (Pedersen et al., 1978; Vodušek, Janko and Lokar, 1983). However, in some cases the reflex can be weak when mechanical stimulation is used. This applies in particular to elderly people in whom the reflex can be elicited only by electrical stimulation and even then often at a much higher stimulation intensity than required in younger subjects.

This reflex has its afferent and efferent pathway in the pudendal nerve and uses the sacral segments S1–S4. This is in accordance with the original demonstration in dogs and with the finding that efferent fibres from S1 to S4 control the external anal sphincter (Tørring et al., 1983). The behaviour of the reflex, with long and stimulus-dependent latency and response characteristics, and with some tendency to habituation, indicates a polysynaptic reflex.

In suprasegmental lesions of the central nervous system, particularly of the spinal cord, typically resulting in uninhibited neurogenic bladder and bowel, and spasticity of the pelvic floor and the legs, the minimum latency of the anal reflex did not differ from that observed in normal subjects. The reaction was, however, usually more pronounced, sometimes with a duration of up to a few seconds, a behaviour similar to that of the flexor withdrawal reflex (Pedersen, 1954; Pedersen et al., 1978; Tørring, Pedersen and Klemar, 1981).

By perianal electrical stimulation, Henry and Swash (1978) demonstrated a short latency reaction with a mean latency of 8.3 ms (s.d. 1.7) in 13 normal subjects. The existence of such early reactions was confirmed by Pedersen et al. (1982), who found such reactions in some but not all, with a first reaction in the range of 2–8 ms and the second with a latency of 13–18 ms, and by Vereecken et al. (1982), with a delay of about 10 ms in some cases. Later, Vodušek, Janko and Lokar (1983) found an early response with typical latencies of 5 and 13 ms in the external anal, urethral and bulbocavernosus muscles.

The early responses have a very constant latency (*Figure 6.2*) and a uniform electrical pattern when a certain placement of stimulation and recording electrodes is used and generally they show no sign of fatigue. The reaction with a latency of 2–8 ms is too short for a spinal reflex (Pedersen et al., 1982; Swash, 1982). The reaction has been attributed to direct activation of the efferent nerves to the anal sphincter (Vodušek, Janko and Lokar, 1983), but the latency is such that very slow conducting fibres should be in operation, since efferent nerves with a conducting velocity of approximately 60 m/s were demonstrated by a reaction in the anal sphincter 7 ms after electrical stimulation of the conus medullaris (Marsden, Merton and Morton, 1982). The short latency reaction is probably due to direct nerve stimulation, causing an antidromic volley in the efferent nerve travelling to a point of branching, then travelling anterogradely in the collateral division of the pudendal nerve. This would be in accordance with both the high threshold level found and the very constant latency and uniformity of electrical pattern when a certain placement of stimulating and recording electrodes was used. It would also be consistent with the lack of habituation, the strictly ipsilateral appearance and the persistence of the response seen with epidural anaesthesia (Pedersen et al., 1982). The nature of the second response to perianal stimulation, with a latency of

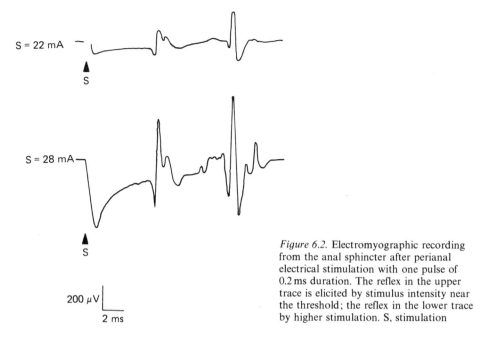

S = 22 mA

S

S = 28 mA

S

200 μV

2 ms

Figure 6.2. Electromyographic recording from the anal sphincter after perianal electrical stimulation with one pulse of 0.2 ms duration. The reflex in the upper trace is elicited by stimulus intensity near the threshold; the reflex in the lower trace by higher stimulation. S, stimulation

13–18 ms, is not quite clear. The latency could allow an oligosynaptic spinal reflex in some of the cases, but other explanations, e.g. for antidromic stimulation with interaction between neighbouring motoneurons, must also be considered. Such a transmission of impulses has been observed between α-motoneurons in the cat (Gogan *et al.*, 1977) (*Figure 6.3*).

Anal sphincter reflex reactions elicited from other sites

By stimulation of the glans penis or clitoris, a reflex reaction is provoked in the bulbocavernosus muscle with a latency in the range of 35–40 ms; this is the classical bulbocavernosus reflex (Rushworth, 1967). A simultaneous response can be picked up from the external anal and urethral sphincters (Bors and Blinn, 1959; Allert and Jelasic, 1974; Bilkey, Awad and Smith, 1983). The latency of this reflex is also dependent on the intensity of stimulation. The minimum latency is in the range of 30–40 ms, e.g. for men 36.8 ms (s.d. 5.2) and for women 38.6 ms (s.d. 4.0) in normal subjects when recorded from the external anal sphincter after electrical stimulation by single high-voltage shocks up to 200–300 V in the case of men and for women up to 80 V (Bilkey, Awad and Smith, 1983). In this investigation the minimal latency was found to be shorter in patients with suprasegmental lesions, in contrast to similar studies by Ertekin and Reel (1976), who found a normal latency in these patients. The minimal latency of this reflex elicited from the glans or clitoris is thus shorter than that of the comparable perianally elicited anal reflex and it shows little or no habituation.

Stimulation of the mucosa of the urethra, bladder and rectum can also provoke reflex reaction in the external anal sphincter. A reflex reaction from the bladder neck to the external anal sphincter with a latency between 50 and 80 ms was described by Bradley (1972).

It has been demonstrated that the pelvic sphincters are connected to the flexor

(a)   (b)

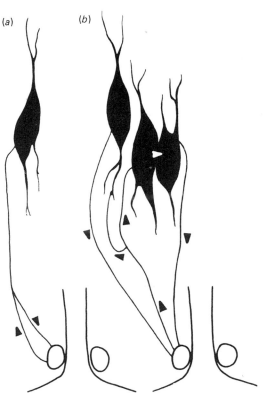

Figure 6.3. Arrows indicating possible routes of the impulses in the first (*a*) and second (*b*) fast response. In (*a*) the impulse travels antidromically to the point of branching and then down the other collateral to the muscle; in (*b*) the impulse reaches the spinal cord antidromically through the efferent fibre and can then pass from the first to the second motoneurons either at sites of direct apposition or by spinal collaterals

muscles and flexor reflexes of the legs (Mai and Pedersen, 1976; Jolesz *et al.*, 1982). Reflex reactions from the external anal and urethral sphincters can also be recorded after mechanical or electrical stimulation of the plantar skin or by electrical stimulation from surface electrodes over the posterior tibial nerve behind the malleolus (Pedersen, 1954), an electrode placement often used in provoking the flexor reflex of the leg (*Figure 6.4*).

Lesions of the segmental pathways

The normal function of reflexes is dependent on the integrity of the segmental pathways including afferent and efferent peripheral nerves and their spinal connections. Such spinal pathways are utilized by the reflex reactions in the external anal sphincter, typically recorded with a minimum latency around 35 ms after glans or clitoris stimulation and around 50 ms after perianal stimulation. These reflexes are always present in normal subjects, although their elicitation in old people requires the use of electrical stimulation. Absence of these reflexes is therefore an indicator of a defect in the reflex pathway, as is the prolongation of the latency and the reduction of the reaction.

The short latency reactions, typically with a latency of 5–8 ms, probably reflect activity in the efferent peripheral nerves and not in the nerve roots or the spinal segment, as demonstrated by their survival in sacral anaesthesia. An increased latency of these responses is therefore assumed to indicate impairment of the efferent nerves.

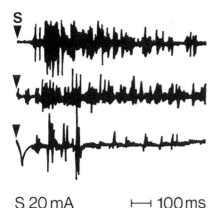

S 20 mA   ⊢—⊣ 100 ms

Figure 6.4. Reflex elicited in spastic patients by electrical stimulation over the posterior tibial nerve behind the malleolus and the response recorded by EMG with needle electrode from the anal sphincter (upper trace), external urethral sphincter with needle electrode (middle trace), and from the tibialis anterior muscle with surface electrodes. S, stimulation

However, the short latency reactions are not constantly present and their absence is therefore of dubious significance.

Absence or depression of the long latency reflexes can be caused by a central lesion in the conus medullaris, by congenital lesions such as myelomeningocele, or by acquired lesions such as infectious, traumatic and expanding lesions. Multiple sclerosis only depresses the reflexes in those unusual cases with conus lesions. The anal reflex can be absent in spinal shock but, as demonstrated by Riddoch as early as 1917, the anal reflex is the first to return after spinal shock (Riddoch, 1917), a finding which has been confirmed by electrophysiological studies (see, for example, Pedersen *et al.*, 1978).

In some patients with absence of reflex anal reactions after perianal stimulation, peripheral stimulation over the posterior tibial nerve can result in an anal response. As the difference between the two reflex elicitations is on the afferent side of the reflex, this would point to a lesion of the afferent sacral nerves.

Neuropathy of the peripheral nerves involved in the reflex arc can increase the latency. Thus, following stimulation of the glans penis of a patient with polyneuritis, Rushworth (1967) found reflexes with a latency of 120 ms which could be shortened to a minimum of 105 ms as compared with normal values of 35–40 ms. Similar delays can be found in cases where disc protrusions have caused a cauda equina syndrome where latencies after perianal stimulation of up to 200 ms can be found (Pedersen *et al.*, 1978).

Traumatic lesions caused by stretch injury of the pudendal nerve have been considered a cause of idiopathic faecal incontinence, in which denervation of the external anal sphincter has been found by histological and electrophysiological methods. Henry and Swash (1978) found a delay of the early reactions in such cases, whereas Bartolo, Jarratt and Read (1983a, 1983b) did not find the early reactions significantly different from the control subjects despite EMG signs of neuropathy. They did not find any difference for the late component, but they were unable to record distinct reactions for this reflex.

It is not surprising that the reflex cannot be used to reveal any neuropathy in the nerves involved. The literature about the early reaction is limited and in the case of the late reactions only the minimum latency and the threshold for stimulation and not the reaction itself can be compared with normal controls. Supplementary investigations are therefore necessary, especially when reflex values are within normal ranges. These should include EMG (duration of motor units, number of polyphasic, denervation) and measurement of conduction velocity in the motor innervation of the pelvic floor muscles (see Chapter 7).

References

ALLERT, M. L. and JELASIC, F. (1974). *Diagnostik neurogener Blasenstörungen durch Elektromyographie.* Stuttgart; Georg Thieme Verlag

BARTOLO, D. C. C., JARRATT, J. A. and READ, N. W. (1983a). The cutaneo-anal reflex: a useful index of neuropathy? *British Journal of Surgery*, **70**, 660–663

BARTOLO, D. C. C., JARRATT, J. A. and READ, N. W. (1983b). The use of conventional electromyography to assess external sphincter neuropathy in man. *Journal of Neurology, Neurosurgery and Psychiatry*, **46**, 1115–1118

BILKEY, W. J., AWAD, E. A. and SMITH, A. D. (1983). Clinical application of sacral reflex latency. *Journal of Urology*, **6**, 1187–1189

BORS, E. and BLINN, K. A. (1959). Bulbocavernosus reflex. *Journal of Urology*, Baltimore, **82**, 128–130

BRADLEY, W. E. (1972). Urethral electromyography. *Journal of Urology*, **108**, 563–564

ERTEKIN, C. and REEL, F. (1976). Bulbocavernosus reflex in normal bladder and/or impotence. *Journal of the Neurological Sciences*, **28**, 1–15

GOGAN, P., GUERITAUD, J. P., BOSSAVIT, G. H. and TYC-DUMONT, S. (1977). Direct excitatory interactions between spinal motoneurones of the cat. *Journal of Physiology*, **272**, 755–767

HENRY, M. M. and SWASH, M. (1978). Assessment of pelvic-floor disorders and incontinence by electrophysiological recording of the anal reflex. *Lancet*, **1**, 1290–1291

JOLESZ, F. A., CHENG-TAO, X., RUENXEL, P. W. and HENNEMAN, E. (1982). Flexor reflex control of the external sphincter of the urethra in paraplegia. *Science*, **216**, 1243–1245

KLEMAR, B., PEDERSEN, E. and TØRRING, J. (1981). A new electronic device for quantitation of EMG activity. *EEG Clinical Neurophysiology*, **51**, 114–116

MAI, J. and PEDERSEN, E. (1976). Central effect of bladder filling and voiding. *Journal of Neurology, Neurosurgery and Psychiatry*, **39**, 171–177

MARSDEN, C. D., MERTON, P. A. and MORTON, H. B. (1982). The latency of the anal reflex. *Journal of Neurology, Neurosurgery and Psychiatry*, **45**, 857–858

PEDERSEN, E. (1954). Studies on the central pathway of the flexion reflex in man and animal. *Acta Psychiatrica et Neurologica Scandinavica*, Supplement 88

PEDERSEN, E. (1978). Electromyography of the sphincter muscles, in *Contemporary Clinical Neurophysiology*, EEG Suppl. No. 34, pp. 406–416 (W. A. Cobb and H. Van Duijn, Eds). Amsterdam; Elsevier

PEDERSEN, E., HARVING, H., KLEMAR, B. and TØRRING, J. (1978). Human anal reflexes. *Journal of Neurology, Neurosurgery and Psychiatry*, **9**, 813–818

PEDERSEN, E., KLEMAR, B., SCHRØDER, H. D. and TØRRING, J. (1982). Anal sphincter responses after perianal electrical stimulation. *Journal of Neurology, Neurosurgery and Psychiatry*, **45**, 770–773

RIDDOCH, G. (1917). The reflex functions of the completely divided spinal cord in man, compared with those associated with less severe lesions. *Brain*, **40**, 264–402

ROSSOLIMO, G. (1891). Der Analreflex, seine Physiologie und Pathologie. *Neurologisches Centralblatt*, **10**, 257–259

RUSHWORTH, G. (1967). Diagnostic value of the electromyographic study of reflex activity in man. *Electroencephalography and Clinical Neurophysiology*, Supplement 25

SWASH, M. (1982). Early and late components in the human anal reflex. *Journal of Neurology, Neurosurgery and Psychiatry*, **45**, 767–769

TØRRING, J., PEDERSEN, E. and KLEMAR, B. (1981). Standardisation of the electrical elicitation of the human flexor reflex. *Journal of Neurology, Neurosurgery and Psychiatry*, **44**, 129–132

TØRRING, J., SØGAARD, I., PEDERSEN, E. and KLEMAR, B. (1983). Selective sacral rootlet neurotomy in the treatment of hyperactive neurogenic bladder in MS, in *Actual Problems in Multiple Sclerosis Research*, pp. 162–164 (E. Pedersen, J. Clausen and L. Oades, Eds). Copenhagen; FADL's Forlag

VEREECKEN, R. L., DE MEIRSMAN, J., PUERS, B. and VAN MULDERS, J. (1982). Electrophysiological exploration of the sacral conus. *Journal of Neurology*, **227**, 135–144

VODUŠEK, D. B., JANKO, M. and LOKAR, J. (1983). Direct and reflex responses in perineal muscles on electrical stimulation. *Journal of Neurology, Neurosurgery and Psychiatry*, **46**, 67–71

Chapter 7

Nerve stimulation techniques

A. Pudendal nerve terminal motor latency, and spinal stimulation

S. J. Snooks and M. Swash

Introduction

A detailed clinical examination may be sufficient to establish a diagnosis in many patients with pelvic floor neuromuscular disorders, but quantitative assessments are needed when a patient is treated medically or surgically, or when it is decided to observe the natural history of a patient's symptoms. For research, quantitative methods are a basic requirement. The techniques of nerve stimulation we describe here contribute substantially to management and research by providing an objective assessment of neuromuscular function as well as, more precisely, identifying the anatomical site of the nerve or muscle lesion. These techniques require relatively little technical expertise and employ apparatus which is standard and readily available in most centres. In this chapter, we shall describe each of the techniques we use in our laboratory at St. Mark's Hospital, and shall discuss their clinical applications. The methods we use can be broadly classified as techniques used for the evaluation of the distal motor innervation of the perianal and periurethral striated sphincter muscles, and techniques by which the proximal part of the innervation of these muscles can be studied (*Figure 7.1*).

Pudendal and perineal nerve stimulation

Pudendal and perineal nerve stimulation techniques assess the distal motor innervation of the pelvic floor musculature, i.e. the innervation of the external anal sphincter and periurethral striated sphincter muscles. The pudendal nerve consists of inferior rectal branches that innervate the external anal sphincter muscle, and perineal branches that innervate the periurethral striated sphincter musculature (*Figure 7.2*). By recording selectively from these two muscles, conduction in the motor nerve fibres innervating them can therefore be separately assessed, utilizing stimulation of the pudendal nerve on either side of the pelvis and measuring the latency from pudendal nerve stimulation to the onset of the electrical response in the muscle under study on an oscilloscope. Pudendal nerve stimulation is achieved using an intrarectal, glove-mounted technique. These nerve stimulation techniques may be used in conjunction with conventional and single fibre needle electromyography (Neill and Swash, 1980) of the external anal

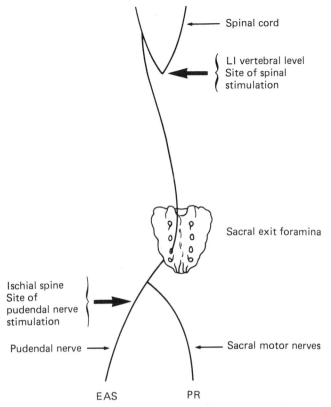

Spinal cord

LI vertebral level
Site of spinal
stimulation

Sacral exit foramina

Ischial spine
Site of
pudendal nerve
stimulation

Pudendal nerve ⟶

⟵ Sacral motor nerves

EAS   PR

Figure 7.1. Sites of proximal and distal nerve stimulation. EAS, external anal sphincter; PR, puborectalis

sphincter muscle which determines the presence or absence of reinnervation (see Chapter 5).

Pudendal nerve terminal motor latency

Pudendal nerve stimulation (Kiff and Swash, 1984a), performed transrectally, has been developed from the technique of electro-ejaculation introduced by Brindley (1981) for use in patients with paraplegia. The stimulating device consists of a rubber finger-stall having two base metal stimulating electrodes at its tip and two steel circular surface recording electrodes mounted 3 cm distant at its base, for recording the evoked contraction response of the external anal sphincter muscle (*Figure 7.3*). The cathode of the stimulating electrodes was made smaller than the anode to improve stimulus localization. The patient is grounded with a large thigh ground electrode and lies in the left lateral position. The device is inserted into the rectum mounted on the examiner's index finger and the ischial spine on one side is palpated. Square wave stimuli of 0.1 ms duration and 50 V are given via the tip-mounted stimulating electrodes at 1 s intervals, and by slowly moving the tip of the device the optimum position for pudendal nerve stimulation is found, recognized by a maximum amplitude of the evoked external anal sphincter muscle response on the oscilloscope of the electromyographic (EMG)

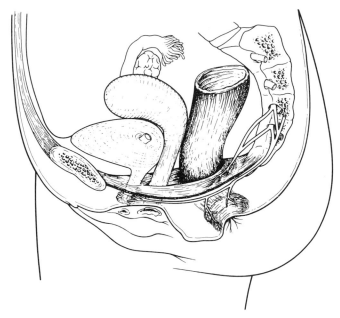

Figure 7.2. Pudendal nerve innervation of the external anal sphincter and periurethral striated sphincter muscles. The sacral motor innervation of the puborectalis is also shown

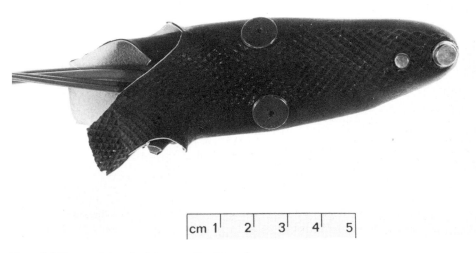

Figure 7.3. Transrectal pudendal nerve stimulator glove

apparatus. This procedure is performed on both sides of the pelvis in order that both pudendal nerves are stimulated. Standard EMG amplifier filter settings are used.

The latency of the external anal sphincter muscle response is measured on the paper print-out of the EMG apparatus from the onset of the stimulus to the onset of the response (*Figure 7.4*). This measurement represents the terminal motor latency of the pudendal nerves to the external anal sphincter muscle. Normal values of the mean (right and left sides) and range of pudendal nerve terminal motor latency in a group of

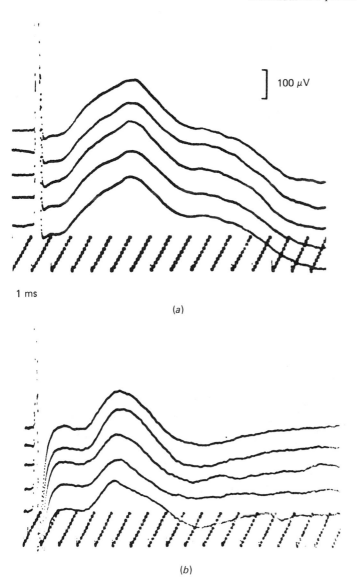

100 μV

1 ms

(a)

(b)

Figure 7.4. Pudendal (*a*) and perineal (*b*) evoked responses in the external anal sphincter and the periurethral striated sphincter muscles, respectively, in a normal subject

control subjects are shown in *Table 7.1*. In this group of control subjects, no correlation was found between the mean pudendal nerve terminal motor latency and age.

Perineal nerve terminal motor latency

Stimulation of the pudendal nerve is performed in exactly the same way, using the same stimulating device as described for the determination of the pudendal nerve terminal motor latency measurement. Using identical nerve stimulation parameters, the terminal motor latency of the perineal nerve is measured by recording the response

TABLE 7.1. Distal nerve latencies—control subjects*

Nerve	n	Mean age (yr)	Age range (yr)	Terminal nerve motor latency (ms)
Pudendal	40	50	25–75	2.1 ± 0.2
Perineal	20	42	25–60	2.4 ± 0.2

* All subjects female.

of the periurethral striated sphincter muscle using an intra-urethral electrode (DISA 21L11) mounted on a Foley catheter. This intra-urethral electrode has two platinum recording surfaces each of 5 mm diameter separated by 3 mm. Measurement of the perineal nerve terminal motor latency is performed from paper recordings in the same manner as that employed for measurement of the pudendal nerve terminal motor latency (*Figure 7.4*). Normal values for the mean (right and left sides) and range of the perineal nerve terminal motor latency in a group of control subjects are shown in *Table 7.1*. In this group of control subjects, as for the pudendal nerve terminal motor latency, no correlation was found between the mean perineal nerve terminal motor latency and increasing age.

Relation between pudendal and perineal nerve terminal motor latencies

In normal subjects there is a linear relation between the terminal motor latencies in these two innervations (*Figure 7.5*). The perineal nerve terminal motor latency is invariably slightly greater than the pudendal nerve terminal motor latency, indicating the greater length of the former from the point of stimulation. Although the curving course of the pudendal nerve through the pelvis does not exactly follow that of the examiner's finger, the stimulation and recording sites are fixed by the construction of the digitally mounted stimulation device, so that results of a constant latency are

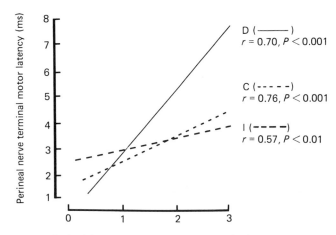

Figure 7.5. Regression analysis lines for 20 female control subjects (C), 20 women with faecal incontinence (I) and 20 women with double incontinence (D) between the perineal and pudendal distal nerve terminal motor latencies

obtained that can be compared from patient to patient (Kiff and Swash, 1984a, 1984b; Snooks and Swash, 1984a, 1984b, 1984c, 1985; Snooks, Henry and Swash, 1985; Snooks *et al.*, 1984; Snooks, Barnes and Swash, 1984).

Transcutaneous cervicolumbar spinal stimulation

The measurement of latency times to evoked pelvic floor muscle contraction can be achieved from the level of the cauda equina, and from spinal cord stimulation in the cervical region, using a modification of the technique of transcutaneous electrical stimulation of the central nervous system devised by Merton *et al.* (1982). This technique thus enables motor conduction to be assessed in the spinal cord, cauda equina and that part of the lower motor neuron proximal to the site of pudendal nerve stimulation (ischial spines). If the recording electrodes are located in the external anal sphincter, this technique assesses conduction in the motor innervation of this muscle. Transcutaneous spinal stimulation used in conjunction with pudendal nerve stimulation therefore enables assessment of both proximal and distal motor conduction in the nerve supply of the pelvic floor musculature.

Transcutaneous lumbar spinal stimulation

Transcutaneous spinal stimulation can be achieved using the method described by Merton *et al.* (1982). A single impulse of 800–1500 V, decaying with a time constant of 50 μs, is delivered through two 1 cm diameter saline-soaked gauze pads, 5 cm apart, held firmly with the cathode over the spinous process of the first lumbar (L1) or fourth lumbar (L4) vertebrae, and with the anode placed cranially. The evoked contraction response of the pelvic floor muscles can be recorded in three muscles—the puborectalis, the external anal sphincter and the urethral striated sphincter musculature. The latter consists of the periurethral striated sphincter and intramural striated sphincter muscles (Gosling, 1979).

Puborectalis response

The latency of the response in the puborectalis muscle after transcutaneous spinal stimulation can be recorded by using a pair of 1 cm diameter steel electrode plates, mounted 1 cm apart on the tip of a rubber finger-stall (*Figure 7.6*). The latter can be held by the examiner's index finger in contact with the puborectalis muscle bar on the posterior wall of the anorectal angulation. In preliminary studies, the origin of this intra-anal surface-recorded response from the puborectalis muscle was verified by recordings using a needle electrode inserted into the muscle percutaneously. The response is recorded and displayed on a standard EMG apparatus. The onset of the stimulus triggers the oscilloscope of the EMG machine, and the latency of the evoked response in the puborectalis muscle can be measured on the paper print-out of the EMG amplifier, from the onset of the stimulus to the onset of the response (*Figure 7.7*).

External anal sphincter response

Using exactly the same technique as that used for recording the response of the puborectalis muscle, the response in the external anal sphincter muscle can be recorded

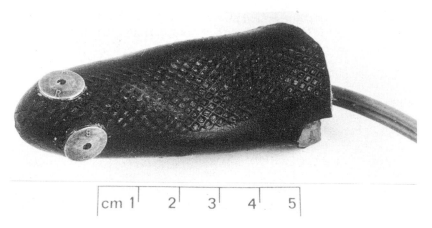

Figure 7.6. The glove surface electrode for transrectally recording the evoked contraction responses of the puborectalis muscle to transcutaneous spinal stimulation

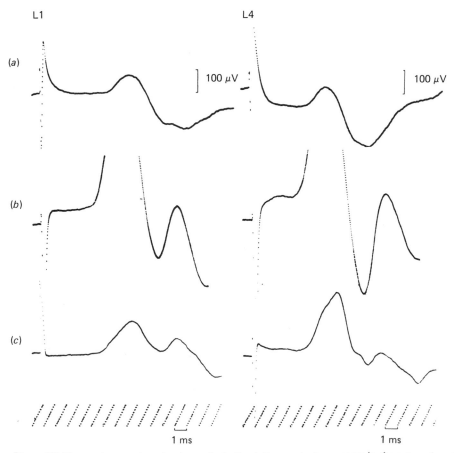

Figure 7.7. Transcutaneous translumbar spinal stimulation evoked responses in the external anal sphincter (*a*), puborectalis (*b*) and the urethral striated sphincter musculature (*c*) in a normal subject

TABLE 7.2. Translumbar spinal latencies—control subjects

Muscle	n	Mean age (yr)	Age range (yr)	Spinal latency (ms) L1	L4
Puborectalis	21*	42	20–78	4.8 ± 0.4	3.7 ± 0.5
External anal sphincter	21*	42	20–78	5.5 ± 0.4	4.4 ± 0.4
Urethral striated sphincter	16	41	20–63	4.8 ± 0.3	4.1 ± 0.3

* Same groups (all subjects female).

through two poles of a 3 cm long, three-pole, telephone-jack plug electrode, situated in the anal canal (*Figure 7.7*). The third pole of the electrode is connected to the ground. The latency of the response in the external anal sphincter muscle is recorded, displayed and measured in the same way as that for measuring the latency of the puborectalis muscle. The normal values from L1 and L4 stimulation are shown in *Table 7.2*.

Urethral striated sphincter musculature response

The response in the urethral striated sphincter musculature can be recorded using an intra-urethral electrode (DISA 21L11) mounted on a Foley catheter. The latency of the response in the urethral striated sphincter musculature is recorded, displayed and measured in the same way as that for the puborectalis and external anal sphincter muscles (*Figure 7.7*). The normal values of the mean spinal latencies from the L1 and L4 vertebral level spinal stimulation sites to the puborectalis, external anal sphincter and urethral striated sphincter muscles are shown in *Table 7.2*.

Spinal latency ratio

The spinal latency ratio (SLR) is represented by:

$$SLR = \frac{\text{Latency to puborectalis after spinal stimulation at L1}}{\text{Latency to puborectalis after spinal stimulation at L4}}$$

The SLR thus represents a comparison of these two latencies from different vertebral levels of transcutaneous spinal stimulation. A similar comparison can be carried out for external anal and urinary sphincter responses. In the presence of distal motor conduction delay, both L1 and L4 latencies increase similarly, since the abnormal zone of nerve conduction is contained in both measurements, and therefore the SLR will remain roughly constant. However, in the case of proximal motor conduction delay, the L1 latency will be more increased compared with the L4 latency, and consequently the SLR value will be increased. Stimulation at two vertebral sites can thus be used to determine whether there is conduction delay within the lumbar spinal canal or distal to the cauda equina, without the necessity of introducing uncertain correction factors for height, i.e. measuring the distance from the site of spinal stimulation to the anal verge (Snooks and Swash, 1984c).

Proximal and distal nerve latency correlations

The spinal latencies to the puborectalis and external anal sphincter muscles are significantly correlated in control subjects and less so in patients with idiopathic anorectal incontinence (*Figure 7.8*). Similarly, there are significant correlations between

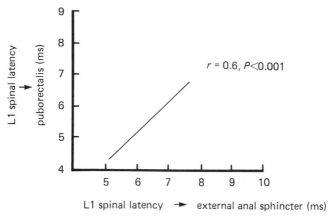

Figure 7.8. Regression analysis line for 21 female control subjects, showing the relationship between the two spinal latencies—external anal sphincter and puborectalis

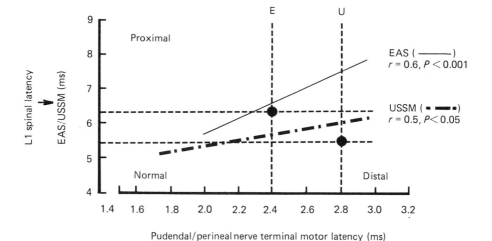

Figure 7.9. Regression analysis line for 21 female control subjects, showing the relationship between two sets of spinal and distal nerve latencies. Areas representing proximal and distal lesions are shown

L1 spinal latencies recorded at the external anal sphincter muscle, and pudendal nerve terminal motor latency, and the L1 spinal latency recorded at the urethral striated sphincter musculature and the perineal nerve terminal motor latency (*Figure 7.9*). This latter relationship is useful for plotting patients' results in order to identify the site of motor conduction delay (Snooks and Swash, 1984c).

Cauda equina conduction velocity

Since the recordings are made from two sites of stimulation, at L1 and L4, measurement of the distance between these stimulation sites allows conduction velocity to be measured directly in the cauda equina by subtraction of the two latencies, using any of the three muscles discussed above for recording the evoked response. In 21 normal subjects, the motor conduction velocity in the cauda equina was $57.9 + 10.3$ m/s.

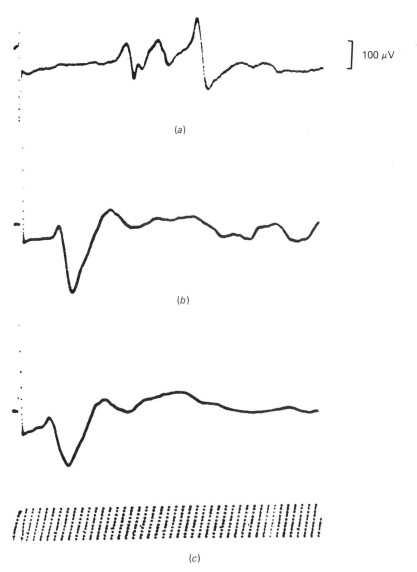

100 μV

(a)

(b)

(c)

Figure 7.10. Transcutaneous cervicolumbar spinal stimulation evoked responses in the puborectalis muscle in a normal subject from (a) C6, (b) L1 and (c) L4. Time base calibration 1 ms

Transcutaneous cervical spinal stimulation

Using exactly the same technique as that used for transcutaneous lumbar spinal stimulation, the spinal cord can be directly stimulated at the sixth cervical (C6) vertebral level. Spinal latency measurements can then be recorded in the puborectalis muscle using the finger-stall recording electrode (*Figure 7.6*), from C6 (*Figure 7.10*), L1 and L4 vertebral level transcutaneous spinal stimulation sites. Measurement of the distances between the C6 to L1 and L1 to L4 vertebral levels thus enables calculation of the conduction velocity between each of these vertebral levels

TABLE 7.3. Transcervicolumbar spinal latencies and conduction velocities—control subjects*

Vertebral level	Spinal latency to puborectalis (ms)	Conduction velocity (m/s)
C6	11.0 ± 1.5	
		† C6 to L1 = 67.4 ± 9.1
L1	5.3 ± 0.5	
		† L1 to L4 = 57.9 ± 10.3
L4	3.8 ± 0.6	

* $n = 21$; mean age = 55; age range = (22 75); all subjects female.
† Significant difference between two velocities $P < 0.01$.

representing motor conduction in the spinal cord (C6 to L1) and the cauda equina (L1 to L4), respectively. Measurement of the distances between C6 to L1 and L1 to L4 can be achieved with reasonable accuracy, unlike measurement from the spine to the anal verge. The stimulus electrodes, situated on the skin overlying the spinal cord or equina, are several centimetres distant from the underlying excitable nervous tissue, so that the precise point of stimulation of cord or nerve roots is not necessarily represented by the surface marking of the cathode. However, we presume this error is similar at the three stimulation sites, so is eliminated during calculation of conduction velocity.

Recording the evoked contraction response of the puborectalis muscle enables stimulation of the S3 and S4 sacral motor nerve roots to be recognized, so that motor conduction in the whole length of the spinal cord, including the sacral cord, can be assessed. Recording evoked contraction of a lower limb muscle, e.g. tibialis anterior (L4 and L5 myotomes) enables lateralization of the response to be assessed, but omits the sacral cord from the study.

The normal values for spinal cord and cauda equina conduction velocities are shown in *Table 7.3*, with spinal latency measurements from C6, L1 and L4 vertebral levels to the evoked contraction response in the puborectalis muscle. This method promises to be of great value in elucidating lumbosacral spinal causes for incontinence, and in the study of patients with neurological disorders involving the spinal cord, such as spinal tumours, and demyelinating diseases, e.g. multiple sclerosis (Snooks and Swash, 1985).

Clinical application

These nerve stimulation techniques are used in our laboratory in the investigation of patients with pelvic floor disorders to examine pathogenesis and to provide objective assessment.

Anorectal incontinence

Slowed distal conduction in the pudendal nerves innervating the external anal sphincter muscle, i.e. an increased pudendal nerve terminal motor latency, has been demonstrated in patients with idiopathic anorectal incontinence (Kiff and Swash, 1984a). Snooks, Barnes and Swash (1984) have showed that slowed distal conduction is present in 80 per cent of patients with idiopathic anorectal incontinence. Similarly, patients with complete rectal prolapse associated with idiopathic anorectal incontinence have been shown to have slowed distal conduction in the pudendal nerves, innervating the external anal sphincter, implying that rectal prolapse in these patients occurs as a secondary event to denervation of the pelvic floor musculature (Snooks, Henry and Swash, 1984). The spinal latencies from L1 and L4 stimulation to the puborectalis and external anal sphincter muscles have been shown to be increased in patients with anorectal incontinence (Snooks, Henry and Swash, 1984) due to distal lesions (Kiff and Swash, 1984a, 1984b). This technique enables differential assessment of the innervation of the puborectalis and external anal sphincter muscles to be achieved. This is important as these two muscles probably have different nerve supplies (Percy *et al.*, 1982; Snooks, Henry and Swash, 1984). The majority of patients with idiopathic anorectal incontinence have distal conduction delay; in these patients motor conduction is normal in the cauda equina using the technique of transcutaneous spinal stimulation at L1 and L4 vertebral levels (Kiff and Swash, 1984b). However, 20 per cent of patients with idiopathic anorectal incontinence have both proximal (cauda equina) and distal (pudendal nerve) conduction delay (Snooks and Swash, 1984c), indicating that in these patients there is a proximal cause for denervation of the pelvic floor muscles. Patients with demonstrable proximal conduction delay may require lumbar myelography. Motor conduction delay in the cauda equina can be easily recognized by the increase in the SLR to the puborectalis muscle (normal SLR, 1.3 ± 0.1) (Snooks and Swash, 1984c).

Transcutaneous lumbar spinal stimulation is useful in determining the site of motor conduction delay in patients with idiopathic anorectal incontinence, and investigating the differential innervation of the two major muscles of anorectal continence—the puborectalis and external anal sphincter.

Double incontinence

Patients with anorectal and urinary incontinence have been shown to have slowed conduction in both the perineal branch of the pudendal nerve innervating the periurethral striated sphincter muscle and the pudendal nerve innervating the external anal sphincter muscle (Snooks, Barnes and Swash, 1984). The degree of damage to the perineal nerve is greater in patients with double incontinence compared with those patients with anorectal incontinence alone (Snooks, Barnes and Swash, 1984) (*Figure 7.5*).

Transcutaneous spinal stimulation is also useful in investigating the innervation of the urethral striated sphincter musculature (Snooks and Swash, 1984b). These results are consistent with the findings of Gosling (1979); the intramural striated muscle and periurethral striated muscle components of the urethral striated sphincter musculature are innervated by pelvic efferent nerves, and by the perineal branch of the pudendal nerve, respectively. Both these innervations can be damaged either separately or together, thus contributing to urethral incompetence (Snooks and Swash, 1984b).

Neurological disorders

Transcutaneous lumbar spinal stimulation performed at the L1 and L4 vertebral levels has been used to demonstrate slowed proximal motor conduction in the cauda equina in patients with myelographic evidence of lumbar canal stenosis, cauda equina tumour, arachnoiditis and sacral agenesis (Snooks and Swash, 1984c). Proximal motor conduction delay can be demonstrated by the calculation from two spinal latency measurements—an increased SLR (Snooks and Swash, 1984c). This technique therefore has particular application to the selection of patients for myelography with suspected cauda equina lesions.

Measurement of motor conduction in the spinal cord probably represents conduction in the fastest fibres in the pyramidal tract in the cord. This technique has wider potential applications in the management and investigation of patients with neurological disorders, especially intrinsic cord diseases such as multiple sclerosis, in addition to its role in the investigation of patients with incontinence and other sphincter disorders due to central nervous system disease.

Obstetric practice

Slowed distal conduction in the pudendal nerves has been demonstrated in 20 per cent of women after vaginal delivery, and is reversible in 15 per cent (Snooks *et al.*, 1984). None of the women studied had sustained division of the external anal sphincter muscles during childbirth. These observations suggest that damage to the pelvic floor innervation is a common and often unrecognized result of vaginal delivery. In the older literature a variety of intrapelvic lumbosacral plexus lesions were recognized, causing obturator, femoral or sciatic nerve palsies (Bianchi, 1867; Lambrinudi, 1924; Noica and Zaharescu, 1933), and incontinence was recognized as a feature of some of these syndromes (Hertz, 1909).

In recent years, faecal and urinary incontinence developing after vaginal delivery has been thought to be due to muscle stretch, or damage to the perineal body, but nerve latency studies (Snooks, Barnes and Swash, 1984) suggest that in the majority of cases this incontinence results from damage to the innervation of the pelvic floor sphincter muscles, especially puborectalis and external anal sphincter muscles (Parks, Swash and Urich, 1977; Neill, Parks and Swash, 1981; Kiff and Swash, 1984a; Snooks, Barnes and Swash, 1984). This often seems to have been initiated by childbirth, although this is not the only cause of this syndrome (Parks, Swash and Urich, 1977). The major predisposing factors are multiparity, vaginal delivery with forceps assistance, prolonged labour and a previous history of pelvic floor injury. In multiparae, it is probable that this nerve damage is cumulative, so that the risk of irreversible nerve damage increases with successive pregnancies. Attention should be turned to obstetric techniques that may protect the pelvic floor musculature and its nerve supply from injury during vaginal deliveries, especially in multiparae, in order to reduce the frequency of anorectal and urinary incontinence in women.

Childbirth is a common cause of external anal sphincter muscle division (Parks and McPartlin, 1971). Damage to the pudendal nerves in addition to the external anal sphincter muscle has been known to occur in 60 per cent of women with evidence of division of the external anal sphincter muscle (Snooks, Henry and Swash, in preparation). Women who have sustained both modes of injury to the external anal sphincter musculature may not be helped by sphincter reconstruction alone (Browning and Motson, 1983).

Conclusions

Nerve stimulation techniques have improved our understanding of disorders of the pelvic floor by showing that nerve damage is an important factor. The techniques offer a quick, relatively non-invasive means of assessing nerve conduction and the site of conduction delay.

B. Electrical stimulation through the scalp of pyramidal tract fibres supplying pelvic floor muscles

P. A. Merton

Introduction

The development of a convenient technique for single-shock electrical stimulation of the motor cortex through the intact scalp in conscious subjects by Merton and Morton (1980) has made possible clinical investigations which were previously out of the question. The first fruits of this have been the demonstration by Marsden's group that the threshold of the motor cortex is normal in severe Parkinson's disease (Berardelli *et al.*, 1984; Dick *et al.*, 1984) and their measurement of conduction delays in the pyramidal pathway in multiple sclerosis (Cowan *et al.*, 1984).

Two years ago we were surprised to find that the external sphincter ani was as accessible to cortical stimulation as the average limb muscle (Merton *et al.*, 1982). So far, this fact has not been exploited. The technique and the few results obtained are described here in the hope that what may be called the 'higher proctology' will prove to have a place in understanding the control of pelvic floor muscles and in diagnosing the causes of their troubles. It is appropriate to recall that my interest in the pelvic floor was first aroused in conversation with Alan Parks, to whom this book is dedicated.

Methods

As compared with ordinary stimulators found in neurological departments for making conduction velocity measurements on peripheral nerve, a stimulator suitable for cortical (or spinal) work has a higher output voltage, 500 V or more, and in particular has to be capable of delivering larger peak currents, i.e. it must have a low output resistance. This is because the structures to be stimulated are deep, so that unusually large currents have to flow between surface electrodes if the fraction of current that reaches down to the brain is to reach threshold. Discomfort and pain depend on current density through the skin and are minimized for the same total current by increasing the area of contact of the stimulating electrodes. We increased the area by sticking on a row of three EEG electrodes, the leads connected together, at each site. They were filled with ordinary salt-containing electrode jelly. The skin underneath should not be abraded, but the hair is parted. It is also the case that brief pulses (50–100 µs) are less apt to stimulate pain fibres than long ones, but the briefer they are the higher the voltage necessary and it is this fact which pushes up the peak voltages required.

For safety, and to get rid of stimulus artefact when recording, the stimulus is passed through an isolating output transformer, which has to be specially designed to pass large currents. Otherwise, the stimulator is a conventional condenser discharge circuit using a high charging voltage. We later used a Digitimer Ltd, D160 stimulator, designed by Mr H. B. Morton to meet the above requirements. The recording was with standard electromyography (EMG) equipment. The amplifier 3 dB points were 32 kHz and 3.2 Hz. Cortical stimulation has now been performed in three laboratories in London on many normal subjects and patients, without ill-effects.

BRINDLEY, G. A. (1981). Electroejaculation: its technique, neurological implications and uses. *Journal of Neurology, Neurosurgery and Psychiatry*, **44**, 9–18

BROWNING, G. G. P. and MOTSON, R. G. (1983). Results of Parks operation for faecal incontinence after anal sphincter injury. *British Medical Journal*, **286**, 1873–1875

COWAN, J. M. A., ROTHWELL, J. C., DICK, J. P. R., THOMPSON, P. D., DAY, B. L. and MARSDEN, C. D. (1984). Abnormalities in central motor pathway conduction in multiple sclerosis. *Lancet*, **ii**, 304–307

DICK, J. P. R., COWAN, J. M. A., DAY, B. L., BERARDELLI, A., KACHI, T., ROTHWELL, J. C. and MARSDEN, C. D. (1984). The corticomotoneurone connection is normal in Parkinson's disease. *Nature*, **310**, 407–409

GOSLING, J. A. (1979). The structure of the bladder and urethra in relation to function. *Journal of Urology*, **6**, 31–38

HERTZ, A. F. (1909). *Constipation and Allied Intestinal Disorders*, pp. 110–114. London; Oxford University Press

KIFF, E. S. and SWASH, M. (1984a). Slowed conduction in the pudendal nerves in idiopathic (neurogenic) faecal incontinence. *British Journal of Surgery*, **71**, 614–616

KIFF, E. S. and SWASH, M. (1984b). Normal proximal and delayed distal conduction in the pudendal nerves of patients with idiopathic (neurogenic) faecal incontinence. *Journal of Neurology, Neurosurgery and Psychiatry*, **47**, 820–823

LAMBRINUDI, C. (1924). Nerve traction injuries. *British Journal of Surgery*, **12**, 554

MARSDEN, C. D., MERTON, P. A. and MORTON, H. B. (1981). Maximal twitches from stimulation of the motor cortex in man. *Journal of Physiology*, **312**, 5P

MERTON, P. A., HILL, D. K., MORTON, H. B. and MARSDEN, C. D. (1982). Scope of a technique for electrical stimulation of human brain, spinal cord, and muscle. *Lancet*, **ii**, 597–600

MERTON, P. A. and MORTON, H. B. (1980). Stimulation of the cerebral cortex in the intact human subject. *Nature*, **285**, 227

NEILL, M. E., PARKS, A. G. and SWASH, M. (1981). Physiological studies of the anal sphincter musculature in faecal incontinence and rectal prolapse. *British Journal of Surgery*, **68**, 531–536

NEILL, M. E. and SWASH, M. (1980). Increased motor unit fibre density in the external anal sphincter muscle in ano-rectal incontinence: a single fibre EMG study. *Journal of Neurology, Neurosurgery and Psychiatry*, **43**, 343–347

NOICA, A. and ZAHARESCU, N. (1933). Paralysie puerpuerale du nerf sciatique poplité externe due coté gauche. *Nouvelle Iconographie Salpetriere*, **xxvi**, 230–233

PARKS, A. G. P. and McPARTLIN, J. G. (1971). Late repair of injuries of the anal sphincter. *Proceedings of the Royal Society of Medicine*, **64**, 1–3

PARKS, A. G., SWASH, M. and URICH, H. (1977). Sphincter denervation in anorectal incontinence and rectal prolapse. *Gut*, **18**, 656–665

PERCY, J. P., NEILL, M. E., SWASH, M. and PARKS, A. G. (1982). Electrophysiological study of motor nerve supply of the pelvic floor. *Lancet*, **i**, 16–17

SNOOKS, S. J., BARNES, R. P. H. and SWASH, M. (1984). Damage to the voluntary anal and urinary sphincter musculature in incontinence. *Journal of Neurology, Neurosurgery and Psychiatry*, **47**, 1269–1273

SNOOKS, S. J., HENRY, M. M. and SWASH, M. (1984). Anorectal incontinence and rectal prolapse: differential assessment of the innervation to puborectalis and external anal sphincter muscles. *Gut* (in press)

SNOOKS, S. J., SETCHELL, M., SWASH, M. and HENRY, M. M. (1985). Injury to the innervation of the pelvic floor musculature in childbirth. *Lancet*, **ii**, 546–550

SNOOKS, S. J. and SWASH, M. (1984a). Perineal nerve and transcutaneous spinal stimulation: new methods for investigation of the urethral striated sphincter musculature. *British Journal of Urology*, **56**, 406–409

SNOOKS, S. J. and SWASH, M. (1984b). Abnormalities of the urethral striated sphincter musculature in incontinence. *British Journal of Urology*, **56**, 401–405

SNOOKS, S. J. and SWASH, M. (1984c). The application of translumbar spinal stimulation in the investigation of patients with idiopathic anorectal incontinence and suspected cauda equina disease (submitted for publication)

SNOOKS, S. J. and SWASH, M. (1985). Motor conduction velocity in the human spinal cord: slowed conduction in multiple sclerosis and radiation myelopathy. *Journal of Neurology, Neurosurgery and Psychiatry* (in press)

Chapter 8

Histopathology of the pelvic floor muscles

M. Swash

Introduction

Understanding of the pathogenesis and management of pelvic floor disorders must be based on both pathological and physiological data. However, the nature of the physiological disturbance of bladder and bowel function in many cases remains poorly understood; indeed, knowledge of the anatomical and physiological basis of normal continence and of the processes of micturition and defaecation are still incomplete. Incontinence and prolapse may occur in patients with denervation of the pelvic floor muscles, for example with cauda equina lesions (Butler, 1954) and incontinence is a well-known feature of many diseases of the central and peripheral nervous system, for example in multiple sclerosis and in diabetic neuropathy. However, the more common variety of faecal incontinence and urinary incontinence, stress incontinence, has no such clear pathogenesis.

Anal continence

Anal continence depends on the interaction of several factors (Duthie, 1971; Parks, 1975; Swash, 1980, 1982). The rectum and anal canal are normally empty of faeces and rectal filling, produced by increased colonic peristaltic activity, is one of the factors leading to defaecation in normal subjects. The rectum itself is situated above the pelvic floor and the anal canal lies below this level. The anorectal junction thus lies at the level of the levator ani muscles and, at this point, there is a sharp angulation, called the anorectal angulation (Parks, 1975). The anorectal angulation (*Figure 8.1*), together with resting tonic contraction of the internal and external anal sphincter muscles, are the three important factors in the maintenance of continence. Of the three, the normal anorectal angulation is the most important (Parks, Porter and Melzack, 1962; Parks, Porter and Hardcastle, 1966; Parks, 1975). This angulation is maintained by the pull of the muscular sling formed in this region by the puborectalis muscles (Thompson, 1899; Kerremans, 1969; Duthie, 1971). The latter muscles are situated at the apex of the funnel-like muscular floor of the pelvis formed by the paired levator ani muscles (*Figure 8.1*).

   The puborectalis muscles form a sling of fibres originating on the two sides from the

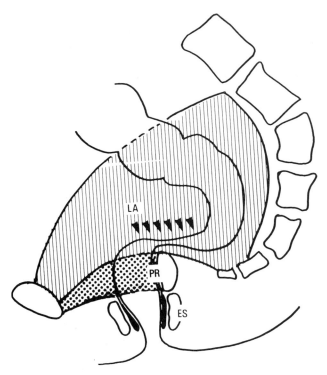

Figure 8.1. The flap-valve mechanism of the anorectal angle. The valve is closed by the intra-abdominal pressure (arrowheads) acting against the pull of the puborectalis (PR) muscles. ES, External sphincter; LA, levator ani

pubis and passing backwards to the posterior wall of the anorectal junction (*Figure 8.1*). They are composed of two parts (Lawson, 1974). These are the pubo-analis sling consisting of fibres of the pubo-analis muscle which decussate behind the anal canal to form a sling, and the pubo-anal sphincteric sling, situated slightly caudally, in the region of the external anal sphincter muscle. The latter consists of deep superficial and cutaneous parts. The upper portion of the external anal sphincter muscle is histologically similar to the puborectalis muscle (Kerremans, 1969; Beersiek, Parks and Swash, 1979) and shows marked differences from the levator ani muscle, suggesting that the former two muscles form a functional unit separate from the levator ani itself. The circular external anal sphincter muscle has often been regarded as playing only a minor role in the maintenance of faecal continence (Kerremans, 1969; Duthie, 1971; Schuster, 1975), but this view is probably an oversimplication. The internal anal sphincter muscle is particularly important in controlling continence to flatus, but in normal subjects it is probably of little importance in the maintenance of faecal continence itself (Bennett and Duthie, 1964).

Anorectal angle

The relatively acute anorectal angle maintains a flap-valve mechanism between the longitudinal axes of the lower rectum and of the anal canal (*Figure 8.1*). The mucosa of the lowest part of the anterior rectal wall thus closes off the upper end of the anal canal. The higher the intra-abdominal pressure, the more securely is continence maintained, provided that this anorectal angulation remains intact (Parks, Porter and Melzack, 1962; Parks, Porter and Hardcastle, 1966; Parks, 1975). The anorectal angle is itself maintained by the pull of the muscular sling formed in this region by the puborectalis muscles (Thompson, 1899; Kerremans, 1969; Duthie, 1971).

In the past there has been some controversy as to the anatomical separation of the puborectalis and external anal sphincter muscles (Thompson, 1899; Goligher, Leacock and Brossy, 1953; Kerremans, 1969) and clarification of this controversy has not been made easier by lack of agreement about the nomenclature of the various muscles, and their component parts, in this region (Lawson, 1974; see also Chapter 1 of this volume). Our own studies have shown differences in the anatomy of these two muscles, but there are close similarities and these suggest that they have a similar function (Beersiek, Parks and Swash, 1979). The levator ani, which forms the funnel-like muscular base of the pelvic floor, is anatomically discrete from the puborectalis muscles, being separated by a fascial plane, although its lowermost fibres are apposed to the latter muscle (*Figure 8.2*).

Innervation of the pelvic floor musculature

It is generally considered that the pelvic floor muscles derive their nerve supply from two distinct sources; these are the pudendal nerve, and a direct branch from the S3 and S4 motor roots. The pudendal nerve arises from the anterior primary rami of the second, third and fourth sacral nerves. Its inferior rectal branches cross the ischiorectal

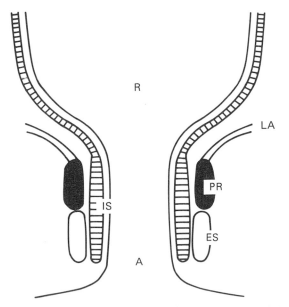

Figure 8.2. The muscles of the funnel-like pelvic floor. IS, Internal sphincter; ES, external sphincter; LA, levator ani; PR, puborectalis; R, rectum; A, anal canal

fossa to reach the external anal sphincter muscles and its perineal branches pass forwards to innervate the periurethral striated musculature and thus to control urinary continence. Other branches of the third and fourth sacral roots reach the pelvic floor via its visceral surface (Stelzner, 1960; Williams and Warwick, 1973; Lawson, 1974). The standard textbook descriptions of the motor innervation of the pelvic floor suggest that the pudendal nerve is the more important of these two innervations, and that the direct branch from S3 and S4 usually supplies only the more peripheral parts of the pelvic floor musculature. The direct branch of S3 and S4 also carries sensory fibres originating in the posterior urethra and in the anal canal. The motor supply to the puborectalis, the most important muscle for the maintenance of faecal continence, has been considered in these accounts to travel with the pudendal nerve.

Our histological studies of patients with anal incontinence suggest that this standard description of the innervation of these muscles is incorrect and, in an electro-physiological study of the motor nerve supply to these muscles, we found that the puborectalis was innervated by a branch of the sacral nerve (S3 and S4) which lies above the pelvic floor. The pudendal nerve, on the other hand, supplied the ipsilateral external anal sphincter muscles, but not the puborectalis muscles (Percy et al., 1981). The puborectalis and the external anal sphincter muscles are thus innervated by different motor nerves, although both originate in the same spinal cord segments. Cross-innervation from side to side has not been studied in the puborectalis, but in the external anal sphincter muscles an experimental study in the monkey (Wunderlich and Swash, 1983) has shown substantial overlap in the pudendal innervation on the two sides. This is related to interdigitations of muscle fascicles across the midline anteriorly in this circular muscle. This functionally overlapping innervation enables reinnervation to be partially accomplished from the opposite side when there is pudendal nerve damage, an important aspect of the histological features of the muscle in incontinent patients.

The internal anal sphincter muscles are smooth muscles which receive autonomic innervation through the pelvic plexus. It is probable that this consists not only of cholinergic nerve terminals but of catecholaminergic nerve terminals. The functional interrelationships of the different types of autonomic innervation in this muscle and their physiological interaction with the somatic innervation of the puborectalis and external anal sphincter muscles, have not yet been fully studied.

External anal sphincter, puborectalis and levator ani muscles

The clinical features of idiopathic anorectal incontinence suggest that the anal sphincter and pelvic floor musculature is abnormal. An opportunity to examine these muscles histologically arose during surgical correction of incontinence. The postanal approach to this operation introduced by Parks (1975) was used and during the operation biopsies of the external anal sphincter, puborectalis and levator ani muscles were taken. Biopsies of these three muscles have been studied in 96 patients. The histological features of these muscles have been described, in previous publications, in 51 of these patients (Parks, Swash and Urich, 1977; Beersiek, Parks and Swash, 1979; Parks and Swash, 1979; Neill, Parks and Swash, 1981), and histometric analysis has been carried out in 16 cases (Beersiek, Parks and Swash, 1979). Standard enzyme histochemical techniques were used, using small pieces of biopsies of each of these muscles, snap-frozen in isopentane–liquid nitrogen.

In one of these studies (Beersiek, Parks and Swash, 1979) the biopsies of these three muscles in 16 patients aged 19–69 yr (mean 48 yr) with anorectal incontinence and in 15 normal subjects aged 17–76 yr (mean 47 yr) were studied. The latter subjects were studied at autopsy: there was no anorectal disorder in these subjects and death had occurred from a variety of causes. None was cachectic. The muscle samples were obtained 7–70 h after death (mean 32 h) and satisfactory histological preparations were obtained in 41 of the 51 muscle samples in this group of 15 normal subjects. In these 33 normal and incontinent subjects, the lesser diameters of all the muscle fibres, of both histochemical types, were measured in at least five separate microscope fields, at a magnification of 100 D, using an eyepiece micrometer. Eighty-two muscle biopsies, containing 19 564 muscle fibres, were studied in this way and the mean muscle fibre diameters of Type 1 and Type 2 fibres were determined in each muscle. These diameters, with their standard deviations in the grouped data of normal and incontinent subjects, were compared using Student's two-tailed t-test. In this way, the abnormality in these muscles was quantified (see 'Histometric observations', p. 143).

Histological observations

In longitudinal sections of the anal canal in normal subjects, the puborectalis and external anal sphincter muscles are usually separated by a layer of connective tissue. This plane of tissue separation could not be recognized in patients with incontinence.

Histological abnormalities were found in all the incontinent patients, although they varied in degree from case to case. The external anal sphincter was always the most abnormal of the three muscles and the levator ani was usually the least affected; in some cases, the levator ani muscle appeared normal. The abnormalities found in the external anal sphincter muscle differed slightly from those found in the puborectalis muscle; in particular, muscle fibre hypertrophy was much more marked in the puborectalis muscles than in the external anal sphincter or levator ani muscles (*Table 8.1*).

TABLE 8.1. Summary of histometric abnormalities in pelvic floor muscles in faecal incontinence

Muscle	Muscle fibre type	Increase in diameter in incontinent patients (per cent)	Type 1 fibre predominance (per cent)	
			Control	Incontinence
External anal sphincter	Type 1	36	78	85
	Type 2	54		
Puborectalis	Type 1	132	75	82
	Type 2	135		
Levator ani	Type 1	21	69	68
	Type 2	61		

External anal sphincter and puborectalis muscles

In the most abnormal of the external anal sphincter and puborectalis muscles, the biopsy contained a few scattered striated muscle fibres embedded in fibrous and adipose tissue (*Figure 8.3*), situated adjacent to the smooth muscle fibres of the internal anal sphincter muscle (*Figure 8.4*). In other, less abnormal biopsies, the muscle fibres were arranged in groups of 10–60 fibres separated from each other by bands of fibrous or adipose tissue (*Figures 8.4* and *8.5*). In these groups, the fibres were often of

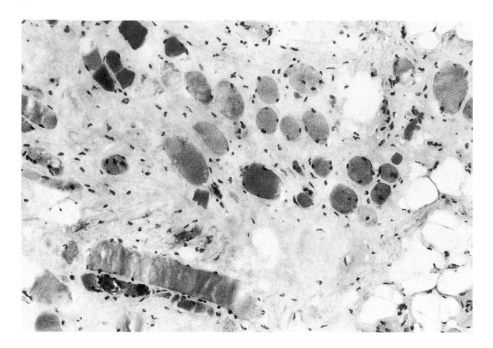

Figure 8.3. External anal sphincter. Haematoxylin and eosin, × 140. Incontinence. There is marked fibrosis and fat replacement. The few remaining muscle fibres are markedly hypertrophied. Scattered tiny atrophic fibres are present

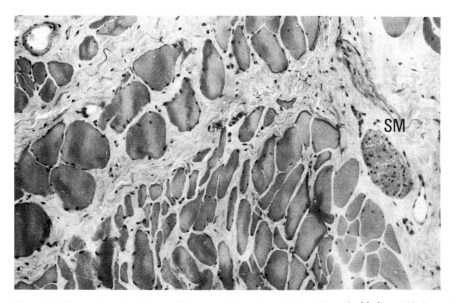

Figure 8.4. External anal sphincter. Haematoxylin and eosin (paraffin embedded), × 140. Incontinence. Groups of fibres of varying size are separated by fibrous tissue. Marked fibre-type hypertrophy is present, but fibres in individual groups tend to be of similar size. A part of the non-striated internal sphincter is included in the biopsy. SM, smooth muscle

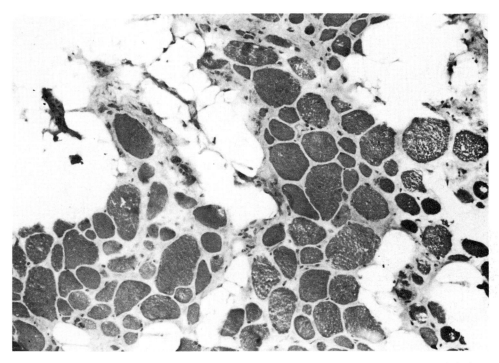

Figure 8.5. Puborectalis. Haematoxylin and eosin, × 200. Incontinence. Groups of fibres are relatively isolated from each other. In several regions there are groups of small atrophic fibres consistent with denervation atrophy

approximately uniform size (*Figure 8.4*). In ATPase and NADH tetrazolium reductase preparations these fibres were of uniform histochemical type (*Figure 8.6*), indicating that reinnervation had occurred, resulting in fibre type grouping. Fibre-type grouping was also noted in muscles in which less marked destructive changes had occurred (*Figure 8.7*). Minor degrees of reorganization of the normal mosaic distribution of Type 1 and Type 2 fibres were found as almost the only abnormality in these muscles in patients with less severe incontinence (*Figure 8.8*). Small atrophic fibres were found scattered in the biopsies, consistent with denervation atrophy (*Figures 8.9* and *8.10*). In the most severely abnormal biopsies, such extensive muscle destruction had occurred that it was not always possible to recognize histological features of reinnervation. These features were noted, however, in about 80 per cent of the biopsies of these two muscles.

Two other features were noted in these muscles. First, there was marked hypertrophy of the remaining fibres, an abnormality which was found in both Type 1 and Type 2 fibres (compare *Figures 8.3–8.10* with *Figures 8.11* and *8.12*). This was especially marked in the puborectalis biopsies. Secondly, myopathic changes were very prominent in some biopsies (*Figure 8.10*). Fibrosis and fatty replacement of muscle fibres were prominent and the remaining muscle fibres showed marked variability in fibre size, with prominent centrally located nuclei. Splitting, or fragmentation of individual muscle fibres, was a feature in many biopsies (*Figure 8.13*) and rare basophilic regenerating fibres were seen. Scattered necrotic fibres, some undergoing phagocytosis (*Figure 8.14*) were sometimes found, often close to the larger fibres in a

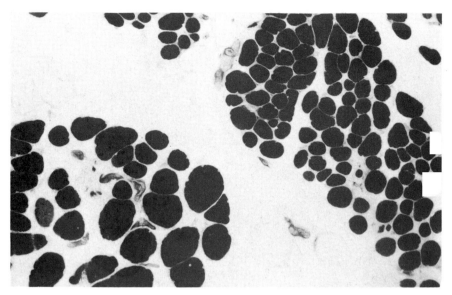

Figure 8.6. Puborectalis. ATPase, pH 4.3, ×140. Incontinence. The groups of fibres consist almost exclusively of Type 1 fibres. Fibre hypertrophy is evident

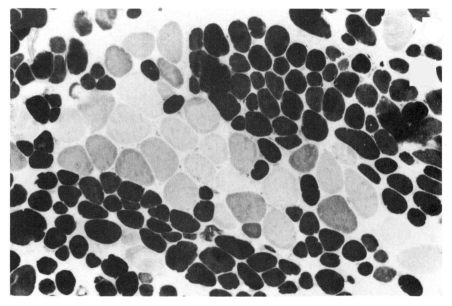

Figure 8.7. Puborectalis. ATPase, pH 4.3, ×140. Incontinence. There is fibre hypertrophy with both Type 1 and Type 2 fibre grouping

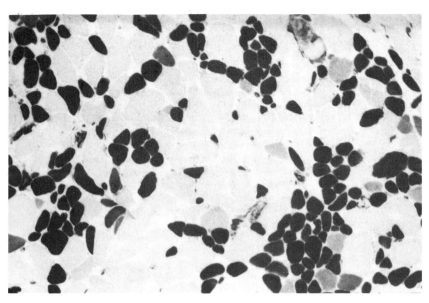

Figure 8.8. External anal sphincter. ATPase, pH 4.3 × 140. Incontinence. There is some hypertrophy of both fibre types, most marked in Type 2 fibres, and reorganization of the fibre-type mosaic has begun, but fibre-type grouping is not yet well developed. There are a few scattered atrophic Type 1 fibres

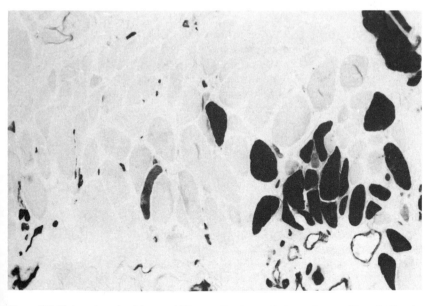

Figure 8.9. External anal sphincter. ATPase, pH 4.3, × 140. Incontinence. There is fibre hypertrophy, and atrophy, with marked Type 1 and Type 3 fibre grouping

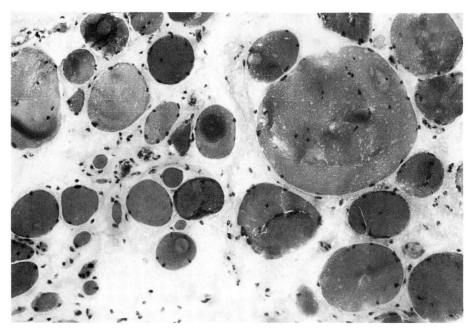

Figure 8.10. Puborectalis. Haematoxylin and eosin, × 140. Incontinence. Fibre hypertrophy is sometimes a very marked feature of the remaining fibres in this muscle. Atrophic fibres can also be seen

biopsy. A few fibres showed degenerative changes of ragged-red fibre type (Engel, 1971). Individual fibres containing scattered rod bodies in their sarcoplasm were found in about 30 per cent of puborectalis biopsies, but rather less frequently in external anal sphincter biopsies (*Figure 8.15*). Ultrastructural studies confirmed that these rod bodies were derived from Z-band material (*Figure 8.16*). These rod bodies were located in clusters in regions of focal myofibrillar degeneration and were often associated with accumulations of lipid droplets. Rod bodies and ragged-red fibres represent non-specific abnormalities in chronic neuromuscular disorders; neither of these abnormalities was present in the distribution or frequency found in the specific neuromuscular disorders with which they are usually associated (Swash and Schwartz, 1981, 1984).

Levator ani muscle

The levator ani muscle biopsies usually showed only mild abnormalities such as disseminated neurogenic atrophy. Grouped denervation atrophy was found in some cases. Fibre hypertrophy was also a feature, but it was not so prominent as in the puborectalis and external anal sphincter muscles. Myopathic abnormalities were rarely found and accumulations of rod bodies were uncommon.

Other features

Muscle spindles were found occasionally in each of the three muscles examined. They usually appeared normal, but in the external anal sphincter and puborectalis muscles

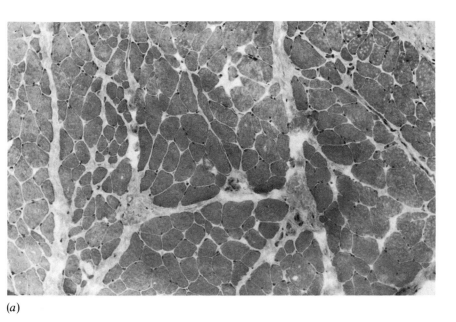

(a)

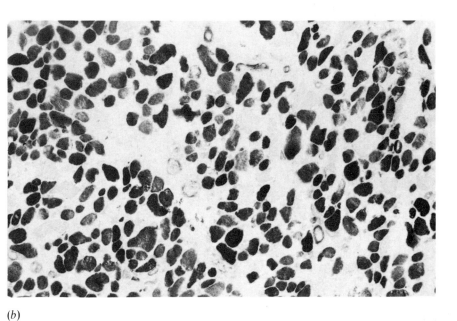

(b)

Figure 8.11. External anal sphincter. Normal subject. (a) Haematoxylin and eosin, ×140. The muscle fibres are small, closely packed and arranged in fascicles. (b) ATPase, pH 4.3, ×140. A mosaic of Type 1 and Type 2 fibres is present, with Type 1 fibre predominance

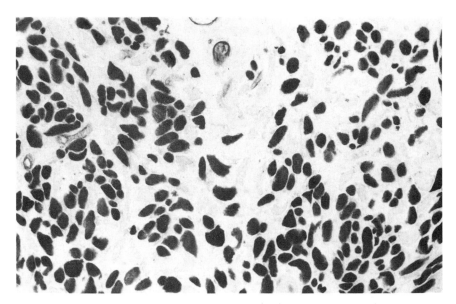

Figure 8.12. Puborectalis. ATPase, × 140. Normal subject. This muscle closely resembles the external anal sphincter

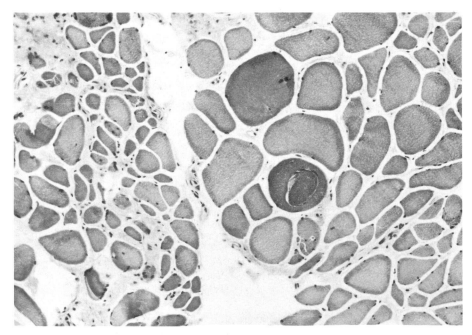

Figure 8.13. Puborectalis. Haematoxylin and eosin, × 140. Incontinence. Groups of fibres of varying size. Fibrous tissue is prominent. One large fibre contains a separate central region and, in an adjacent fibre, splitting has occurred

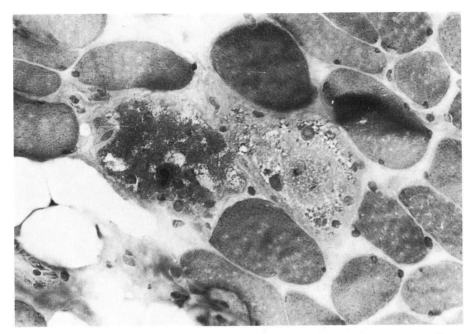

Figure 8.14. Puborectalis. Gomori trichome, × 350. Incontinence. Two vacuolated necrotic fibres, containing macrophages

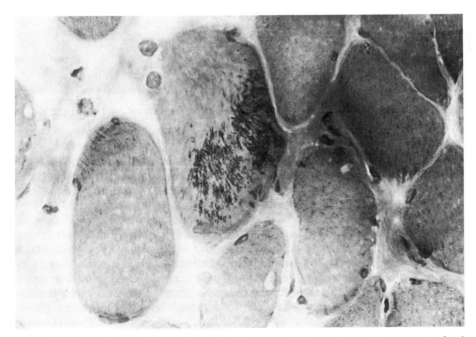

Figure 8.15. External anal sphincter. Gomori trichrome, × 560. Incontinence. An aggregate of rod bodies. Other nearby fibres do not contain rod bodies. Note that the rod bodies are *not* located in the subsarcolemmal region, as in nemaline myopathy

Pathogenesis of idiopathic faecal incontinence

The puborectalis and external anal sphincter muscles bear the brunt of the histological changes observed in idiopathic anorectal incontinence, but fibre hypertrophy is far more prominent in the puborectalis than in the external anal sphincter muscles. Type 1 fibre predominance, a normal feature of these two muscles, and of the levator ani muscles, is increased to a similar degree in both the puborectalis and the external anal sphincter muscles in patients with incontinence.

No histological differences have been observed in relation to the presence of a history of defaecation straining, or to the presence of perianal sensory impairment which was found in a few patients. However, those patients who had experienced difficult or precipitate childbirth accounted for most of the cases in which a severe abnormality was found without clear evidence of fibre-type grouping. Fibre-type grouping, evidence of reinnervation of a muscle, was found in about 80 per cent of the puborectalis and external anal sphincter muscle biopsies examined in patients with faecal incontinence.

Type 1 fibre predominance is a characteristic feature of muscles with a tonic, postural function, for example, soleus and tibialis anterior (Johnson et al., 1973). It may also occur in certain neuromuscular disorders (Dubowitz and Brooke, 1973), but there were no features of such disorders in our incontinent subjects. Type 1 muscle fibres, dependent on oxidative metabolic pathways, have relatively slow twitch characteristics, and are capable of sustained contraction (Burke et al., 1971). The external anal sphincter has been shown to be in a state of continuous partial activity, even during sleep (Floyd and Walls, 1953; Porter, 1962), a characteristic consistent with Type 1 fibre predominance.

In patients in whom the external anal sphincter and puborectalis muscles have been virtually destroyed, as in most of our patients with faecal incontinence, continence must depend on the caudal fibres of the levator ani muscle. When damage occurs to the external anal sphincter and puborectalis muscles, whatever its cause, continence can be maintained only if the remaining innervated fibres of these muscles can contract sufficiently strongly, both to maintain the anorectal angulation and to close the anal canal. There is thus an increased functional load on the remaining fibres in these muscles. This leads to fibre hypertrophy (Edgerton, 1970; Schwartz et al., 1976). However, this may itself lead to secondary degenerative changes in muscles (Swash and Schwartz, 1977), and thus to failure of compensation.

In those patients in whom histological abnormalities in the external anal sphincter and puborectalis muscles were gross, it was not possible to be certain of the cause of the abnormality. Anorectal incontinence is clearly a syndrome with more than one cause and denervation is not a factor in all cases. Direct trauma to the puborectalis and external anal sphincter muscles during childbirth, associated with various surgical procedures, with inflammatory bowel disease or as a result of fistula formation, is also an important causative factor. We have suggested (Parks, Swash and Urich, 1977) that damage to the nerve supply to these muscles may result from obstetric trauma (see Snooks et al., 1984), and from repeated stretch injury to the pudendal nerves during perineal descent, itself induced by excessive defaecation straining (see also Porter, 1962; Parks, Porter and Hardcastle, 1966). The changes found in small nerve branches innervating the external anal sphincter and puborectalis muscles are consistent with this hypothesis. Normal nerves are vulnerable to stretching forces greater than about 12 per cent of their length (Sunderland, 1978), and the combination of nerve entrapment in the pelvis with perineal descent induced during defaecation straining might be sufficient to lead to recurrent injury to the pudendal nerves, and so to progressive denervation atrophy of the muscles supplied by these nerves. This process seems often to be initiated by injury sustained in childbirth (Snooks *et al.*, 1984) but, in addition, it is possible that hormonally dependent changes may occur in the pelvic floor muscles after the menopause and that these may also be a factor in the remarkable preponderance of incontinence among women. Ageing itself, which is associated with loss of neurons in the spinal cord (Gardner, 1940), and with increasing neurogenic damage to the pelvic floor sphincter muscles (Neill and Swash, 1979; Percy *et al.*, 1982), may also be important.

Studies of related anorectal disorders

Perineal descent and rectal prolapse are major associated features of many patients with the syndrome of idiopathic anorectal incontinence. The relation between these features and the incontinence itself is therefore important in formulating concepts of pathogenesis.

Perineal descent

The syndrome of the descending perineum (see Chapter 14) was described by Parks, Porter and Hardcastle (1966). In this syndrome, the position of the anorectal angle with respect to the bony pelvis is changed, both at rest, and especially during coughing, sneezing or defaecation straining, so that it lies at a lower level than in the normal. The syndrome is often associated with painful discomfort in the perineum, sometimes due to mucosal prolapse, and a sensation of inadequate defaecation, leading to persistent straining at stool. Some degree of faecal incontinence occurs in about half the patients with this syndrome, and abnormal descent of the perineum during straining is observed in nearly all the patients with idiopathic faecal incontinence. An extreme form of the disorder occurs in cauda equina lesions, e.g. tumours, in which the perineal musculature is denervated (Butler, 1954). In a series of patients with this syndrome of perineal descent, we found that the anal reflex latency is prolonged in those patients who also suffer from some degree of faecal incontinence, and that there was hypertrophy of both Type 1 and Type 2 fibres in the external anal sphincter muscle to a similar degree to that found in patients with incontinence (Henry, Parks and Swash, 1982). However, features of denervation of this muscle were not prominent in those patients in whom incontinence was not a symptom. These investigations suggest that the descending perineum syndrome is a symptom complex which may precede the development of frank incontinence, and that this syndrome is itself associated with, and may be causally related to, features of damage to the nerve supply to the anal sphincter musculature (Henry, Parks and Swash, 1982).

Rectal prolapse

A similar series of investigations, both histological and physiological, has been carried out in patients with rectal prolapse (see Chapter 15), a disorder which is sometimes also associated with descent of the perineum and with incontinence (Neill, Parks and Swash, 1981). In these studies, two groups of patients with rectal prolapse were identified. In one group, in which rectal prolapse was associated with incontinence, there was electrophysiological evidence of denervation of the external anal sphincter and puborectalis muscles, and in the other, in which rectal prolapse was rarely associated with incontinence, no electrophysiological or morphological abnormality was found in these muscles.

Haemorrhoids

Teramoto, Parks and Swash (1981) found a marked degree of hypertrophy of both Type 1 and Type 2 fibres in the external anal sphincter muscles in patients with haemorrhoids (see Chapter 11). In addition, these muscles showed increased Type 1 fibre predominance. These histological studies did not reveal evidence of reinnervation or denervation of this muscle in this disorder. The findings were interpreted as evidence for an increased workload of the external anal sphincter in these patients. This is consistent with the high anal resting pressure found in patients with this disorder, and there is evidence that this might be due to reflex contraction of the external anal sphincter muscle complex induced by the stimulus of the presence of a haemorrhoidal bolus within the anal canal.

It is, thus, evident that muscle fibre hypertrophy in the external anal sphincter muscle is not a pathognomonic feature of patients with incontinence, but rather that it occurs in a number of different disorders in which an increased workload falls upon this and the puborectalis muscles, either from abnormalities in function or because damage to these muscles leads to an increased load on the remaining functioning muscle fibres.

Urinary incontinence

Most patients with anorectal incontinence are not incontinent of urine. However, similar prolapse of the anterior pelvic floor is observed in many women with idiopathic urinary incontinence, and studies of the striated sphincter musculature of the urinary bladder similar to those we have performed on the anal sphincter musculature might have revealed similar abnormalities (Snooks and Swash, 1984). The innervation of the striated urinary sphincter muscle is similar to that of the anal sphincter in that it is derived from branches of the pudendal nerves. The role of direct branches from the pelvic branches of S3 and S4 in the innervation of the external urinary sphincter is less certain. The detrusor smooth muscle of the bladder wall receives a complex innervation from autonomic afferents and efferents and there is controversy as to the function of this innervation both in normal urinary continence and micturition, and in patients with urinary incontinence (Bradley, Logothetis and Timm, 1973; Anderson and Bradley, 1976; Staunton, 1977). Further studies are needed to answer these questions.

References

ANDERSON, J. T. and BRADLEY, W. E. (1976). Abnormalities of detrusor and sphincter function in multiple sclerosis. *British Journal of Urology*, **48**, 193–198

BEERSIEK, F., PARKS, A. G. and SWASH, M. (1979). Pathogenesis of ano-rectal incontinence: a histometric study of the anal sphincter musculature. *Journal of the Neurological Sciences*, **42**, 111–127

BENNETT, R. C. and DUTHIE, H. L. (1964). The functional importance of the internal anal sphincter. *British Journal of Surgery*, **51**, 355–357

BRADLEY, W. E., LOGOTHETIS, J. L. and TIMM, G. W. (1973). Cystometric and sphincter abnormalities in multiple sclerosis. *Neurology*, Minneapolis, **23**, 1131–1139

BURKE, R. E., LEVINE, O. N., ZAJAC, F. E., TSAIRIS, P. and ENGEL, W. K. (1971). Mammalian motor units; physiological/histochemical correlation in three fibre types in cat gastrocnemius muscle. *Science*, **174**, 709–712

BUTLER, E. C. B. (1954). Complete rectal prolapse following removal of tumours of the cauda equina. *Proceedings of the Royal Society of Medicine*, **47**, 521–522

CIHAK. R.. GUTTMANN. E. and HANZLIKOVA. V. (1970). Involution and hormone-induced persistence of the M sphincter (levator) ani in female rats. *Journal of Anatomy*, London, **106**, 93–101

DUBOWITZ. V. and BROOKE. M. H. (1973). *Muscle Biopsy—A Modern Approach*. London; Saunders

DUTHIE, H. L. (1971). Progress report: anal continence. *Gut*, **12**, 844–852

EDGERTON. V. R. (1970). Morphology and histochemistry of the soleus muscle from normal and exercised rats. *American Journal of Anatomy*, **127**, 81–87

ENGEL. W. K. (1971). Ragged red fibres in ophthalmoplegia syndromes and their differential diagnoses, in *Proceedings of 2nd International Congress on Muscle Diseases*, p. 237. Perth; ICS. Amsterdam; Excerpta Medica

FLOYD. W. F. and WALLS. E. W. (1953). Electromyography of the sphincter ani extremus in man. *Journal of Physiology*, London, **122**, 599–609

GARDNER. E. (1940). Decrease in human neurones with age. *Anatomical Record*, **77**, 529–536

GOLIGHER. J. C.. LEACOCK. A. G. and BROSSY. J. J. (1953). The surgical anatomy of the anal canal. *British Journal of Surgery*, **43**, 51–61

HENRY. M. M.. PARKS. A. G. and SWASH. M. (1982). Electrophysiological and histological studies of the pelvic floor in the descending perineum syndrome. *British Journal of Surgery*, **69**, 470–472

JOHNSON. M. A.. POLGAR. J.. WEIGHTMAN. D. and APPLETON. D. (1973). Data on the distribution of the fibre types in thirty-six human muscles: an autopsy study. *Journal of the Neurological Sciences*, **18**, 111–129

KERREMANS. R. (1969). *Morphological and Physiological Aspects of Anal Continence and Defaecation*. Brussels; Editions Arscia

LAWSON. J. O. N. (1974). Pelvic anatomy (i), pelvic floor muscles (ii), anal canal and associated sphincters. *Annals of the Royal College of Surgeons of England*, **54**, 244–252, 288–300

NEILL. M. E.. PARKS. A. G. and SWASH. M. (1981). Physiological studies of the anal sphincter musculature in faecal incontinence and rectal prolapse. *British Journal of Surgery*, **68**, 531–536

NEILL. M. E. and SWASH. M. (1979). Is faecal incontinence in the elderly neurogenic? *Lancet*, **2**, 364

PARKS. A. G. (1975). Anorectal incontinence. *Proceedings of the Royal Society of Medicine*, **68**, 681–690

PARKS. A. G.. PORTER. N. H. and HARDCASTLE. J. (1966). The syndrome of the descending perineum. *Proceedings of the Royal Society of Medicine*, **59**, 477–482

PARKS. A. G.. PORTER. N. H. and MELZACK. J. (1962). Experimental study of the reflex mechanism controlling the muscles of the pelvic floor. *Diseases of the Colon and Rectum*, **5**, 407–414

PARKS. A. G. and SWASH. M. (1979). Denervation of the anal sphincter causing idiopathic ano-rectal incontinence. *Journal of the Royal College of Surgeons of Edinburgh*, **24**, 94–96

PARKS. A. G.. SWASH. M. and URICH. H. (1977). Sphincter denervation in ano-rectal incontinence and rectal prolapse. *Gut*, **18**, 656–665

PERCY. J. P.. NEILL. M. E.. KANDIAH. T. K. and SWASH. M. (1982). A neurogenic factor in faecal incontinence in the elderly. *Age and Ageing*, **11**, 175–179

PERCY. J. P.. NEILL. M. E.. SWASH. M. and PARKS. A. G. (1981). Electrophysiological study of motor nerver supply of pelvic floor. *Lancet*, **1**, 16–17 (see also *Lancet*, 1981, **1**, 999–1000)

POLGAR. J.. JOHNSON. M. A.. WEIGHTMAN. D. and APPLETON. D. (1973). Data on fibre size in thirty-six human muscles: an autopsy study. *Journal of the Neurological Sciences*, **19**, 307–318

PORTER. N. H. (1962). A physiological study of the pelvic floor in rectal prolapse. *Annals of the Royal College of Surgeons of England*, **31**, 379–401

SCHUSTER. M. M. (1975). The riddle of the sphincters. *Gastroenterology*, **69**, 249–262

SCHWARTZ. M. S.. SARGEANT. M. K. and SWASH. M. (1976). Longitudinal fibre splitting in neurogenic muscular disorders; its relation to the pathogenesis of 'myopathic' change. *Brain*, **99**, 617–636

SNOOKS. S. J. and SWASH. M. (1984). Abnormalities of the innervation of the urethral striated sphincter musculature in incontinence. *British Journal of Urology*, **56**, 401–405

SNOOKS. S. J.. SWASH. M.. SETCHELL. M. and HENRY. M. (1984). Injury to innervation of pelvic floor sphincter musculature in childbirth. *Lancet*, **2**, 546–550

STAUNTON. S. (1977). *Female Urinary Incontinence*. London; Pitman Medical

STELZNER. F. (1960). Über die Anatomie des analen Sphincterorgans, wie sie der Chirurg Sieht. *Zeitschrift für die Anatomische Entwicklungsgeschamte*, **121**, 525–535

SUNDERLAND. S. (1978). *Nerve and Nerve Injuries*, 2nd edn, pp. 62–66. Edinburgh; Churchill-Livingstone

SWASH. M. (1980). Idiopathic faecal incontinence: histopathological evidence on pathogenesis, in *Recent Advances in Gastrointestinal Pathology*, pp. 71–89 (R. Wright, Ed.). London; Saunders

SWASH. M. (1982). The neuropathology of idiopathic faecal incontinence, in *Recent Advances in Neuropathology 2*, pp. 243–271 (W. T. Smith and J. B. Cavanagh, Eds). Edinburgh; Churchill-Livingstone

SWASH. M. and SCHWARTZ. M. S. (1977). Implications of longitudinal fibre splitting in neurogenic and myopathic disorders. *Journal of Neurology, Neurosurgery and Psychiatry*, **40**, 1152–1159

Using video recording, we have tried to assess the differences in behaviour between the expulsion of a water-filled balloon and a semi-solid bolus. It would appear that the balloon gives less information. Its contained fluidity tends to hide minor protrusions or indentations of the rectal wall during defaecation. Small infoldings of the mucosa are not seen. Its position in the rectum is also below the level at which intussusceptions start, and the balloon may be expelled prior to the formation of an intussusception, so that internal intussusceptions will be missed. There is also no indication as to the overall emptying of the rectum. Some patients with gross incontinence are unable to retain the balloon, which then has to be strapped in. Changes in the anorectal angle are then difficult to estimate, as the patient expels the balloon on the slightest attempt at straining.

We regard dynamic imaging as essential to a proper understanding of defaecation. Defaecography with a semi-solid bolus of contrast appears to be the easiest way of obtaining the most physiologically representative examination, with the greatest detail in changes of rectal contour.

Mechanics of continence and defaecation

Sphincteric contraction can be maintained only for a short period, so that some other means of long-term continence must exist. The 'flap' valve theory was proposed by Parks, Porter and Hardcastle (1966) (see p. 44), but this mechanism is not apparent at proctography, perhaps due to complete filling of the rectum, which as Parks indicated is one of the factors that may unlock the valve.

One of the problems in radiology is relying on a two-dimensional image to interpret three-dimensional anatomy. To overcome this, Phillips and Edwards (1966) performed proctography in both lateral and AP planes. By doing so, they demonstrated that the anal canal is flattened from side to side rather than circular; also that after the rectum had been filled with contrast and the patient allowed to move around, an 'empty segment' develops. This is about 1.5 cm in length, situated at the anorectal junction. This was thought to be a 'flutter' valve, analogous with the cardia, maintained by the intra-abdominal pressure collapsing the bowel just above the pelvic floor.

Voluntary contraction, or coughing, elevates the pelvic floor making the anorectal angle more acute, whereas bearing down produces pelvic floor descent with straightening out of the anorectal angle. The normal anorectal angle is 92° ($\pm$1.5) at rest and 137° ($\pm$1.5) on straining (Mahieu, Pringot and Bodart, 1984a, 1984b). The relationship between the position of the pelvic floor and the anorectal angle confirms the dependence of the angle on the tone of the puborectalis (Parks, Porter and Hardcastle, 1966).

Defaecation screened in the AP projection (Phillips and Edwards, 1965) shows that as the pelvic floor descends, the distal rectum opens out to a 'funnel'. This extends into the anal canal, which then opens and fills during evacuation. The pelvic floor should not descend by more than 2 cm during defaecation (Mahieu, Pringot and Bodart, 1984a, 1984b). At the end of defaecation the process reverses, with the funnel closing, the pelvic floor rising and restoration of the normal anorectal angle. How the rectal contents are expelled remains unclear. Active rectal contraction has been postulated, but is difficult to prove. Observation during proctography shows apparent contraction of the rectum, with prominent curves forming mainly on the superior border. Whether this is due to actual contraction or not is uncertain.

Although the exact nature of the mechanism of continence may remain unclear, there is good evidence radiologically that the tone of the pelvic floor muscles affects the configuration of the anorectal junction in such a way as to prevent rectal contents entering the anal canal, and to maintain continence with sudden changes of intra-abdominal pressure, without voluntary sphincteric contraction. A change in tone, coupled with straining and voluntary sphincteric relaxation, allows pelvic floor descent and defaecation to occur.

Descending perineal syndrome

Descent of the perineum was defined originally by measuring radiologically the drop in the anorectal junction on straining (Parks, Porter and Hardcastle, 1966). Films were taken with the patients lying on their side, with barium-soaked gauze outlining the rectum and anal canal. The distance between the anorectal junction and the pubococcygeal line was measured at rest and on straining. Out of 100 patients attending a rectal clinic, only 23 per cent had symptoms of excessive straining with <2.5 cm descent, compared with 83 per cent with >2.5 cm descent.

An absolute measurement for the anorectal junction is that it should lie <1.8 cm below a line from the tip of the coccyx to the front of the pubic symphysis (*Figure 9.15*) (Hardcastle and Parks, 1970). In none of these studies was the pelvic floor stressed in any way. However, although the resting position of the junction may vary when the patient is sitting on the commode with the rectum filled with barium (*Figure 9.16*), the descent on straining should still be <2 cm (*Figures 9.17a* and *9.17b*) (Mahieu, Pringot and Bodart, 1984a, 1984b).

Perineal descent is now a clinical diagnosis. The value of defaecography is to

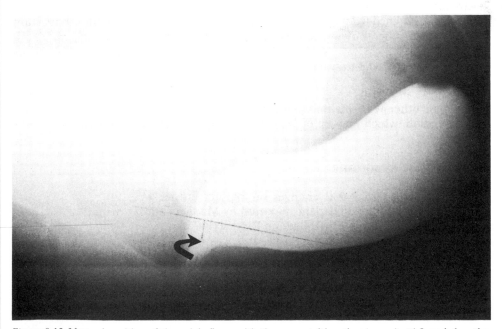

Figure 9.15. Normal position of the pelvic floor, with the anorectal junction (arrow) <1.8 cm below the pubococcygeal line

170

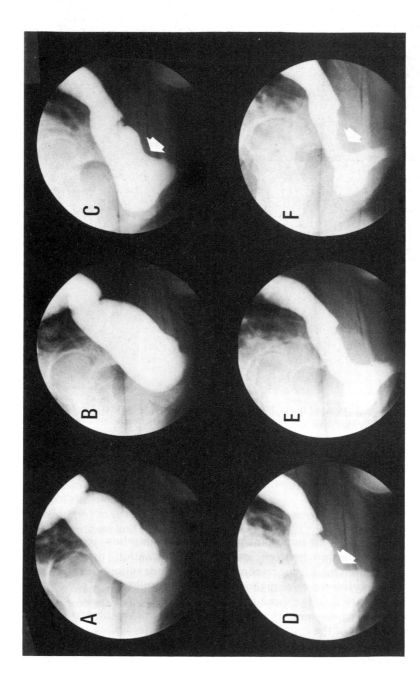

Figure 9.20(a). Accentuation of the puborectalis impression during defaecation. A. At rest, the anorectal angle is normal. B. Initiation of defaecation with pelvic descent and slight opening of the anal canal. C.D. Sudden increase in the puborectalis tone (arrow). E. Cessation of defaecation and rectocele formation. F. In spite of repeated straining there is no further evacuation and the impression due to the puborectalis becomes more pronounced (arrow) (From Mahieu, Pringot and Bodart (1984a, 1984b), by permission of the publishers)

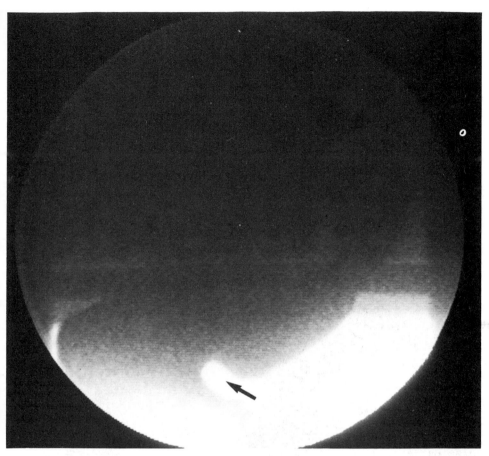

Figure 9.20(b). Prominent infolding of the mucosa at the level of the puborectalis in a patient with the solitary ulcer syndrome (From Mahieu, Pringot and Bodart (1984a, 1984b), by permission of the publishers)

puborectalis, to lie either intra-anal or extra-anal (Mahieu, Pringot and Bodart, 1984a, 1984b). Loss of the normal way the rectum fits into the sacral curve has been noted in complete rectal prolapse (Ripstein and Lanter, 1963). The rectum takes up a vertical course, displaced away from the sacral curve, which can be shown by taking films in the squatting position with the patient straining (Ripstein, 1965). Following operative fixation, the rectum returns to a more normal configuration, and on straining is pushed back into the sacral curve (Ripstein, 1965). Ivalon rectopexy does not affect the level of the pelvic floor. There was no significant change in the position of the anorectal junction, anorectal angle or post-rectal space in 11 patients following ivalon rectopexy for complete rectal prolapse (unpublished data).

Defaecography shows that almost all intussusceptions start 6–8 cm up the rectum, at the level of the main rectal fold. The intussusception begins as an infolding of the rectal wall (Broden and Snellman, 1968), which is anterior in 60 per cent (*Figure 9.23*), annular in 32 per cent (*Figure 9.24*) and posterior in 8 per cent (Mahieu, Pringot and Bodart, 1984a, 1984b). The fold deepens and descends forming the intussusception, which may either remain internal or pass through the anal canal to become an external rectal

172

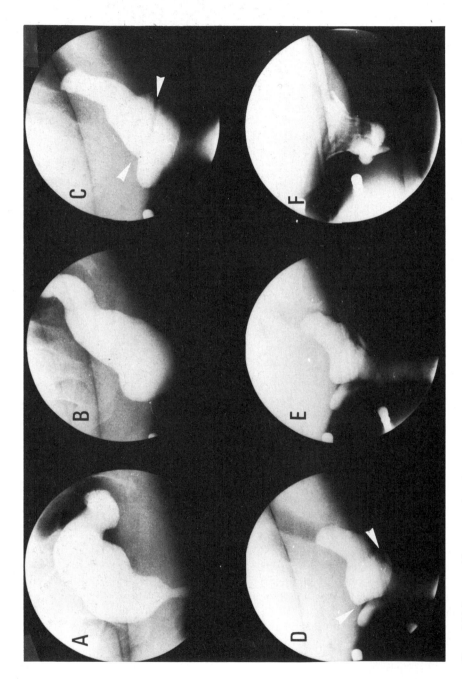

Figure 9.21. Intra-anal intussusception. A. Normal appearance at rest. B. Commencement of evacuation. C. Annular fold (arrowheads) forms at the level of the main rectal fold. D. This fold deepens and invaginates downwards (arrowheads). F. At the end of defaecation the intussusception lies within the anal canal

TABLE 9.1. Defaecography in the solitary ulcer syndrome

1. Intussusception	
(a) external prolapse	12
(b) intra-anal	1
(c) rectal	2
(d) rectal + rectocele	2
2. Rectal stricture	1
3. Accentuation anorectal angle	2
4. Inability to evacuate	1
5. Normal	1
Total cases	22

After Mahieu *et al.* (1981).

prolapse. An intussusception arose within the anorectal junction region in only two of Broden and Snellman's cases and in one of Mahieu's (*Figure 9.25*). It is therefore rare for the anal canal and distal rectum to be involved in prolapse.

Opacification of the small bowel with oral barium prior to defaecography has been used to investigate the relationship of enterocele to prolapse. It had been suggested that a deep pouch of Douglas was a contributory factor to the development of a prolapse. However, the small bowel enters the pouch in a large prolapse only after the prolapse has formed, so that enterocele and a deep pouch of Douglas are only secondary manifestations of prolapse.

Intussusception is usually a gradual process, but can occur suddenly in the final stages of defaecation (*Figure 9.26*). It is therefore important to continue recording until the rectum is completely empty. Intussusception may be divided radiologically into three types: (a) internal–rectal; (b) internal–intra-anal, where the intussusception reaches the anal canal (*Figure 9.27*); (c) external, where the apex of the intussusception passes through the anal canal (*Figure 9.28*).

A rectocele may be associated with intussusception (*Figures 9.23, 9.24* and *9.29*). This can act as a diverticulum with contrast collecting within it when the patient strains, only to flow back into the rectum on relaxation (*Figure 9.30*). As a result, complete evacuation may require several attempts.

Incontinence

In primary incontinence, changes in the pelvic floor result in displacement of the anal canal posteriorly and inferiorly (Parks, 1975). The anorectal junction is > 1.8 cm below the pubococcygeal line, the anorectal angle increased with shortening of the anal canal and a significant increase in the anopubic distance, as shown on lateral proctograms (*Figures 9.31* and *9.32*) (Hardcastle and Parks, 1970). The posterior displacement of the anal canal is confirmed by balloon proctography, where a considerable increase in the anococcygeal distance was found in constipation compared with incontinence, namely 11.0 ± 4 to 6.4 ± 0.5 cm (Preston, Lennard-Jones and Thomas, 1984). In patients with prolapse, there is a significant difference in the anorectal angle, depending on whether the patient is continent. Generally, incontinence is associated with an anorectal angle in excess of 130° (Mahieu, Pringot and Bodart, 1984a, 1984b; Preston, Lennard-Jones and Thomas, 1984). Probably a combination of abnormal radiological parameters is required before incontinence occurs. Widening of the anorectal angle by itself may not

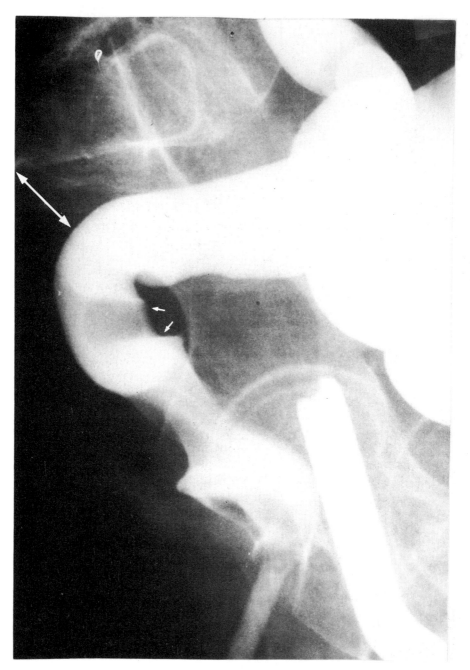

Figure 9.22. Lateral pelvic view during barium enema, showing changes that may be seen in association with rectal prolapse. Note the generalized narrowing of the rectum, widening of the post-rectal space (double arrow) and thickening of the rectal fold (small arrows)

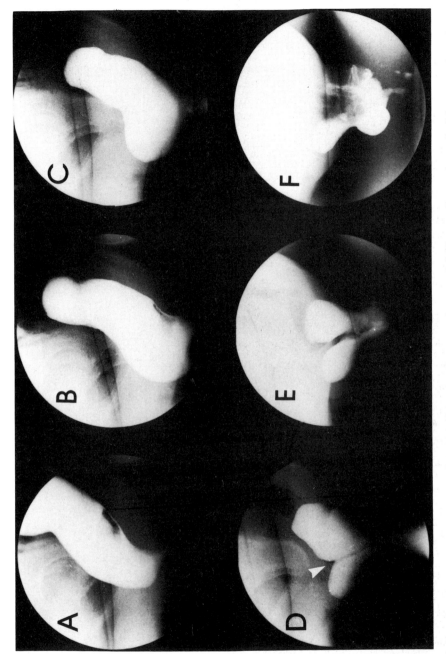

Figure 9.23. Defaecography demonstrating external rectal prolapse, starting as an infolding on the anterior wall of the rectum (arrow)

176

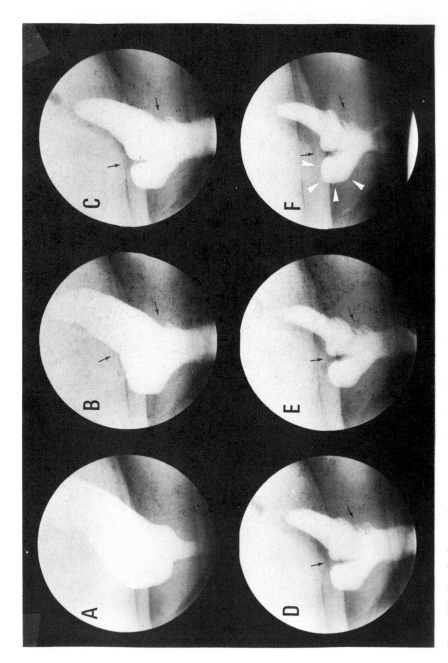

Figure 9.24. Annular internal intussusception (arrows) with rectocele formation (white arrowheads) (From Mahieu, Pringot and Bodart (1984b), by permission of the publishers)

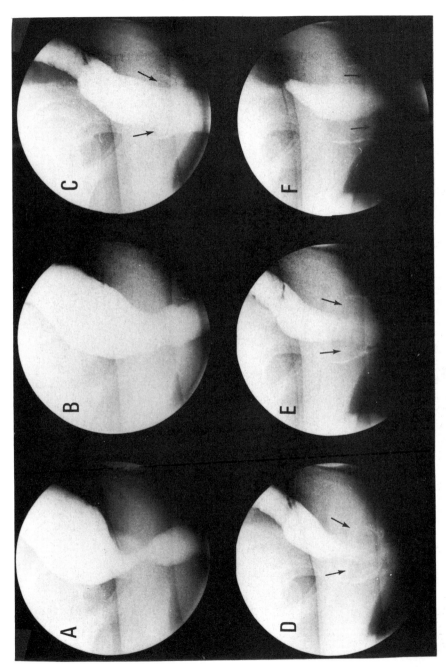

Figure 9.25. External rectal prolapse arising from the distal part of the rectum (arrows)

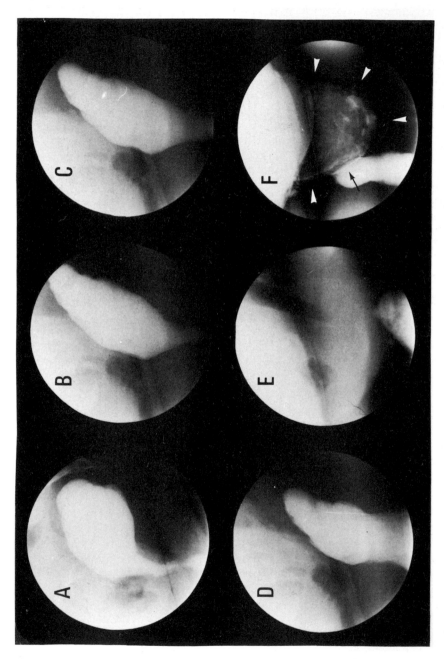

Figure 9.26. External intussusception arising suddenly at the end of defaecation. B. Rectum almost empty. Note the absence of any infolding of the mucosa. F. Sudden appearance of the prolapse (arrowheads). Eccentric position of the anal orifice noted (black arrow)

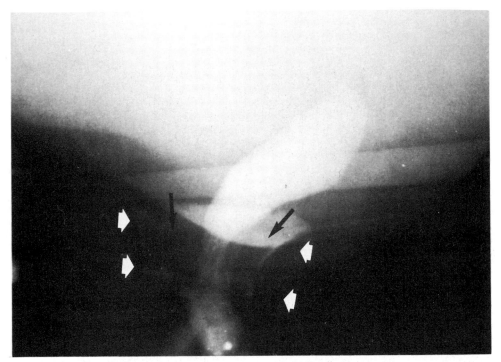

Figure 9.27. Intra-anal intussusception at the end of defaecation. The head of the intussusception (black arrows) is seen within the anal canal (white arrows)

be enough (Hardcastle and Parks, 1970). No significant difference has been found in these parameters when comparing incontinence to solids or liquids (Read, Bartolo and Read, 1984).

Proctography has been used to show how the anatomy is restored to normal by post-anal repair (Hardcastle and Parks, 1970). The anorectal angle is reduced from 135 ± 4.4 to $103 \pm 4.1°$, and the pelvic floor descent from 4.6 ± 0.4 to 3.1 ± 0.4 cm following surgery (Preston, Lennard-Jones and Thomas, 1984).

Haemorrhoids

Single contrast barium enemas did not show the rectum well, as the density of the barium obscured any small lesion that was not viewed exactly in profile. The double contrast barium enema is quite different and small lesions are readily visible.

Internal haemorrhoids can be seen deforming the three columns of Morgagni, provided films are taken when the rectal tube has been removed. The commonest appearance is of multiple nodules. A single nodule is less common (*Figure 9.33*) and a polypoid or varicoid mass unusual. Radiologically, the main differential diagnosis is carcinoma. These present as an irregular polypoid mass, with fixation of the wall causing incomplete distension (*Figure 9.34*) and asymmetry, which is never seen with haemorrhoids (Theoni and Venbrux, 1982).

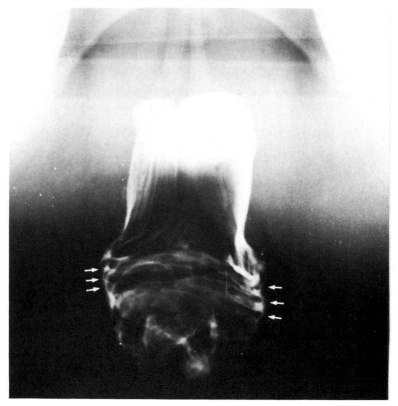

Figure 9.28. En face view of a large external prolapse showing the transverse mucosal folds (arrows) at the head of the intussusception

Conclusions

Defaecography is a relatively specialized investigation, performed at present in only a few proctological units, and it remains to be seen whether it will become amalgamated into routine clinical practice. As with all radiological examinations, this will depend on its ability to demonstrate abnormalities that cannot be detected clinically, which will significantly alter the patient's management. Much will depend on future developments, but at present only some broad indications can be given for defaecography. It is particularly useful in:

1. The solitary ulcer syndrome, where dysfunction of the puborectalis or small internal intussusceptions will be shown.
2. Evacuation problems, where there is arrest of defaecation or a feeling of incomplete evacuation, to show internal intussusceptions or rectoceles.
3. Suspected prolapse.

The role of defaecography in incontinence and constipation is more uncertain, but it may be helpful to determine the degree of pelvic floor descent, changes in the anorectal angle and to exclude intussusception.

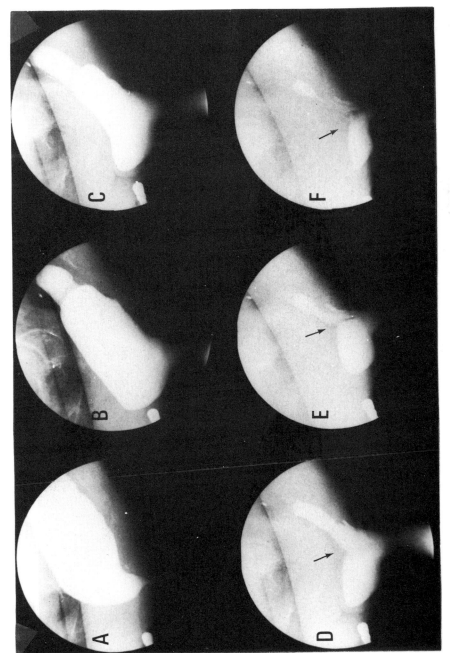

Figure 9.29. Rectocele with small anterior internal intussusception. E. F. There is some emptying of the rectocele when the rectum empties completely

anal sphincter muscles between the tributaries of the superior, middle and inferior rectal veins were also demonstrated, indicating a site of portosystemic anastomosis.
Radiological and serial section histological techniques demonstrated arteriovenous communications by means of tiny arterioles connecting with the venous dilatations, presumably explaining why haemorrhoidal bleeding is often bright red in colour.
W. Thomson (1975a) showed that the submucosal smooth muscle is derived partly from the internal sphincter and partly from fibres of the longitudinal muscle passing between the fasciculi of the internal sphincter. This smooth muscle, which is also found to be mixed with some elastic tissue, forms a network of connective tissue around the haemorrhoidal venous plexuses and probably supports the anal lining during defaecation. It is also attached to the perianal skin and some fibres rejoin the longitudinal muscle by passing around the distal border of the internal sphincter.
The anal cushions are found in the left lateral, right posterior and right anterior positions of the anal canal, and consist of venous dilatations together with a network of smooth muscle, elastic and fibrous tissue and the overlying epithelium. These structures were found in infants and asymptomatic people and are regarded as normal structures.
W. Thomson (1975a) considers the nature of haemorrhoids to be due primarily to a laxity of the anal canal epithelium which by sliding downwards causes distal displacement of the anal cushions. This is especially liable to occur where there is a history of constipation or prolonged straining at stool, leading to stretching or disruption of Treitz's muscle together with venous engorgement. Once displaced, a tight internal sphincter (Hancock and Smith, 1975) is liable to perpetuate the venous engorgement. Haas, Fox and Haas (1984) comment, in addition, that ageing further weakens the connective tissue support and this may result in further venous dilatation.

Appearance of haemorrhoids

Based on the above description of the pathoanatomy, the clinical findings in patients with haemorrhoids should not be too difficult to detect and understand.
The sites of the three primary haemorrhoids are the left lateral, right posterior and right anterior aspects of the anal canal—the sites of the three anal cushions. When the primary haemorrhoids are large, secondary haemorrhoids will develop in between them in the left anterior, left posterior and right lateral positions and the ultimate appearance may be similar circumferentially.
There are two components to each haemorrhoid, one above (internal) and one below (external) the line of the anal valves (dentate line), corresponding to the two venous plexuses. The distinction between the external and internal components is clearly marked by a groove (*Figure 11.1*) and by the different epithelial covering.
The epithelium of the external component is skin and the stratified squamous epithelium of the pecten (sometimes breached by a concurrent fissure-in-ano). That of the internal component is usually columnar epithelium. However, in patients with a long history of prolapse, not only may the columnar epithelium be reddened (traumatic proctitis), but areas of it may undergo squamous epithelial change (*Figure 11.1*).

Pathophysiology

Recently, relatively simple methods of assessing the function of the anal canal have been developed, and these have resulted in an upsurge of interest in anal physiology, not

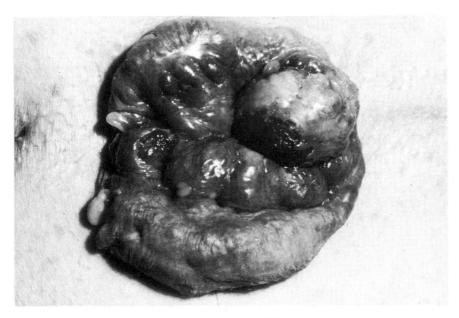

Figure 11.1. Large prolapsed haemorrhoids. Note the different epithelial covering over the internal and external components together with the groove separating them. Squamous epithelial change is present on the right anterior internal component

only of disturbances of function, such as incontinence, but also the so-called 'common anal problems'.

Internal anal sphincter

Hancock and Smith (1975) have demonstrated an increase in internal sphincter activity in some patients, but not all, with haemorrhoids (*Figure 11.2*). Although there is a significant difference in the resting anal canal pressure between the normal controls and those with symptomatic haemorrhoids, there is a considerable overlap in the results, with some patients with haemorrhoids having relatively normal pressures. Furthermore, the pattern of anal canal motility differed in that ultra-slow waves of contraction (variations of more than 25 cmH$_2$O) were noted in more than one-third of patients with haemorrhoids. The patients with haemorrhoids who had ultra-slow waves had greater resting anal canal pressures than those without. Hancock and Smith (1975) concluded that these latter observations indicated excessive internal sphincter activity, as they were noted again when the patients were anaesthetized with striated muscle paralysis. Hancock (1977) also concluded that an internal sphincter abnormality may be an aetiological factor in some patients with haemorrhoids, although the exact mechanism was difficult to explain. A similar conclusion was reached by Arabi, Alexander-Williams and Keighley (1977).

Hancock (1977) felt that there must be other factors, especially as there was no significant relationship between sphincter activity and duration of symptoms, predominant symptoms, severity of symptoms or the size of the haemorrhoids. However, while Leicester, Nicholls and Thomson (in preparation) confirmed the

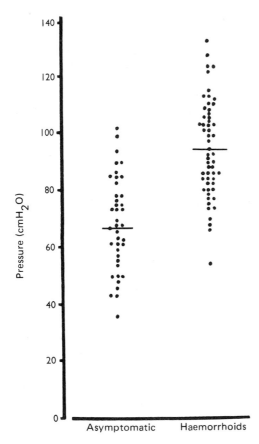

Figure 11.2. Resting anal canal pressures measured by means of a water-filled balloon attached to a 7 mm probe in 40 asymptomatic people and 56 patients with haemorrhoids (From Hancock and Smith (1975), by permission of the authors and publishers)

findings of increased resting anal canal pressures in patients with haemorrhoids, they found that there was a return to normal pressures after the passage of a proctoscope, suggesting that it might be the presence of the haemorrhoidal cushion that produces increased sphincter activity—the passage of the proctoscope having decompressed the venous dilatation within the upper anal canal. Read *et al.* (1982) also noted raised resting anal canal pressure and ultra-slow waves in patients with haemorrhoids. In addition, they found that after haemorrhoidectomy, whether there was an accompanying anal stretch (four fingers) or not, resting pressures were significantly lower and that ultra-slow waves were absent. They also suggested that this preoperative increased sphincter activity is an effect of the presence of haemorrhoidal masses rather than the cause.

Hancock and Smith (1975) found that by performing a Lord's procedure (maximal anal dilatation) as treatment (Lord, 1969), the majority of patients had a satisfactory outcome with regard to symptoms and that resting anal canal pressure and the incidence of ultra-slow waves were also significantly reduced. This treatment aims at disrupting internal sphincter fibres and so will inevitably reduce internal sphincter activity.

External anal sphincter

Evidence that striated muscle hypertrophy is present in the external anal sphincter in patients with haemorrhoids has been provided in a histometric study by Teramoto, Parks and Swash (1981). Fibre size was increased when compared with a control group. However, there was no relationship with age, degree of haemorrhoidal change, length of history, history of straining or constipation or perineal descent. They concluded that this muscle hypertrophy, representing an increased workload, could be the result of increased reflex stimulation due to the presence of the haemorrhoids within the anal canal, or to the effort required to prevent haemorrhoidal prolapse. They felt that the altered external sphincter function might also contribute to the raised anal canal pressures.

There is definitely a relevance of the internal and external anal sphincters in patients with haemorrhoids, but its true nature, that is whether it is cause or effect, still requires further work and evaluation.

Patterns of defaecation

Burkitt (1972) highlighted the possible role of the refined Western diet and constipation in the genesis of haemorrhoids, by drawing attention to the rarity of this condition in rural African communities.

In their recent study of 100 consecutive patients presenting with haemorrhoids, Leicester, Nicholls and Thomson (in preparation) have found that while four-fifths of patients have at least one bowel movement a day, more than half the patients do pass hard stools and need to strain at defaecation, thus indicating a degree of constipation. However, laxatives are only taken on a regular basis by 1 in 10 patients. Continence is impaired in just under 10 per cent of patients, but only for loose or liquid stools and flatus. Hancock (1977) had previously shown that 31 per cent of patients with haemorrhoids had a bowel frequency of less than once a day, and had shown a similar incidence of straining at defaecation.

Predisposing factors

Heredity

There is no doubt that there is a familial incidence of haemorrhoids; Leicester, Nicholls and Thomson (in preparation) report an incidence of 42 per cent.

Pregnancy

Haemorrhoidal symptoms often begin during pregnancy and may be considerably aggravated during labour. Recent work has suggested that certain hormones such as follicle stimulating hormone (FSH), prolactin and glucocorticoids may be responsible for initiating some of these symptoms in female patients (Saint-Pierre, Treffot and Martin, 1982).

Pelvic tumours

It is well established that occasionally haemorrhoids are due to pelvic tumours such as an ovarian cyst or fibromyomata of the uterus. Carcinoma of the rectum is often cited as a cause of haemorrhoids. It is probable that their relationship is coincidental rather than causal, as both conditions are common and will therefore from time to time occur together.

It must be recognized, however, that in the majority of patients no explanation for the onset of symptoms due to haemorrhoids can be found.

Clinical features

Age

It is very unusual for haemorrhoids to present before the third decade. Thereafter, they occur at all ages (*Table 11.1*).

Sex

Haemorrhoids occur in patients of either sex, and despite the predisposing factor of pregnancy, haemorrhoids predominate in men (*Table 11.1*).

Length of history

As with other patients presenting with anorectal symptoms, in patients with haemorrhoids there is often a long history before advice is sought and maybe a long delay before a firm diagnosis is made. Hancock (1977) quotes some interesting figures for patients with bleeding and prolapse (*Table 11.2*).

Symptoms

The symptoms of haemorrhoids may resemble those of serious colorectal disease, namely cancer and inflammatory bowel disease. It is always very important, therefore, that full

TABLE 11.1. Haemorrhoids—age and sex incidence

Series	Number	Age (yr)		Sex	
		Range	Mean ± s.d.	M	F
Arabi, Alexander-Williams and Keighley (1977)	145	20–92	46.0 ± 12.8	101 2.3	44 : 1
Leicester, Nicholls and Thomson (in preparation)	100	20–74	44.3 ± 14.5	59 1.4	41 : 1

TABLE 11.2. Length of history

First symptom	Number	Mean (± s.d.) duration of symptoms (yr)
Bleeding	44	7.3 ± 7.5
Prolapse	31	10.5 ± 9.0

After Hancock (1977).

TABLE 11.3. Traditional classification of haemorrhoids

Classification	Symptom
First degree	Bleeding
Second degree	Prolapse at defaecation (with or without bleeding) with spontaneous return to anal canal
Third degree	Prolapse (with or without bleeding) requiring replacement

TABLE 11.4. Symptoms of haemorrhoids—an analysis in 100 patients

Symptom	Overall	First symptom	Most troublesome symptom	
			Actual number	Percentage of total with symptom
Bleeding	81	39	35	43
Discomfort	64	13	17	27
Pruritus	62	8	6	10
Prolapse	50	20	21	42
Swelling	47	11	1	2
Pain	35	9	19	54
Discharge	29	0	1	3

From Leicester, Nicholls and Thomson (in preparation).

attention be paid to patients with anorectal symptoms and steps taken to establish an accurate diagnosis.

The traditional classification of haemorrhoids (*Table 11.3*) is based on two symptoms only: bleeding and prolapse. *Table 11.4* summarizes the symptoms in a consecutive group of 100 patients with a definitive diagnosis of haemorrhoids attending two of the outpatient clinics at St Mark's Hospital (Leicester, Nicholls and Thomson, in preparation). While it will be noted that bleeding and prolapse are indeed important symptoms, others of perhaps more significance to the patient do occur. It must also be emphasized that many patients with anatomical haemorrhoids of varying size remain asymptomatic.

Anorectal bleeding

This is without doubt the most prominent symptom of haemorrhoids and is the first and most troublesome symptom (*Table 11.4*) to most patients. The blood is usually bright red and without clots. It is noted more commonly in the lavatory pan, into which it may drip or spurt after defaecation, than on the paper used for wiping clean (cf. fissure-in-ano). Seldom does bleeding occur between acts of defaecation. Another characteristic of the bleeding is that it tends to be intermittent in episodes of a few days, rather than continuously at every act of defaecation (*Table 11.5*). It is for this reason that iron deficiency anaemia is very unusual in patients with haemorrhoids (1 per cent).

The mechanism of bleeding must be either trauma to the internal component of the haemorrhoid, by the passage of a hard stool, or the straining efforts during defaecation, or to engorgement of a prolapsed internal component. The latter is the most likely explanation for the spurting of blood which frequently occurs. That the blood is usually bright red and therefore well oxygenated is probably due to the arteriovenous

TABLE 11.5. Characteristics of haemorrhoidal bleeding

At defaecation	
on paper	39.5 per cent
in pan	55.6 per cent
In between stools	4.9 per cent
Bright red	92.6 per cent
Dark red	7.4 per cent
Clots	Nil
Intermittent	93.8 per cent
Continuous	6.2 per cent

From Leicester, Nicholls and Thomson (in preparation).

anastomoses which occur in the anal cushion. One possible explanation for haemorrhoids being the cause of dark bleeding is that the blood passes from the haemorrhoid into the rectum, where it stays until the next act of defaecation.

The differential diagnosis of anorectal bleeding includes many of the pathologies which affect the large intestine, but especially important are neoplastic disease and inflammatory bowel disease. In a series of patients attending a rectal clinic, Williams and Thomson (1977) found 54 per cent of the patients who presented with bleeding had haemorrhoids, and 18 per cent had fissure-in-ano, 6.5 per cent had a tumour (4.2 per cent malignant, 2.3 per cent benign) and 5.0 per cent had inflammatory bowel disease. This means that approximately 1 in 8 patients had a serious or potentially serious problem, and indicates the importance of a thorough clinical assessment in all patients with anorectal bleeding, even if they are thought only to have haemorrhoids.

Discomfort and pain

These are really different degrees of the same symptom and, contrary to what is often taught, are relatively common in patients with haemorrhoids (*Table 11.4*). Hancock (1977) indicates an incidence of pain in 42 per cent of patients, but there was no difference in basal anal canal pressure in those with and those without pain. In most patients it is due to engorgement of the external haemorrhoidal component, with stretching of the sensitive overlying skin. Pain may be due to some of the complications of haemorrhoids; namely a fissure-in-ano, thrombosis of the external venous plexus, or a clotted venous saccule (*vide infra*). It is hardly surprising that this is relatively the most troublesome symptom (*Table 11.4*) that haemorrhoids can produce.

Pruritus ani

This usually means itching in the perianal area, producing an intense desire to scratch, but it can develop, in the presence of excoriation, into actual soreness and pain, especially when the perianal area moves such as in walking. Pruritus ani is a symptom with many different causes. One prominent cause is poor hygiene after defaecation, resulting in faecal matter persisting on the perianal skin, and possibly with faecal soiling of the underwear. This is especially likely to occur in patients with large external haemorrhoids, skin tags and prolapsed haemorrhoids with or without a mucous discharge, as the irregular contour of the anal area may lead to considerable difficulty in achieving perfect cleansing. The patient may report that, after defaecation, many sheets of paper are required to wipe away faecal matter and often the process is abandoned before complete cleansing is achieved! In the series of Leicester, Nicholls and Thomson (in preparation) 9 per cent of the patients were found to have faecal matter on the perianal skin and 22 per cent had staining of the underwear (in itself a distressing happening for a patient). While other causes of pruritus must always be considered, it is not unreasonable to ascribe the symptom to faecal soiling if it is present. Faeces contain many bacteria, some of which may produce endopeptidases, among the most powerful itch-producing substances known.

Prolapse

This is defined as something slipping through the anus at the time of defaecation, or at other times of exertion, which reduces spontaneously or requires replacement by hand. The differential diagnosis is shown in *Table 11.6*. The haemorrhoid is due to the internal component slipping downwards once the supporting smooth submucosal muscle fibres have been stretched. An associated external haemorrhoidal venous engorgement is nearly always also present (*Figure 11.1*).

TABLE 11.6. Differential diagnosis of anorectal prolapse

Site	Diagnosis
Anal canal	Haemorrhoids
	Hypertrophied anal papillae
	Fibrous anal polyps
	Condylomata acuminata
Rectum	Mucosal prolapse
	Complete rectal prolapse
	Adenomas—pedunculated and sessile
Colon	Adenomas (intussusception)

Swelling

A swelling at the anal margin may be the way a patient describes prolapse, but more usually it is due to engorgement with blood of the external component of the haemorrhoid. Such a swelling can reach a considerable size, particularly if there has been straining at stool and there is a tight sphincter. After defaecation, the swelling will decompress spontaneously or may require digital pressure to empty it of its blood. It is therefore evident why it may be confused not only by the patient but also the surgeon with prolapse. Other causes of swelling may be anal skin tags, thrombosis of the external component or a clotted venous saccule.

Discharge

Discharge occurs when there is excessive mucus production. The internal component of the haemorrhoid is covered with columnar epithelium, at least in part. If this mucosa is subjected to trauma in the form of recurrent prolapse, it will become inflamed (traumatic proctitis) and produce more mucus. This may cause a constant feeling of dampness around the anus or soil the underwear, and be confused with faecal soiling. Furthermore, it may contribute to pruritus ani.

Physical signs

In all patients a full rectal examination, consisting of inspection, palpation, sigmoidoscopy and proctoscopy is essential.

Inspection will indicate much about the extent of a patient's haemorrhoidal problems. There may be a skin tag, engorgement (*Figure 11.3*) or thrombosis (*Figure 11.4*) of the external haemorrhoidal venous plexus, a clotted venous saccule (*Figure 11.5*) or permanent prolapse of the internal component with engorgement of the external haemorrhoidal venous plexus (*Figure 11.1*). Evidence of a long history of prolapse is provided by squamous epithelial change on the internal component and also reddening of the remaining columnar epithelium covered mucosa. Next, the perianal skin should be wiped with a damp piece of white cotton wool to determine if there is any faecal soiling (it will become yellow-brown!); this is especially relevant in the patient with pruritus ani when excoriation of the skin may also be present. Then, the anal margin should be gently parted to determine whether or not a fissure is present (*Figure 11.6*). Finally, the patient should be asked to strain (Valsalva manoeuvre) to determine what probably happens to the external and internal venous plexuses during defaecation and perhaps at other times of exertion.

The occurrence of these signs in the series of Leicester, Nicholls and Thomson (in preparation) is shown in *Table 11.7*. That only 23 were demonstrated to have prolapse when 50 patients complained of this symptom (*Table 11.8*) must mean that either the examination failed to demonstrate prolapse that normally occurs during defaecation, or that it is distension of the external haemorrhoidal venous plexus that is producing the symptom. In addition, some guidance may be obtained as to the state of the pelvic floor and as to whether there is any evidence of the descending perineum syndrome.

On *palpation* some estimate of the tone of the anal sphincter can be made. Any

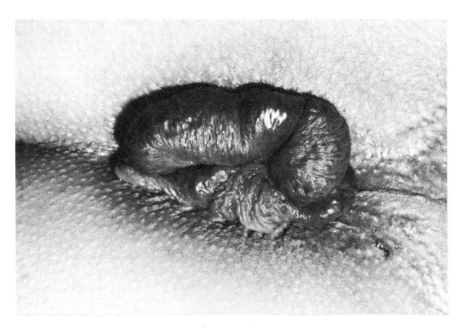

Figure 11.3. Engorgement of the external venous plexus alone

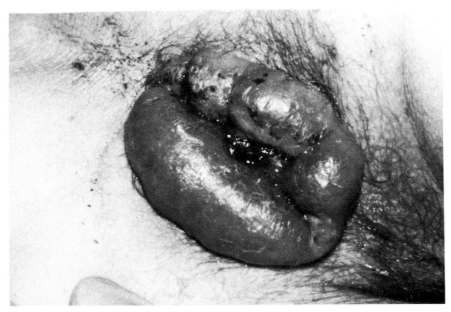

Figure 11.4. External plexus thrombosis

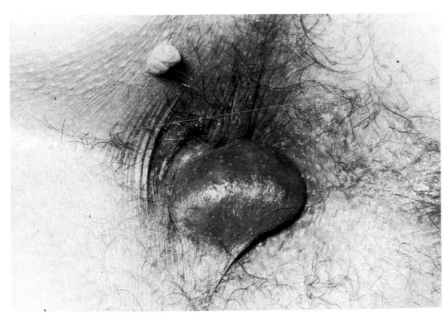

Figure 11.5. Clotted venous saccule (perianal haematoma)

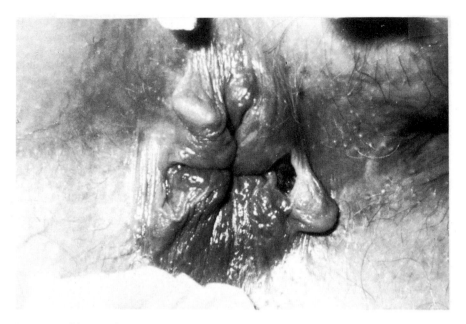

Figure 11.6. The anus is gently parted — the finger grip being aided by dampened cotton wool. There is a prominent external venous plexus and an anterior skin tag concealing a fissure

TABLE 11.7. Occurrence of signs noted on inspection in a series of 100 consecutive patients with haemorrhoids

Physical sign	n
Distensible external haemorrhoidal venous plexus	60
Skin tags	50
Prolapse	23
Skin excoriation	16
Fissure-in-ano	14
Clotted venous saccule	12
Soiling	9
Thrombosis	2

TABLE 11.8. Ability to diagnose prolapsing haemorrhoids

Number of patients complaining of prolapse	50
Number diagnosed on *inspection*	23 (46 per cent)
Number diagnosed after *proctoscopy*	44 (88 per cent)

From Leicester, Nicholls and Thomson (in preparation).

thrombosed areas will feel indurated, but it should be emphasized that uncomplicated haemorrhoids are not palpable.

Sigmoidoscopy is always the next part of the examination which is aimed not at assessing the haemorrhoids, but to exclude other, perhaps more serious, problems. It must always be remembered that more of the rectum can be felt with the finger than seen with the proctoscope (*vide infra*), so it is therefore logical to pass the sigmoidoscope after the finger. The presence of inflammatory bowel disease will modify one's approach to any haemorrhoids that may require treatment, and tumours must be excluded. Haemangioma of the rectum may be detected. It is noteworthy that abnormalities were found on sigmoidoscopy in 7 patients in the series of Leicester, Nicholls and Thomson (in preparation): 3 patients with inflammatory bowel disease, 1 patient with threadworms, 1 with a metaplastic polyp, 1 with an adenomatous polyp and 1 with a carcinoma—a significant yield!

Proctoscopy follows next and, after assessment of the haemorrhoids, certain 'office' therapeutic procedures can readily be undertaken, e.g. injection sclerotherapy, infrared coagulation, elastic band ligation and cryotherapy. This examination may be used to detect enlargement of the anal cushions, reddening of the mucosa, squamous epithelial change (occurring in approximately 35 per cent of patients), hypertrophy of anal papillae and anal polyps (occurring in approximately 20 per cent of patients). Finally, if the patient is asked to strain as the instrument is withdrawn, the ability to diagnose prolapse is considerably increased (*Table 11.8*). While it is often assumed that haemorrhoids only occur in three well-defined zones (left lateral, right posterior and right anterior), it must be remembered that it is not always as clear cut as this and secondary haemorrhoids in between do occur.

Anal manometry

It was suggested by Arabi, Alexander-Williams and Keighley (1977) that anal manometry might be of value in selecting treatment for a given patient. While this has not been widely adopted, others, as has been previously mentioned, have measured anal canal pressure and attempted to relate the observations to the clinical findings. Hancock (1977) found that there was no difference in the resting anal canal pressure in those patients with haemorrhoids with symptoms and those without. Furthermore, he found that there were no differences in pressure in those with differing degrees of haemorrhoids, and with varying lengths of history. In addition, he found that the various symptoms, e.g. bleeding, pain and prolapse, could not be separated on the basis of manometry.

These findings were confirmed by Leicester, Nicholls and Thomson (in preparation), who also showed that the fall in pressure after successful treatment to normal levels was similar to that after the passage of a standard proctoscope. There is therefore doubt about the suggestion of Arabi, Alexander-Williams and Keighley (1977) that routine manometry has a relevance in planning treatment. This is clearly another area where much more work is needed.

Differential diagnosis

As previously mentioned, the symptoms of haemorrhoids may be mimicked by several serious large intestinal problems. Great care must be exercised in excluding these conditions before accepting the final diagnosis of haemorrhoids.

There are two conditions, both very rare, which may be confused with haemorrhoids: varices due to portal hypertension and haemangioma of the rectum and anal canal—presenting usually in the first and second decade of life, with anorectal bleeding and haemorrhoid-like swellings.

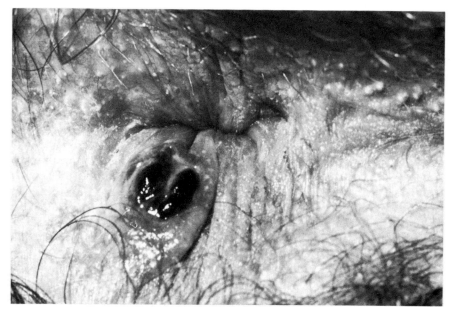

Figure 11.7. The 'clot' extruding spontaneously after ulceration of the skin overlying a clotted venous saccule ('perianal haematoma')

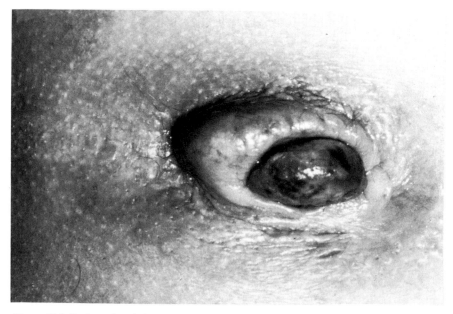

Figure 11.8. Prolapsed and thrombosed right posterior haemorrhoid. Note the groove between the internal and external components

Complications

Thrombosis within the venous dilatations occurs not infrequently and may result in severe pain and anal sphincter spasm. This complication may give three distinct clinical situations. Thrombosis may occur in the external venous plexuses, where the venous dilatations are sometimes quite large, and this may involve the whole circumference of the anal canal (*Figure 11.4*) or be very localized (*Figure 11.5*). This latter condition was called 'perianal haematoma', but now it is regarded as a thrombosis in a large venous dilatation as it has a complete endothelial surround, rather than a ruptured vein. Thomson (1982) has called the condition 'clotted venous saccule'. This concept is in line with the known fact that after evacuation of the 'clot' surgically or spontaneously (*Figure 11.7*), massive haemorrhage, presumably from the opened venous dilatation, may occur.

If the internal component prolapses then this too can become thrombosed, but the groove between the internal and external components is always clearly visible. Thrombosed prolapsed haemorrhoids have often incorrectly been referred to as strangulated haemorrhoids. Again the process can involve one haemorrhoidal site (*Figure 11.8*) or the whole circumference of the anal canal.

Should there be necrosis of the overlying skin or mucosa, it is theoretically possible for infection within the thrombosis to occur, but this is exceedingly rare. Portal pyaemia as a complication of this is also described, but few have seen it.

Other complications include an associated fissure-in-ano (*Figure 11.6*), an anal polyp and skin tags often, but by no means always, the result of external thrombosis.

The subject of haemorrhoids is therefore receiving much attention. This is especially so in the context of altered physiology of the pelvic floor. How this relates to therapy and maybe to prophylaxis will be the focus of interest for many years to come.

B. Treatment

R. W. Beart, Jr

Introduction

The number and the continued evolution of new treatments for haemorrhoidal disease is a testimony to the controversy that surrounds the management of this common ailment. When numerous alternatives exist, one probably should be suspicious that there is no effective management, and such may be true for haemorrhoids. If patients are carefully selected, however, most can be relieved of their symptoms with minimal morbidity or mortality. This chapter places into perspective the most commonly discussed alternatives: medical management, sclerotherapy, rubber band ligation, anal dilatation, surgical excision, cryotherapy and phototherapy.

General guidelines

As with most diseases, the least treatment that is effective should be offered to the patient, consistent with the nature and extent of the symptoms. All available therapies

TABLE 11.9. Staging of haemorrhoidal disease

Stage	Symptoms
First—Haemorrhoid maintained with proper level in anal canal	Bleeding
Second—Prolapse with bowel movements, but spontaneously reduce	Bleeding, prolapse, discharge, pruritus, discomfort
Third—Prolapse out of anal canal and require manual reduction	Bleeding, prolapse, discharge, pruritus, discomfort, mass
Fourth—Prolapsed and incarcerated	Bleeding, pain, necrosis, ulceration, discharge, pruritus, mass, thrombosis

for haemorrhoids have side effects. Complications from treatment range from flatulence to death. Therefore, the experienced physician will avoid treatment, when reasonable. Haemorrhoids are normal anatomical structures (Thomson, 1975b) and should not be removed unless symptoms warrant. Occasional bleeding that does not alter a patient's life-style or cause excessive concern frequently requires nothing more than firm reassurance that there is not a more serious underlying disorder. Symptoms of pressure or chronic aching are rarely caused by non-prolapsing haemorrhoids, and treatment of the haemorrhoids is unlikely to relieve these symptoms. Bleeding and prolapse in the absence of other pathological changes are true haemorrhoidal symptoms and require attention if bothersome to the patient.

Haemorrhoids are treated in response to symptoms, and for this reason some physicians have minimized the value of a staging system (Marino, 1980). However, we have found, at the Mayo Clinic, that a staging system is valuable in assessing the results of treatment, particularly when comparing various therapeutic alternatives. Staging also helps in counselling the patient on what to expect after the operation. *Table 11.9* reflects the staging system used at the Mayo Clinic.

Medical management

For minor bleeding, conservative therapy consisting of reassurance and stool bulking is favoured. The patient should consume at least 15 g of fibre each day. A sudden increase in dietary fibre content may be associated with excessive flatulence, and the patient should be advised to add 5 g of fibre each week, until satisfactory stool consistency is achieved. In addition to the fibre, the patient should consume at least eight 8 oz (0.2 l) glasses of water each day. Fibre in the absence of water may aggravate constipation. Although studies by Broader, Gunn and Alexander-Williams (1974) and Webster, Gough and Craven (1978) conflict as to the effectiveness of stool bulking, regardless of symptom resolution, patients are frequently satisfied with this treatment alone. Local emollients and analgesics appear to have little therapeutic effect, although they may offer transient relief of pain and provide the patient with some psychological support.

Prolapse and more significant bleeding are not satisfactorily controlled by dietary measures and require direct therapy. Only ulcerating or necrotic haemorrhoids require treatment during pregnancy, because parturition will be associated with rapid relief of symptoms. Care must be taken in treating the patient who has haemorrhoids that are associated with inflammatory bowel disease. Wounds may heal poorly, and symptoms may become much worse.

Sclerotherapy

Sclerotherapy became used widely as a treatment in the nineteenth century. Andrews (1879) reported on 3295 patients treated before 1879 and estimated that at least 10 000 patients had been treated by injection techniques using carbolic acid. This solution was injected directly into the haemorrhoid and usually caused massive necrosis of the tissue. Complications were frequent and ranged from pain and slough to death. Subsequently, weaker solutions of carbolic acid (5%), glycerine and water, phenol (5%) in almond oil, quinine and urea hydrochloride have had widespread use. Unlike that in the management of varicose veins, the direct injection of solutions into the haemorrhoid is not desirable. Instead, injection just proximal to the haemorrhoidal mass causes sufficient inflammation to induce fibrosis of the haemorrhoids. The injection should be into the submucosa, and within 24 h this causes pronounced oedema and infiltration of fibroblasts. When oil-containing solutions are used, multinucleated giant cells are also seen and an 'oleogranuloma' may form. If the injection is too deep, ulceration may result, and if the injection is too superficial, the solution may escape back into the lumen of the bowel (Anderson and Dukes, 1924; Graham-Stewart, 1962).

Injection therapy is particularly well suited for patients with first-degree haemorrhoids who have minimal bleeding or discharge. Patients with second- or third-degree haemorrhoids rarely obtain prolonged benefit from injection. External haemorrhoids or thrombosed internal haemorrhoids should never be treated by injection. Complications include ulceration, pain, abscess and oleogranuloma, bleeding and rarely bacteraemia (Adami et al., 1981).

There have been few recent reports of sclerotherapy from the USA. In spite of the resurgence of this technique in the USA during the early twentieth century, other alternatives, such as rubber band ligation, seem to have gained more acceptance. However, several reports from the UK continue to support this technique as being satisfactory. In a randomized trial, Greca et al. (1981) concluded that rubber band ligation and sclerotherapy provide similar results, but that ligation is more liable to complications when the operator is inexperienced. Dencker et al. (1973) reported that the results obtained with injection were poor—only 21 per cent of patients being relieved of symptoms. Both these studies demonstrate the importance of physician technique and patient selection in evaluating results. Kilbourne's collective review of 26 262 patients with haemorrhoids treated by injections documents a recurrence rate of 15 per cent within 3 years (Kilbourne, 1934). Milligan (1943) reviewed the 5-year results of injection treatment and found that additional injections were required by 15 per cent of patients with first-degree haemorrhoids, by 38 per cent of patients with second-degree haemorrhoids and by 69 per cent of patients with third-degree haemorrhoids.

Sclerotherapy has not been used at the Mayo Clinic during the past decade. Other alternatives have proved satisfactory, and in spite of the Dencker et al. (1973) review, we believe that rubber band ligation is less subject to physician error. Furthermore, evaluating the patient who has persistent perineal discomfort after injection therapy is difficult.

Rubber band ligation

Rubber band ligation was first described by Blaisdell (1958). The procedure gained greater acceptance with the introduction of the Barron (1963a) ligator. The principle of the procedure is to apply the rubber band to the non-innervated portion of mucosa above the haemorrhoidal mass. This is done through a proctoscope or small anoscope. The tissue within the band becomes necrotic, and within 4–5 d the band drops off. Some bleeding may occur when the band is dislodged and for up to 14 d after ligation. The procedure is generally painless, and multiple sites may be banded at one time.

Complications of this technique, as with injection therapy, are rare. Delayed haemorrhage, which occurs in about 1 per cent of patients, is probably due to localized infection and ulceration. Bleeding may be massive and require hospitalization. If pain occurs (4 per cent), it will occur shortly after application, and this indicates that the band has been placed too near the dentate line. The band may be cut off and replaced at a higher point. Thrombosis of external haemorrhoids may occur distal to the band. It occurs in 2–3 per cent of patients, and patients with such thrombosis should be treated with warm baths and stool softeners (Barron, 1963b). Recently, there have been reports of several deaths after rubber band ligation of haemorrhoids, particularly from the state of California. It had not been recognized that these patients were immunologically suppressed or had unusual bacterial flora. In these cases, the treating physician may have been slow to respond to a complaint of anal pain that was increasing in severity after banding. The delayed onset of pain is extremely unusual and is suggestive of an inflammatory process, which requires careful monitoring.

Neither banding nor injection removes external skin tags, although either may be associated with a decrease in the external component of the haemorrhoidal disease. Generally, banding is more uncomfortable than injection (interferes with daily activity in 2 per cent) (Barron, 1963b), but is equally effective in relieving first-degree haemorrhoid symptoms (Clark, Giles and Goligher, 1967). Reviews by Gehamy and Weakley (1974), Steinberg, Liegois and Alexander-Williams (1975) and Wrobleski et al. (1980) document that 70 per cent of the patients are free of symptoms after banding. A recent review by Jeffery et al. (1980) noted residual symptoms in 69 per cent of patients, but this rate was similar to their experience with haemorrhoidectomy, and they considered this to be satisfactory. The rate seems to be comparable with that after injection, if differences in patient selection are considered. Banding appears to be more effective for second-degree haemorrhoids and may be more effective when only one treatment is given (Corman, 1984).

Anal dilatation

Anal dilatation, as recommended by Lord (1969), has also been used for the treatment of chronic haemorrhoidal disease. It is believed that traumatic disruption of anal fibrotic bands will lower intra-anal pressures and relieve haemorrhoidal congestion. This is now a generally accepted treatment and is used for first- and second-degree haemorrhoids, although Lord has also described using it for third-degree haemorrhoids (Lord, 1969). Success rates are generally similar to those after banding and injections, with 70 per cent of patients noting satisfactory long-term results. Particular success seems to be recorded in patients with high intra-anal pressures (Keighley et al., 1979; Sandilands, Schofield and Sykes, 1981; Kenter and Keeman, 1983). Anal dilatation appears to be less satisfactory for patients with third-degree haemorrhoids or for those with significant mucosal prolapse (Hancock, 1981). Of greatest concern is the complication rate, which approaches 10 per cent. The three most common complications are splitting of the anal canal, mucosal prolapse and anal incontinence. The first two complications are frequently transient or can be managed by subsequent banding, but incontinence may persist and be bothersome. In the Macintyre and Balfour (1972) series, 22 per cent of patients complained of incontinence for flatus and 36 per cent of incontinence for faeces. These symptoms were usually transient.

We have had minimal experience with the Lord procedure. Many US surgeons find such uncontrolled trauma to the sphincter mechanism to be offensive, and probably for this reason the procedure has not enjoyed widespread acceptance in the USA. Nevertheless, the literature suggests that anal dilatation is a viable alternative in the management of patients with first- and second-degree haemorrhoids.

Surgical haemorrhoidectomy

Surgical haemorrhoidectomy remains the standard against which alternatives must be compared. The decreasing frequency of haemorrhoidectomy at most institutions is an indication of the effectiveness and safety of the alternatives (Jeffery *et al.*, 1980). Haemorrhoidectomy would now seem to be reserved for those patients with associated anal pathology requiring surgery: incarcerated haemorrhoids, necrotic haemorrhoids and haemorrhoids with a significant external component.

Individual haemorrhoidal groups should be excised, and the techniques of Milligan *et al.* (1937) and Ferguson and Heaton (1959) have stood the test of time. Open and closed techniques are capable of achieving excellent results and frequently can be carried out with local anaesthesia (McConnell and Khubchandani, 1983). More extensive haemorrhoidectomy, as described by Whitehead (1882), has received much criticism since the report of Andrews (1895). Much of this criticism may have been due to a basic misunderstanding of the surgical technique and a subsequent unacceptable incidence of ectropion formation. Recent reviews by Barrios and Khubchandani (1979) and Hodedadi, Kurgan and Jersky (1979) suggest that clinical results can be excellent and the incidence of ectropion minimized. Indeed, the rapidly accruing experience with the ileo-anal procedure would seem to be the ultimate vindication of the surgical principles that Whitehead proposed and suggest that the ectropion may be more a result of faulty surgical technique than an innate defect of the procedure.

Wolf, Munoz and Rosin (1979) recently completed a survey in the USA to assess the changing trends of haemorrhoid surgery. They received responses from 445 (43.6 per cent) of the membership of the American Society of Colon and Rectal Surgery, reflecting experience with 89 497 procedures. Of the procedures, 42 per cent were open and 58 per cent were closed. There was mucosal prolapse in 90 per cent of the patients. Bleeding and thrombosis were the next most frequent surgical indications. Pruritus as the sole indication for surgery was rarely mentioned. The surgeons used various anaesthetic techniques—general, spinal or caudal. Local anaesthesia was used most commonly by surgeons who preferred the closed technique. Seventy-five per cent of surgeons removed haemorrhoids as groups or in columns, and 95 per cent left mucosal bridges. When surgery was indicated because of associated anal conditions, most surgeons were willing to perform an internal sphincterotomy. Regardless of whether open or closed techniques were used, no statistical differences were found in the average length of stay; incidence of urinary retention; secondary bleeding; time to return to full activity; postoperative fissure, fistula or abscess; incontinence to liquid stool, solid stool or flatus; or incidence of re-operation. However, closed techniques had a greater incidence of dehiscence, shorter healing time, less stenosis and greater postoperative infection.

incontinent patients pose the greatest problem for those who have to care for them at home. There are also other important implications; it is often the reason for admission to hospital, and sometimes earns for the patient an erroneous label 'senile' or 'mental', resulting in placement in a psychogeriatric hospital (Hyams, 1974).

Most geriatricians agree that faecal incontinence is much more likely to stem from some local cause rather than from cerebral deterioration. In fact, the source of the problem is quite commonly undetected faecal impaction. In this context, the high proportion of doubly incontinent people to be found in institutions must lead one to consider the whole subject of bowel management.

Concepts and attitudes

There is little doubt that to many people the management of the bowel is of great importance to the feeling of well-being. Disturbed rhythm can give rise to great concern and anxiety, and if incontinence also occurs the emotional reaction is devastating. Bowel habit, attitudes and practice vary from one individual to another, and are influenced by childhood conditioning in addition to social and cultural factors. Reaction to one's own excreta and its disposal also has a bearing: the subject as a whole is treated in general as a 'dirty' one and is therefore taboo.

Over the centuries the bowel has been the subject of innumerable myths and misconceptions. The cleansing of impurities of both body and mind was thought to be achieved by emptying the bowel; hence the age-old practice of regular purging. The ancient Greek use of cathartic drugs was closely associated with religion; if a man was not ritually cleansed he was thought to be obsessed by impurities which defiled him in the sight of the gods (Talalay, 1964). The use of clysters became popular in Europe throughout the seventeenth and eighteenth centuries. The *New London Dispensary* of 1698 includes a prescription for a clyster 'to cure disorders from sorrow, loss of sense, to ringworm and cancer'. As late as 1840, Louis XI was said to have been cured of apoplexy by the administration of a clyster (Russell, 1932). The development of pharmacology increased the variety of purgative medicines and led on through the nineteenth and early twentieth centuries to the almost universal reliance on patent laxatives. The theory of intestinal intoxication was widely held, and a daily bowel action was considered essential. The remnants of this belief are still found in many elderly patients, and after a lifetime's dependence on Beecham's Pills, Ex-Lax, Eno's Fruit Salts or Andrews Liver Salts, and other over-the-counter remedies, they still believe that 'inner cleanliness comes first'.

Some problems encountered

In a rigidly toilet trained society like ours the stigma of faecal incontinence is immense. Clinical histories reveal the many years that people suffer it before seeking help. In a study 'Faecal incontinence—the unvoiced symptom', conducted at Hope Hospital, Manchester (Leigh and Turnberg, 1982), it was found that out of 76 patients presenting with diarrhoea, 51 per cent had faecal incontinence. Fewer than half volunteered this information and only persistent interrogation by the medical staff enabled the true situation to be assessed—a point that is stressed in the study. This apparent reluctance of patients to complain may be compounded by the reluctance of medical attendants to embarrass patients by asking about it. Emotional inhibition in relation to the subject is not confined to patients.

This inhibition may contribute to the lack of medical interest in the day-to-day functioning of the patient's bowel. The elderly patient presenting to his family doctor with faecal or double incontinence may be admitted to hospital for want of a rectal examination. Undetected faecal impaction with consequent incontinence, accompanied as it sometimes is with restlessness and confusion, is often the last straw for relatives nursing the old person at home. Family disruption may needlessly occur as the result of what one geriatrician describes as the 'recto-cephalic reflex' (Hyams, 1974). Another geriatrician comments on the frequency of finding faecal staining round and under the finger nails of patients. This is not necessarily a sign of mental deterioration, but of physical distress and attempts at self-help to relieve discomfort (Stewart, 1971).

This lack of medical involvement in bowel function is inevitably reflected in nursing practice. Inadequate nursing assessment of individual habit and a haphazard approach to bowel management as a whole can adversely affect anyone of any age when in hospital. A medical colleague, when a patient in a teaching hospital, found after surgery that he required a suppository. The first nurse could not accede to his request as 'she did not believe in it'. He waited and asked another on the next duty, who co-operated. A great deal of discomfort and anxiety could have been caused to a less well-informed and persistent patient.

A young woman with poliomyelitis, paralysed from the neck down, describes her long struggle to manage her own bowels while in hospital (Munn, 1972). For a number of years she was subjected to a routine of four cascara tablets at night and two dessertspoons of liquid paraffin in the morning. She was totally incontinent and sometimes constipated. Eventually she was transferred to a different hospital where a bowel regime was worked out with her co-operation. After some experimentation of dosage and with the eventual inclusion of natural bran in her diet, she became continent and her bowel was no longer a problem to herself and others.

The experience of another colleague admitted to a well-known orthopaedic hospital for a lumbosacral fusion provides another example. With the prospect of bed rest for three weeks and well aware of the risks of potential constipation, she tried but was unable to persuade the staff to follow a preventive regime. The result was faecal impaction followed by manual extraction, causing her intense distress.

Aspects of institutional care

The British have the reputation of being preoccupied with their bowels, unlike the French who are more pleasantly preoccupied with filling the stomach with food. However true these national attributions are, it certainly appears that, in hospitals, some patients are obsessed with bowel function. This is not surprising as there is usually some change of bowel habit after admission, with an accompanying increase of worry and concern. In a study of 660 patients in 43 medical wards in 8 hospitals, bowel habit was monitored and subjective reactions noted (Wright, 1974). In 5 days following admission, 54.7 per cent of patients had fewer bowel actions than when at home. While many of this group took aperients at home and were accustomed to worrying about bowel function, 16 per cent of the total sample became concerned for the first time.

There are certain aspects of institutional care which exacerbate this worry and concern; for instance, it is not common practice to ascertain the patient's normal bowel pattern prior to admission and therefore it may be difficult to maintain it. Recording of subsequent bowel action is often inaccurate and lacking in sufficient detail. Aperients tend to be administered on a routine basis rather than on individual requirement.

Environmental factors are often not conducive to relaxed bowel action, and can result in inhibition of the rectal reflex.

There is too little emphasis on assessment of bowel habit included in nursing practice. The written procedures found in hospital wards are mainly concerned with the mechanical details of administering enemas, etc., rather than with the details of overall bowel care. For instance, a simple checklist (see Appendix below) would be useful. Fortunately, in some geriatric units procedures are becoming more enlightened and apposite. In one, it is stated that 'faecal incontinence in most patients is due to impaction with overflow and is a largely preventable phenomenon even in severely demented patients'. Practical measures are then described in order to achieve this. Incontinent patients are by no means confined to geriatric wards, and more policies along these lines in medical and surgical wards would help to alleviate the problem at source.

The position is at its worst for patients in long-term care. One study (Habeeb and Kallstrom, 1976), in a Veterans' Administration Hospital in California for patients with neurological conditions, revealed that unpredictable faecal incontinence was a major problem for staff. They were discontented and frustrated because of the constant cleaning work and, in consequence, tended to avoid incontinent patients; the patients themselves also became frustrated by this lack of attention. When, however, a planned regimen by physician, nurse and dietition was instituted, it produced positive results. Bowel action was anticipated and both patient and staff morale improved. Not only were relationships better between patients and staff, but between patients themselves. To make such changes in traditional ritualistic routines is a challenge to both medical and nursing staff, who may hitherto have given the matter relatively little thought.

Use of aperients

Considerable quantities of purgatives are bought by the public at large. Consumption is related to age and sex, being greater in the young and the elderly, and more in women than in men. This usage is often based on the assumption that a daily evacuation must be achieved, an idea which is often perpetuated in hospitals, where large quantities of aperients are also used.

Another matter for concern is the type and dosage, a matter which is usually left to the nurse. A number of physicians feel, however, that rather than being available on demand aperients should be prescribed, both to achieve the most effective results and to avoid the consequences of overdosage. Florence Nightingale made this point in 1859 in her *Notes for Nursing*. Such medical involvement implies devoting time and interest to bowel function and management. In establishments where a doctor visits perhaps only once a month this would be impracticable, but an agreed policy of management could be applied if staff were given adequate guidance.

Lavatories and toilets

The inadequacy of toilet facilities in many hospitals and institutions has been well documented. Following the trend towards early patient ambulation, the shortage of lavatories has become increasingly apparent. In the Ministry of Health Building Notes 1961, it was recommended that there should be at least 1 toilet to every 6 patients and that it must be large enough to accommodate a wheelchair.

To the patient, lack of privacy and comfort in the toilet is of great concern. Doors which cannot be locked, low temperatures and lack of cleanliness are all inhibiting factors to natural defaecation. The tendency for staff to have their own toilets and not to use those of the patients is in itself significant.

It is not easy to improve such environmental shortcomings except by long-term planning, but where facilities are inadequate or inaccessible the provision of substitute toilets such as suitably placed commodes is essential. Recognition by the nurse of the patient's bowel pattern, together with ensuring that the bowel can be emptied in privacy at the appropriate time, are simple steps towards the prevention of dyschesia. This is equally true for those cared for in residential homes or even in their own homes.

Policy

As the number of elderly people increases in relation to the population as a whole, this will inevitably be reflected in hospitals and other institutions and in the practice lists of general practitioners. Since faecal incontinence is already a problem in this age group, it will be seen that a diminishing number of younger people will be faced with caring for an increasing number of ageing patients and dependants with 'dirty habits'. A preventive policy is therefore essential, based on a fundamental reappraisal of bowel function and management.

Medical education on the subject of faecal incontinence is at present still scant; the average length of time spent on this subject by medical students during their clinical course totals only 21 minutes (King's Fund Centre, 1983). Neither is there much relevant education and training for the nurse, and existing ward procedures are frequently underinformed and inadequate. It is hardly surprising, therefore, that relatives at home and residential care staff understand even less. I have known untrained care assistants in residential homes, a category of staff only marginally more experienced than that of domestic workers, to be expected to perform manual removal of faeces on patients. An obvious need is improved education and the placing of far greater emphasis on this aspect of care. The body of knowledge which has become available, as this book shows, could and should be incorporated into practice.

Apart from the cost in human terms of allowing the present situation to continue, the financial cost must also be considered. Expenditure on management aids, laundry and disposal services is heavy, quite apart from the general cost of avoidable hospitalization. There is also the diversion of valuable nursing time and skill into such wasteful and unproductive work as 'cleaning up' large numbers of patients whose incontinence is unnecessary.

Appendix: checklist for the management of bowels

Bowel activity or actions can be a source of worry to patients. In order to alleviate these worries and prevent distress and constipation, or worse still faecal incontinence, time spent with the patient on admission to find out normal habits is of value. The following points need to be considered:

1. How regular is the normal bowel habit? This can vary from 3 times a day to 3 times a week. A record is necessary of frequency, nature and number of stools and if there is pain or discomfort on defaecation.
2. When were the bowels last opened?

Stress urinary incontinence is sometimes associated with idiopathic neurogenic anorectal incontinence and, in these patients, abnormalities in motor nerve conduction in the perineal branches of the pudendal nerve that innervates the periurethral striated sphincter musculature have been described (Snooks and Swash, 1984a, 1984b). These resemble the slowed terminal motor conduction found in the inferior rectal branches innervating the anal sphincter musculature. Indeed, in some patients with stress urinary incontinence, EMG abnormalities of neurogenic type have been found in the external anal sphincter muscles (Anderson, 1984). These observations strongly suggest that idiopathic anorectal incontinence, which is itself a form of stress incontinence, and stress urinary incontinence have a similar pathogenesis. Elderly people may be particularly likely to develop these problems because of coincident age-related neurogenic changes in these muscles (Percy *et al.*, 1982).

In earlier work we suggested that entrapment of the pudendal nerves in Alcock's canal might be a factor leading to neurogenic change in the external anal sphincter muscle in idiopathic neurogenic anorectal incontinence, but this hypothesis seems to be excluded by the finding that the puborectalis muscle, which is probably more important than the external anal sphincter in the control of continence in normal people, is innervated largely by direct branches of the sacral plexus, and not by branches of the pudendal nerves. *Table 12.1* gives a classification of the causes of faecal incontinence.

Clinical features

The degree of incontinence should be established at the outset. The management of a patient with minor soiling would differ from that of a patient who wears incontinence pads which require frequent changes during the course of the day. A previous history of obstetric difficulties or of anal surgery should be noted. If the history is comparatively short, includes perineal or low back pain or is associated with motor and sensory symptoms in the legs or buttocks, then an underlying neurological cause should be considered and investigated.

Inspection of the perineum may reveal soiling of the perineal skin, local scarring from previous injury or surgery and, during a straining effort, a complete rectal prolapse may be observed. The cutaneous anal reflex should be tested; if it is absent a pudendal neuropathy or cauda equina lesion is likely to be present (Henry, Parks and Swash, 1982).

Digital examination of the anus is of key importance. Resting anal tone is an indication of internal anal sphincter function and will be reduced if there has been previous anal surgery (e.g. anal dilatation) or if there is a complete rectal prolapse. In the patient with pelvic floor denervation there will be reduced or absent voluntary squeeze contraction in the external anal sphincter, and the posterior bar created by the puborectalis may be deficient or weakened.

An abdominal examination and sigmoidoscopy should always be performed to exclude other pathology which could be responsible for alteration of stool consistency and subsequently for incontinence, e.g. Crohn's disease.

Investigations

Although a large part of this monograph is devoted to the range of investigative methods that have been adopted in pelvic floor disorders, it has to be stated that clinical

TABLE 12.1. Classification of the causes of faecal incontinence

A. *Normal sphincters and pelvic floor*
    Diarrhoea:
        Infective
        Inflammatory bowel disease
        Intestinal resection
        Metabolic (e.g. diabetes mellitus)
    Fistula/colostomy

B. *Abnormal function of sphincters and/or pelvic floor*
    Partial incontinence:
        Internal sphincter deficiency:
          Previous surgery (e.g. anal stretch, sphincterotomy)
          Rectal prolapse
          Third-degree haemorrhoids
        Faecal impaction:
          The elderly
          Generalized neurological disorders (e.g. mental defect)
        Minor external sphincter and pelvic floor denervation
    Major incontinence:
        Congenital anomalies of the anorectum
        Trauma:
          Iatrogenic
          Obstetric
          Fractures of pelvis
          Impalement
        Complete rectal prolapse
        Rectal carcinoma
        Anorectal infection (e.g. lymphogranuloma)
        Idiopathic (primary neurogenic faecal incontinence)
        Drug intoxication (especially in the elderly)
        Neurological:
          Upper motor-neuron lesion:
            Cerebral:
              multiple strokes
              metastases and other tumours
              dementia and other degenerative disorders
              trauma
            Spinal:
              multiple sclerosis
               metastases and other tumours
              degenerative diseases (e.g. B_{12} deficiency)
          Lower motor-neuron lesion:
            Cauda equina (tumour or trauma)
            Peripheral neuropathy (diabetes, multiple sclerosis)
            Tabes dorsalis
            Lumbar meningomyelocele (spina bifida)

evaluation often suffices as a basis for treatment. Most clinicians, however, find it of considerable value to have an objective quantitative assessment of sphincter and pelvic floor function before proceeding with treatment. Anorectal manometry is useful in identifying internal anal sphincter weakness by the finding of reduction of resting anal tone. We find the most accurate means of routine assessment of the external anal sphincter and pelvic floor musculature is by single fibre electromyography (Chapter 5) and by measurement of the pudendal nerve terminal motor latency (Chapter 7). If a cauda equina lesion is suspected, spinal stimulation at L1 and L4 vertebral levels should be carried out before myelography is considered; in our practice, the latter is not commonly indicated.

Treatment

Non-surgical

If incontinence is due to the loose consistency of the stool, perhaps in combination with reduced internal sphincter tone, management should be directed initially at the underlying disorder, that is the diarrhoea should be investigated. In combination with treatment with simple constipating agents, full function may be rapidly restored in the majority of patients within this group.

In contrast, patients who soil because of faecal impaction can be adequately managed by disimpaction, bowel education and, if necessary, the regular use of purgatives.

Patients with established denervation of the pelvic floor and sphincter muscles gain little permanent benefit from pelvic floor faradism. Similarly, treatment by external stimulation either by direct electro-implantation (Caldwell, 1963) or by anal plug stimulation (Hopkinson and Lightwood, 1966) has proved generally disappointing (Duthie, 1971). A technique to improve sphincter function in some patients employing the principle of biofeedback is discussed later in this chapter.

Surgical

The varying techniques which have been developed are discussed in later sections of this chapter. Generally, they are highly successful in restoring continence to the majority of patients such that a colostomy should only rarely be contemplated.

C. Treatment: (i) Postanal repair

M. M. Henry and J. P. S. Thomson

Introduction

The importance of the anorectal angle approximating to a right angle and a closed anal canal in maintaining normal faecal continence has been discussed in Chapter 3. Patients with idiopathic (neurogenic) incontinence have a widening of this angle and shortening of the anal canal. Parks (1975) devised an operation whereby the widened angle could be reduced by moving the anorectal junction upwards and forwards. In the process, the anal canal is lengthened and tightened, with a corresponding improvement in mean resting anal canal and squeeze pressures (Browning and Parks, 1983). This operation is called postanal repair (PAR).

This operation has proved to be of value in those patients with incontinence associated with the descending perineum syndrome, and with incontinence following a successful abdominal rectopexy used as treatment for complete rectal prolapse.

It is our practice to assess sphincter function physiologically prior to operation (Chapter 2), as this permits a quantitative assessment of the situation and may protect against the possibility of performing an operation which could produce little gain to the patient. Furthermore, it permits objective assessment postoperatively.

Preoperative preparation

As it is possible for the bowel to be opened during the dissection, it is sensible for the patient to have a mechanical preparation of the large intestine.

The operation

The patient is anaesthetized and placed in the lithotomy position. A urinary catheter is inserted, and an instrument tray attached to the foot of the operating table is most useful. The subcutaneous tissues to the left and right, and behind the anus, are infiltrated with 1:300 000 Adrenaline in saline solution, as this reduces bleeding in the early stages of the dissection and aids the definition of the lower borders of the anal sphincter muscles. A V-shaped incision is made posterior to the anus, with its apex at the level of the tip of the coccyx (*Figure 12.1*). The flap of skin contained within the incision is then dissected to expose the inferior border of the external anal sphincter— pinky brown in colour—and the lower border of the internal sphincter—pale grey or white in colour (*Figure 12.2*). Identification of the external sphincter can be further aided by the use of an electronic stimulator.

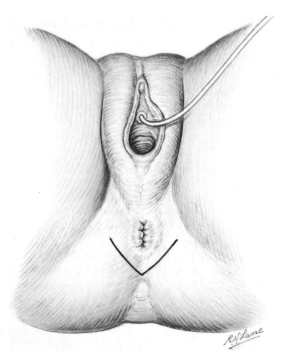

Figure 12.1

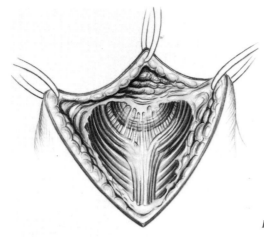

Figure 12.2

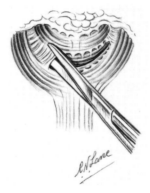

Figure 12.3

The anatomical key to this operation is the intersphincteric space, an avascular space which separates the smooth muscle of the viscus from the somatic musculature of the pelvic floor. Its position is usually more posterior than one would imagine, because of the laxity of the somatic musculature, and can be detected by identifying the emerging longitudinal fibres—the terminal fibres of the longitudinal muscle of the gut tube. These therefore belong to the viscus and it is important to divide these in order to expose the inner aspect of the somatic musculature (*Figure 12.3*). It should now be possible, with a combination of digital and scissor dissection, to open up the intersphincteric space (*Figure 12.4*). This is usually more straightforward at the sides than in the midline posteriorly, which is therefore conveniently done last. At the tip of the external sphincter the puborectalis will be found, and at this site it is often firmly adherent to the visceral structures, so sharp dissection is often required.

In order to expose the upper surface of the levator ani muscles, the thick fascial layer, often called Waldeyer's fascia, will need to be divided (*Figure 12.5*). Care must be taken not to strip this fascia off the sacrum as venous bleeding may be encountered.

Once the muscle has been completely exposed from left to right, suturing begins. A lattice is constructed with 0 polypropylene from one side of the levator ani to the other, as high as possible (ileococcygeus muscle) (*Figure 12.6*). No attempt at this stage must be made to approximate the muscle, as this would result in tension and possible

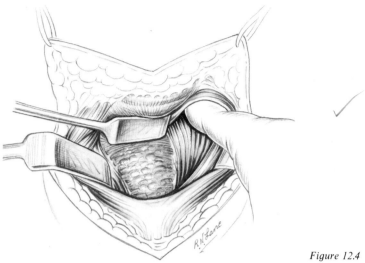

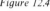

Figure 12.4

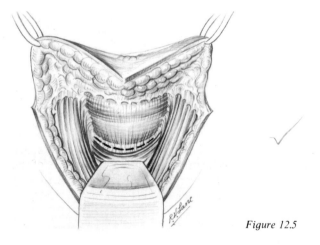

Figure 12.5

necrosis. A second lattice is inserted at a lower level approximating the pubococcygeus muscle fibres (*Figure 12.7*). The third layer approximates the puborectalis muscles, and it is usually possible to approximate these without there being any tension on the muscle fibres (*Figure 12.8*). However, it is important that the knot should not be tied too tightly, as this will cause necrosis of tissue. A small gap may be left between the approximated muscles so that should there be any postoperative swelling, this will not cause tissue necrosis. Finally, the external sphincter is approximated and the skin sutured (*Figures 12.9* and *12.10*). The skin can be sutured in the form of a 'Y', but there is often a redundant piece of skin in the midline posteriorly, which can form a large postoperative tag, making cleaning after defaecation difficult. This can with profit be excised.

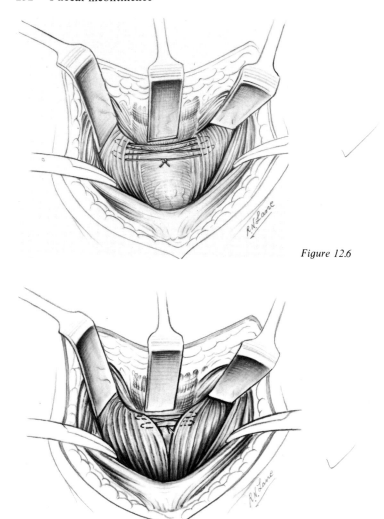

Figure 12.6

Figure 12.7

Postoperative care

It is very important that excessive straining at stool is avoided after operation and that faecal impaction does not occur. The former would result in a breakdown of the suturing and the latter would require disimpaction, which would inevitably disrupt the repair. A regimen of agents to maintain a soft stool is therefore desirable, together with an irritant suppository to induce defaecation.

Results

The published results for this operation are most encouraging, and in the late Sir Alan Parks series of 183 patients, 72 per cent became fully continent for solid and liquid stool

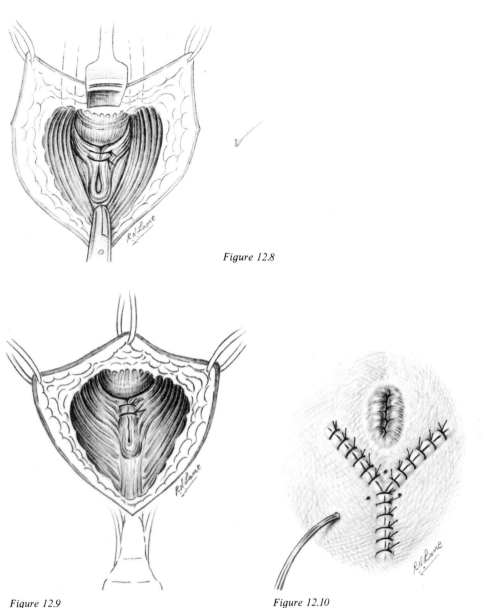

Figure 12.8

Figure 12.9   Figure 12.10

and a further 12 per cent were continent for solid stool only (Browning *et al.*, 1984). Of those who were not helped by this operation, one-quarter in fact had recurrent complete rectal prolapse. It is very important to stress that this operation will not succeed if the muscles are held separated by the presence of complete prolapse.

The reasons, other than technical, for poor functional results after this operation include wound sepsis, destruction of muscle fibres by strangulation with the sutures being tied too tightly, and of course patients with very severe preoperative muscle degeneration. Sometimes the apex of the flap of skin, if it is not excised, becomes ischaemic, and may slough away from the healing wound. However, healing will always eventually occur.

Another problem which may sometimes occur after a successful sphincter repair is that some patients have rectal inertia and are totally unable to expel their rectal contents. In this event, a terminal colostomy is probably the most appropriate treatment.

M. Keighley, of The General Hospital in Birmingham, has recently reported his results in a series of 89 patients (Keighley, 1984). There was a follow-up of at least 6 months after operation. The results are similar, with 63 per cent being continent for solid and liquid stools, and a further 21 per cent who were continent for solid stool only.

It is therefore apparent that this operation does produce satisfactory results in the majority of patients, and it has brought hope to a situation which a few years ago had no useful treatment other than the construction of a colostomy.

Acknowledgement

All the illustrations in this section are taken from Parks and Percy (1983), by permission of the publishers.

C. Treatment: (ii) Gracilis muscle transposition

M. L. Corman

Introduction

The optimal procedure for restoring the sphincter mechanism would be to utilize the muscles in the area, should this be possible. However, if there has been loss of muscle tissue as a result of trauma or disuse, such an approach is usually unsuccessful. Under these circumstances, reconstruction requires supplementing the sphincter mechanism by means of one of several techniques—the transposition of muscle (gluteus, vastus internus, adductor longus, gracilis) or one of the Thiersch procedures (e.g. wire, Teflon, Marlex, Dacron-impregnated Silastic mesh).

Pickrell et al. (1952) developed a procedure using the gracilis muscle as a substitute anal sphincter. I have used this operation when a supplementary sphincter was required and when multiple attempts at direct repair have been unsuccessful (Corman, 1978, 1980, 1984). This operation, however, is not for elderly patients who soil their underclothes. It is a rather esoteric approach to sphincter repair that should be used only in limited circumstances.

Technique

The gracilis muscle is the most superficial muscle in the medial aspect of the thigh. It is broad in the upper thigh, becomes narrow, and tapers to a tendon which inserts below the tibial tuberosity. The major blood supply enters proximally, so that division at the insertion and mobilization of the muscle to the proximal neurovascular bundle usually do not compromise viability.

Patients are placed on a bowel preparation as if for a colon resection. Enemas are administered the morning of surgery until the returns are clear. Intravenous broad-spectrum antibiotics are suggested preoperatively, intraoperatively and post-operatively.

Patients are placed in the perineolithotomy position to expose the thighs and the anus. The side which is selected for transposition is draped so that it can be removed easily from the stirrup.

Three incisions are utilized on the medial aspect of the thigh—upper, mid-thigh and across the knee joint. The muscle is identified initially through the proximal incision. A quarter-inch (6 mm) Penrose drain is passed under the muscle (*Figure 12.11*), and the dissection is carried cephalad to the neurovascular bundle (inset), which is the upper limit of the dissection. The muscle is mobilized to the tendinous insertion (*Figure 12.12*) by incising the investing fascia and by blunt dissection between the skin bridges. The tendon of the gracilis muscle passes under the sartorius muscle, so that the latter structure must be retracted anteriorly in order to identify the gracilis tendon. It is because of this relationship that I have found it rather difficult to proceed with the dissection initially from the distal incision. The dissection proceeds distally as far as possible, and the tendon is divided. The two distal incisions are closed in two layers (subcutaneous tissue and skin) and the muscle delivered through the proximal incision (*Figure 12.13*).

Attention is then turned to the anal dissection. A curvilinear incision is made approximately 1.5 cm from the anal verge anteriorly and posteriorly. If possible, an attempt should be made to preserve the raphes (as illustrated) so that the muscle can be pulled around them as a pulley (*Figure 12.14*). A tunnel is developed between the

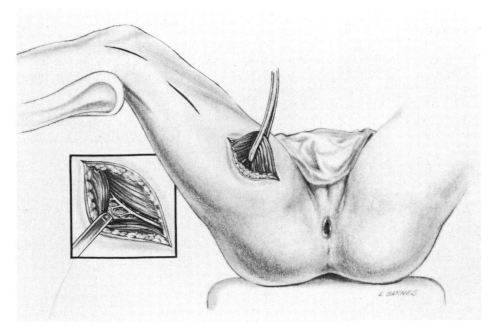

Figure 12.11

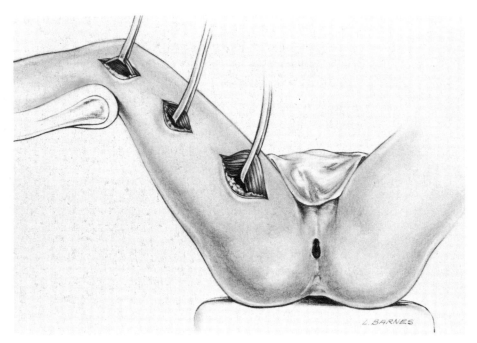

Figure 12.12

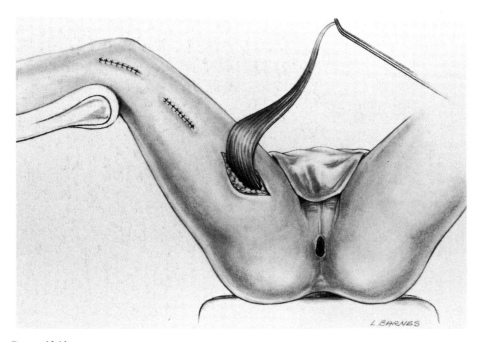

Figure 12.13

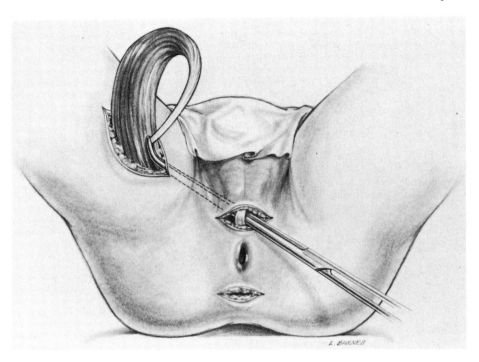

Figure 12.14

proximal thigh incision and the anterior perianal incision, and the tendon is pulled through (*Figure 12.15*).

A tunnel is then created in the extrasphincteric space on either side of the anal canal. The tendon is passed clockwise if the right gracilis muscle is being transposed, or counterclockwise if the left gracilis muscle is utilized (*Figure 12.16*). The thigh incision is then closed.

After the tendon is passed 360° and *behind* the muscle, an incision is made over the contralateral ischial tuberosity. Three monofilament non-absorbable sutures (Prolene) are placed in the gluteal fascia and held in place (*Figure 12.17*). The tendon is pulled through a tunnel developed between the ischial incision and the anterior perianal incision (*Figure 12.18*). At this point, the leg from which the gracilis muscle was taken is removed from the stirrup and adducted (*Figure 12.19*). This is a very important manoeuvre because it releases tension on the muscle. If the tendon were to be anchored without adduction, the substitute sphincter would be too loose, and the results would be unsatisfactory. With maximal adduction, the surgeon pulls the tendon taut. It should be quite snug when the finger is inserted in the rectum. Too tight an anal orifice may be corrected by dilatation. However, if the opening is too wide, surgical failure will result. The sutures are placed into the tendon and secured. All incisions are closed and no drains are employed (*Figure 12.20*). *Figure 12.21* illustrates schematically the final position of the muscle and tendon.

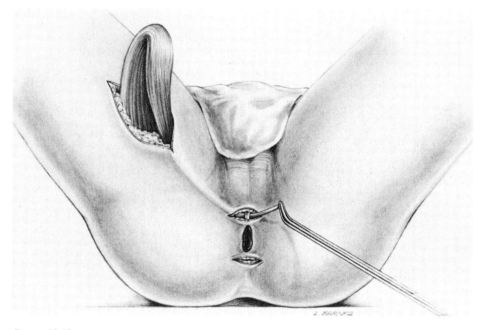

Figure 12.15

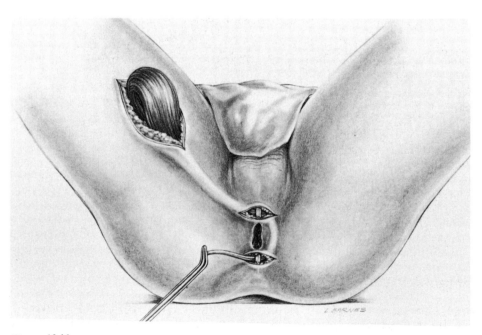

Figure 12.16

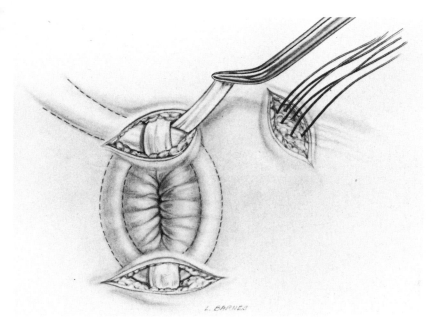

Figure 12.17

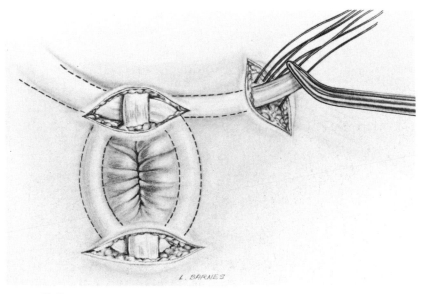

Figure 12.18

Postoperative care

Postoperatively, the bowels are confined for 1 week. The patient is kept at bed rest for 48 h, after which ambulation is permitted. The wounds are gently cleansed 3 times daily, and a topical antiseptic ointment is applied.

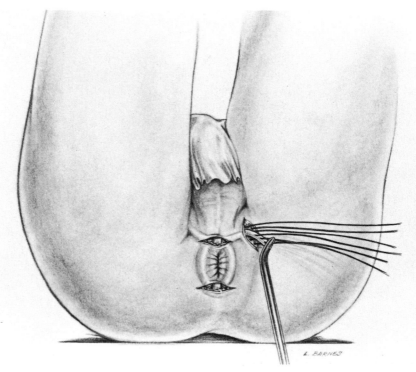

Figure 12.19

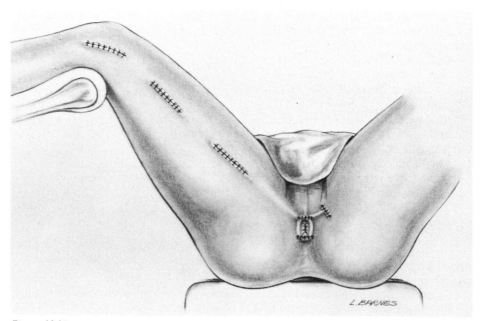

Figure 12.20

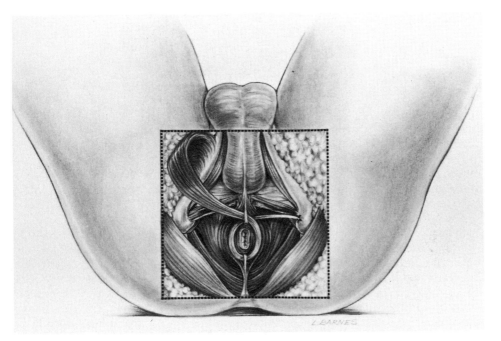

Figure 12.21

The postoperative management of these patients must be vigorous. Lack of success in the past with this procedure may have been the result of insufficient attention to this aspect of treatment. This repair is much like the Thiersch operation in narrowing the anal canal, except that this 'purse-string' is dynamic. The anal orifice can be stretched open, and then it passively closes. I do not believe that patients can be instructed on voluntarily contracting and relaxing the muscle. In fact, the muscle is maximally relaxed when the patient is in the squatting position for defaecation.

The goal in the postoperative period is establishment of a workable time for defaecation. For most patients, this is in the morning. When the patient is eating a regular diet, a suppository (e.g. bisacodyl) is inserted immediately after breakfast. Ideally, the patient will defaecate and remain clean until the next morning when the procedure is repeated. Ultimately, the patient will establish a pattern that should avoid the need for a suppository. Obviously, each patient must be treated individually; some may require laxatives; others, 'slowing' medications.

The gracilis muscle transposition can be advised when sphincter muscle has been lost, or other sphincteroplastic approaches have failed. Relative contraindications include an atonic rectum, neurological deficit, diarrhoea and severe constipation. Elderly patients also should not be submitted to the rigours of this procedure. With careful patient selection and compulsive postoperative care, good to excellent results may be anticipated.

Acknowledgement

All the illustrations in this section are from Corman (1984) and are reproduced with permission of the publishers, Lippincott/Harper and Row.

C. Treatment: (iii) Neonatal and paediatric incontinence

R. C. M. Cook

Introduction

The surgeon caring for an incontinent adult patient is in most instances aiming to restore what has been lost. His paediatric surgical colleague is more likely to be faced with a patient who has no experience of normal continence, in whom there has been a failure of development of the normal anatomy or physiology or of both. The very term incontinence may be hard to define in childhood. The age at which a child is anticipated to be toilet trained varies in different cultures (Fritz and Armbrust, 1982). Continence of faeces in British and North American children is expected by the second birthday; in French and Scandinavian children not until their third birthday; and in some parts of the world it is not considered abnormal for the 6-year-old child to show little evidence of conscious control (Whiting and Child, 1953).

Too early and overzealous 'potty training' has long been recognized as a potential cause of bowel and other problems in later childhood. The age at which the central nervous system is sufficiently mature to co-ordinate the very complex pelvic sensory and motor mechanisms is uncertain. The activity of the external anal sphincter has been studied in normal children by the use of surface electrodes (Molander and Frenckner, 1983). The external sphincter is in tonic continuous activity, maintained by spinal reflexes and augmented by supraspinal centres which increase the tone in response to rectal fulness in children over the age of $2\frac{1}{2}$ years. In infants tested when aged between 2 and 18 months, the tonic continuous activity of the sphincter is lost in response to rectal distension. Such an inhibition reflex is exactly what would be expected from the common observation of defaecation following rectal examination in the small infant who has not achieved functional supraspinal connections.

'Encopresis'

Although much less common than failure of urinary control, faecal incontinence is sufficiently frequent to have earned the title 'encopresis', although the word is probably best reserved for those children with psychogenic soiling for whom the term was first coined (Weisenberg, 1926). It probably affects 1–2 per cent of 7-year-old children (Levine, 1982), and boys outnumber girls five- or six-fold. Although the child usually appears unaware or unconcerned, the soiling has a profound effect on the life of the family and the child. The reaction of parents is usually one of blame, and of peers of ridicule, both of which add to the isolation, denial and psychological damage. The organic causes and consequences, even in the child with considerable psychological problems, must not be overlooked; and where organic causes predominate, skilled psychological help may be needed, as well as good surgery, to achieve acceptable continence and social integration.

Levine (1982) lists the 'potentiation factors' in encopresis at different ages (*Table 12.2*) and, of these, congenital anorectal anomalies will occupy much of our discussion. There must be added neuropathies (spina bifida and sacral agenesis), and trauma (surgical, accidental and non-accidental). Neurodevelopmental delay may play a part in some

TABLE 12.2. Potentiation factors in encopretic children

Age group	Potentiation factor
Infants and toddlers	Simple constipation Colonic inertia Congenital anorectal anomalies Parental over-reaction
2–5 yr	Psychosocial stress during training Coercive or extreme permissive training Toilet fears Painful defaecation
Early school years	Avoidance of school lavatories Gastro-enteritis Short attention span Frenetic life-styles Psychosocial stresses

After Levine (1982).

older children with no obvious pelvic floor problems. Evidence of clumsiness, choreiform or athetoid movements and sensory developmental delay has been found in a proportion of encopretic children (Mikkelsen *et al.*, 1982).

Of more importance is the fact that, whatever other factors may be involved, virtually all (except some of the children with treated developmental anomalies) are chronically constipated, with evidence of faecal retention. Chronic overdistension of the rectum would be expected to lead to accommodation of the rectal proprioceptors, and a reduction in sensory feedback. Low anal resting pressures have been described and attributed to this (Revillon, Jehannin and Arhan, 1979; Loening-Baucke and Younoszai, 1982). Anorectal pressure/volume curves and rectal compliance are normal in children who are 'constipated' without rectal overdistension (Amano, 1980). Metabolic (e.g. hypercalcaemic) and endocrine (e.g. hypothyroid) causes of constipation must, of course, be excluded.

The psychological and physiological consequences of chronic constipation with encopresis remind us of the need for prompt and thorough treatment of the 'normal' child who becomes constipated because of psychological factors, or following a simple illness (especially with dehydration and loss of appetite), or following development of a fissure-in-ano. Early attention to the potentiating factors may prevent the establishment of a habit which is hard to change. Successful treatment needs the child's co-operation over a long period of time, with careful explanations, exoneration from blame, and emptying of the overloaded colon with enemata or suppositories in the initial stages followed by oral aperients. Dietary co-operation is essential, as is adjustment of the family's life-style to permit and encourage regular toiletting (Fritz and Armbrust, 1982; Levine, 1982; Sarahan *et al.*, 1982; Corman, 1983).

These measures in re-education of the child whose encopresis has a small organic and large psychological basis apply equally to the education of the child whose congenital lesion has meant that he has never known continence.

Traumatic incontinence

Developmentally satisfactory neuromuscular mechanisms of continence may be injured surgically by operations on the perineum and pelvic floor (e.g. for Hirschsprung's disease or sacrococcygeal teratomata) or by straddle injuries in the child who climbs and falls. It must always be borne in mind that an all too common cause of severe perineal injury with tears of the sphincters is child abuse and deviant sexual behaviour by adults in whose care the child is placed (Black *et al.*, 1982). Surgical repair should follow the same principles as in adults (Browning and Motson, 1983).

Neurogenic incontinence

Although neuropathy leads to incontinence in children with sacral agenesis and myelomeningoceles, they can usually achieve satisfactory social control by school age. Some attention to the diet is necessary in most of these children, both for weight control and to avoid those things which give them loose stools. The stools are usually small firm scybala which are relatively easily retained. Nixon (1984) postulates that an abnormal colonic action with some internal sphincter tone produces these stools. Regular toiletting, with voluntary effort to evacuate the bowel, possibly with the assistance of suppositories or enemata, will often establish a habit of rhythmic evacuation, and 24 or 48 h periods of confident cleanness. If the stools are persistently loose, carefully graded doses of kaolin or loperamide (Lomotil) usually produce the characteristic and normally hard stools. Anorectal manometry in myelomeningoceles is described (Sakaniwa, Takahashi and Maie, 1981), but probably contributes little to the practical management of the child. Local operations on the paralysed and insensitive pelvic floor would seem doomed to failure, but occasional reports appear of (usually) unsuccessful attempts to use muscle transplants (Brandesky, Geley and Janout, 1984).

Anorectal malformations

One of the most taxing problems that faces a paediatric surgeon is the child with an anorectal malformation. The pathological anatomy in all its variations is well described in the generally accepted international classification agreed in Melbourne in 1970 (Santulli, Kiesewetter and Bill, 1970; Stephens and Smith, 1971). The relationship of the termination of the bowel to the muscular floor of the pelvis (and especially the puborectalis sling) has for a long time been recognized as being a key factor in management, and a guide to prognosis (Louw, 1962; Kiesewetter, 1967; Swenson and Donnellan, 1967; Puri and Nixon, 1977). Where the bowel terminates on the cranial side of the levator muscle, lesions are referred to as 'high' or 'supralevator'; those infants whose bowel extends through the puborectalis sling have 'low' or 'translevator' anomalies; while in a third intermediate group, even though the fistula may be embraced by the puborectalis sling, the bowel proper terminates above it. A working party in Wisconsin in May 1984 (Stephens and Smith, 1984) has attempted to make the 1970 Melbourne classification simpler and more practical, relegating variants and rare forms to a supplementary list, with the core classification containing the common and significant forms of high, intermediate and low anomalies (*Table 12.3*).

Definitions and descriptions

High deformities in the male infant

The most common high deformity in the male in all reported series is anorectal agenesis with a recto-urethral fistula. The levator muscle is usually well formed and normally

TABLE 12.3. 'Wingspread' classification of anorectal malformations—1984

Female	Male

HIGH
1. Anorectal agenesis:
   (a) with rectovaginal fistula
   (b) without fistula
2. Rectal atresia
	HIGH
	1. Anorectal agenesis:
	   (a) with rectoprostatic urethral fistula
	   (b) without fistula
	2. Rectal atresia

INTERMEDIATE 1. Rectovestibular fistula 2. Rectovaginal fistula 3. Agenesis without fistula	INTERMEDIATE 1. Rectobulbar-urethral fistula 2. Agenesis without fistula
LOW 1. Anovestibular fistula 2. Anocutaneous fistula 3. Anal stenosis	LOW 1. Anocutaneous fistula 2. Anal stenosis
CLOACAL MALFORMATION	
OTHER RARE MALFORMATIONS	OTHER RARE MALFORMATIONS

After Stephens and Smith (1984), by permission of the publishers.

innervated, unless there is associated agenesis of three or more sacral vertebrae, and the puborectalis portion of the muscle is wrapped around the posterior urethra caudal to the site of the fistula. The internal sphincter is stated to be absent (Stephens and Smith, 1971), but there may be a condensation of circular fibres in the bowel just proximal to the fistula which show normal sphincteric responses (Kiesewetter and Nixon, 1967). The external sphincter is usually present in the perineum, even if poorly developed. Anorectal agenesis with a rectovesical fistula is a less common, but a much more serious malformation, with a high incidence of associated major malformations which may prove lethal within a few days of birth (Magnus, 1972, 1974). Rectal atresia is a rare condition that is probably acquired later in development than those deformities that are true ageneses. The anus and anal canal are correctly sited and connected to the blind rectum by a cord of tissue that passes through the puborectalis sling. Direct anastomosis via a Stephens approach should lead to the development of good continence (Dias, Santiago and Ferreira, 1982).

Apart from the infant with rectal atresia, the appearance of the perineum in the newborn boy with a high lesion is variable and unrelated to the precise form of the anomaly, except when the absence of a natal cleft, and flat buttocks, points to sacral agenesis. No meconium will be visible, of course, in any anal dimple or prominent raphe that may be present but may be seen issuing from the urethra.

Intermediate deformities in the male infant

The intermediate anomalies are rather more complex in that, although the bowel ends above the levator muscle, any fistula lies within the puborectalis sling. The anal canal is partly or completely absent. The most common form is anal agenesis with a rectobulbar fistula. An abnormal perineum is common, with an absent or weak raphe, hypospadias, cleft scrotum or urethral fistula.

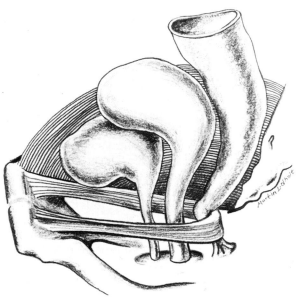

Figure 12.30. Schematic illustration of the normal relations between puborectalis muscle, anal canal and vagina

continence (Scharli and Kiesewetter, 1970). The importance of the puborectalis in maintaining anal continence is paramount and it is probable that the function of the external anal sphincter is limited to containing sudden increases in rectal pressure, and in emptying the anal canal distal to the puborectalis sling.

Free autogenous muscle transplantation

Studitsky (1964) first reported the survival of entire mammalian muscles after transplantation. He removed a muscle and minced it into small fragments. The fragments were replaced into the bed of the removed muscle. A few weeks later the minced muscle was found to be reorganized into a muscle of normal architecture. Studitsky considered that the newly formed muscle consisted of regenerated muscle. Thompson demonstrated the possibility of successful free transplantation of whole muscle bellies, initially in dogs (Thompson, 1971a) and later in patients with facial palsy (Thompson, 1971b). The muscle was transplanted onto a normal muscle from which it was revascularized and reinnervated. He suggested that the muscle fibres survived the transplantation without necrosis and subsequently regenerated. Thompson emphasized that a prerequisite for survival was motor denervation of the graft 2–3 weeks before transplantation. He assumed that the favourable outcome of grafting with this technique was partly a result of a change in enzyme constitution of the muscle fibres following denervation, which gives a more economical level of metabolism, allowing the transplant to survive the period of avascularity before the re-establishment of effective circulation. However, subsequent authors (Sciaffino *et al.*, 1975; Faulkner *et al.*, 1976) have shown that although there is a thin zone of surviving fibres at the periphery of the graft, in the rest of the graft there is regeneration of new muscle fibres following breakdown of the originally transplanted material.

In a series of investigations on denervated cat muscle autotransplants, an analysis was made of vascular supply, reinnervation and metabolism (Hakelius and Nyström, 1975a; Hakelius and Nyström, 1975b; Hakelius, Nyström and Stålberg, 1975). The transplants were placed in close contact with normally vascularized and innervated muscle. It was shown that a new capillary network was established during the first few days after grafting. The first signs of reinnervation could be identified electromyographically after 4 weeks and histochemically after 6 weeks. New motor end-plates on the transplanted muscle fibres were demonstrated from 5 weeks after grafting. The reinnervation took place through collateral nerve sprouting from the terminal nerve twigs in the adjacent normal muscle. There are limitations on the thickness of a muscle it is possible to transplant. If the diameter of the muscle is too great, no regeneration of muscle fibres occurs in the central part of the graft; instead, a central core of fibrosis is formed. My experience is that a graft diameter greater than 15 mm gives this unfavourable central fibrosis. The importance of motor denervation before grafting has also been questioned. Some authors are of the opinion that the results of grafting are equal whether the graft is predenervated or not (Carlsson and Gutmann, 1975). In our experimental work, we have found a better result with prior denervation than without (Hakelius, Nyström and Stålberg, 1975).

To summarize, four conditions must be fulfilled for successful transplantation:

1. The graft must have a diameter below 15 mm.
2. The graft must be placed in direct contact with the recipient muscle bed.
3. The recipient muscle must be innervated.
4. Only limited strength of the graft can be expected.

Free muscle transplantation for anal incontinence

The aim of the operation is to place a muscle graft as a sling around the rectum, so as to mimic the position and function of the puborectalis muscle (*Figure 12.31*) (Hakelius, 1975). The transplant must be in contact with normally innervated levator ani muscles to permit reinnervation. No attempt need be made to reconstruct the external anal sphincter. The procedure is carried out in two stages, with an interval of 2–3 weeks. In the first stage, denervation of the muscle intended as graft is made. In the second, the transplantation is performed. The muscle of choice is the palmaris longus muscle of the forearm. If this muscle is congenitally absent, a part of the sartorius muscle can be used.

Indications

It is important to recognize that the technique of free muscle transplantation cannot be used in patients with anal incontinence of neurogenic origin because a prerequisite for successful results is the presence of normally innervated muscles in the pelvic floor. The huge group of older patients with anal incontinence with laxity of the pelvic floor caused by senile involution or denervation are not suitable for treatment with the operation, probably because there is a low capacity for neural regeneration, and sufficient reinnervation of the graft cannot occur. Patients with anal incontinence in combination with or due to anorectal prolapse should first be managed by correction of their prolapse (Buchmann and Keighley, 1982). The graft will not be strong enough to withstand the pressure from the prolapse. If incontinence remains after rectopexy, transplantation can be used.

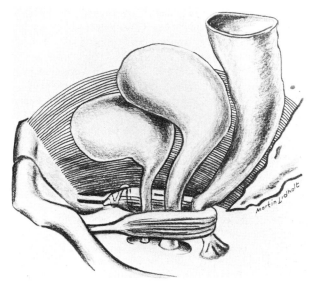

Figure 12.31. Schematic illustration of the palmaris longus transplant in position, with the tendons sutured to the periosteum of the os pubis

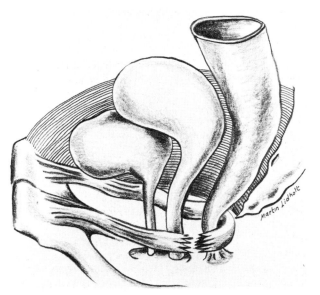

Figure 12.32. Schematic illustration of disturbed function of the puborectalis muscle because of rupture of the muscle

The best results of transplantation are obtained in anal incontinence due to imperforate anus or other congenital malformations, and incontinence of traumatic origin. Trauma may be due to a perineal tear at delivery, or due to operation for anal fistula. An injury to the anal region can disturb the physiological function of the puborectalis sling at least in two ways. First, the continuity of the muscle may be interrupted and the torn ends retracted (*Figure 12.32*). Secondly, the anus and anal

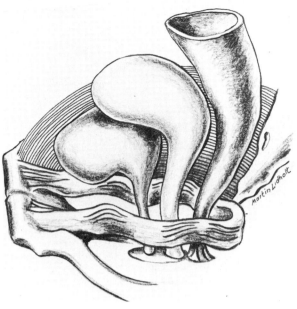

Figure 12.33. Schematic illustration of ineffective contraction of the puborectalis muscle because of ventral displacement of the anal canal

canal may be displaced ventrally, so that the muscle sling then becomes relatively too long and therefore unable to sharpen the anorectal angle acutely enough on contraction (*Figure 12.33*). If the muscle is ruptured, it can be replaced with a free muscle graft. In cases of a deficient perineum with an intact but incompetent puborectalis, the logical approach is to reconstruct the perineum thereby pushing the anal canal backwards and making the incompetent muscle competent (Hakelius, 1979).

In order to select patients suitable for transplantation, an accurate history is essential. In this way it is possible to exclude patients with normal strength and function of the sphincteric apparatus in whom incontinence is due to uncontrolled defaecation due to supra-anal bowel disease. In these cases, anorectal pressure measurements may be useful. Inspection of the anal region and rectal palpation are also most important to select the right cases for grafting. The best way to do this examination is to have the patient lying on the left side, with the hips and knees slightly flexed. In this position it is possible to evaluate the height of the perineum and observe if the normal upwards and forwards movement of the anus occurs when the patient contracts the sphincter. It is also possible to evaluate the sensibility of the perineal skin. If anaesthesia is found in this area, it strongly suggests a neurological cause of the incontinence. Rectal examination in this position makes it possible to evaluate the strength and mobility of the puborectal sling. The sling can be 'hooked up' on the index finger and then if the patient is asked to contract the sphincter this muscle should also contract. It is also easy to recognize scars or disruptions of the continuity of the puborectalis muscle. In cases with a deficient perineum, quite often a compensatory hypertrophy of the puborectalis muscle is found, probably because the muscle cannot adequately sharpen the angle of the ventrally displaced anal canal. Radiographic examinations in the lateral view are helpful not so much for confirming the diagnosis as for controlling the postoperative

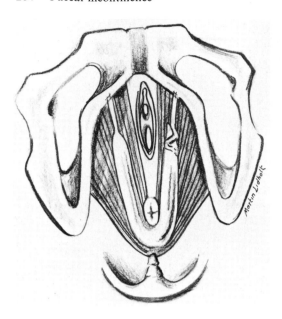

Figure 12.34. Schematic illustration of the operative field with the graft in close contact with the muscular pelvic floor

results. In spite of difficulties in getting reproducible figures in measurements of the pressure in the sphincter region of the anal canal, anorectal manometry can be of value for the same reason.

Surgical technique

Denervation

Palmaris longus.   The operation is carried out with axillary plexus local anaesthesia and a bloodless field. A short transverse incision is made at the wrist over the distal part of the palmaris tendon. The tendon is sectioned near its junction with the palmaris aponeurosis and a haemostat is clamped to the severed proximal end of the tendon. Next an incision is begun 2 cm below the ulnar epicondyle on the volar side of the arm, and is continued in a curved fashion down the ulnar aspect of the forearm for approximately 10 cm. The distal part of the bicipital aponeurosis is divided and the dissection is continued just medial to the ulnar group of muscles down to the median nerve.

The motor nerve of the palmaris longus arises by branching from the median nerve, usually just above the level of the elbow joint. The median nerve is carefully dissected free. Special care is taken not to damage the nerve branches to the ulnar muscle group and to the flexors of the fingers. To identify the nerve that supplies the palmaris longus, electrical stimulation is used. When the correct nerve is stimulated, it is easy to feel the contractions of the muscle, transmitted to the haemostat placed at the severed end of the palmaris tendon. The nerve is then divided. The severed tendon at the wrist is temporarily repaired with a 3–0 non-absorbable suture. This repair not only simplifies identification of the tendon at the second operation, but more importantly it preserves the tension of the muscle. This significantly reduces atrophy of the muscle during the denervation period.

Sartorius.   The sartorius muscle is more difficult to denervate. It receives its motor nerve supply from the femoral nerve usually via three branches. The upper part of the muscle is dissected free and the fascia is opened. The nerve branches are identified outside the sartorius fascia with electrostimulation and simultaneous inspection of the contracting fibres of the muscle. It is important not to damage the branches to the quadriceps muscle and afferent nerve branches also found in this area.

Transplantation

Two to three weeks after denervation, transplantation is performed. Two days prior to surgery, the patient is put on a low bulk diet. The colon is emptied with three water enemas during these two days. No antibiotics are used.

The operation is performed under general anaesthesia and starts with removal of the denervated muscle. When the intended graft is obtained from the palmaris longus, the operation is performed in a bloodless field. The incisions made at the denervation are reopened. If necessary, the proximal incision should be lengthened to expose the entire belly of the palmaris longus. At the wrist, the non-absorbable suture in the tendon is identified. The tendon is severed at the same place as in the denervation procedure. A tendon stripper is used to free the tendon up to the musculotendinous junction. The muscle is then carefully detached from its origin in the intermuscular connective tissue and at the ulnar epicondyle of the humerus. The fascia of the muscle is then carefully removed, because reinnervation is hindered by this layer of fibrous connective tissue (Kugelberg, Edström and Abbruzzese, 1970). The appearance of the palmaris longus varies significantly. Some muscles are attached to the epicondyle by a short tendon, whereas in others the muscle fibres are fixed directly to the bone. In the latter case, the distal half of the tendon is resected and sutured to the tendon-free end of the muscle. In this way, a muscle belly with tendons at each end is constructed. When the sartorius is used, the upper third of the muscle is uncovered. The origin at the iliac spine is detached and the muscle is sectioned approximately 12 cm below the origin. About one-third of the thickness of the muscle is used as graft.

With the patient in the lithotomy position, the next step of the operation starts with an incision in the crena ani from just behind the anus to the tip of the coccyx. By cautious dissection strictly in the midline the incision is deepened just behind the anal canal up to the anorectal angle. At this level, the dissection is continued laterally on both sides, so that the caudal surface of the muscular pelvic floor is identified. In close contact with and partially in these muscles, a tunnel is created by blunt dissection on each side of the anal canal in a direction towards the medial part of the inferior ramus of the pubic bone. Through short incisions on both sides of the labia majora or scrotum, the periosteum of the pubic bone is laid bare at the ends of the dissected tunnels. The transplant is now placed as a U-sling around the rectum at the angle between the anal canal and the rectum. The ends of the transplant are sutured to the periosteum of the pubic bone in slight tension (*Figure 12.34*). For these stitches non-absorbable 3–0 sutures are used. The incisions are sutured in layers without drainage. In adults, the urinary bladder is drained by a urethral catheter.

Postoperative care

The patients are kept strictly in bed for 7 d with the urethral catheter in place. The low bulk diet is continued and morphine is given by mouth. These precautions usually prevent evacuation of the bowel during the first postoperative week. The bladder drainage and the bed rest make optimal relaxation of the pelvic floor possible during the first critical healing period. On the eighth day the urethral catheter is removed and the low bulk diet and bed rest are discontinued. Ordinarily, the first postoperative movements of the bowel occur within 2 d.

Material and results

The patients are considered in two groups; one group of adults (Hakelius, 1981) and one of children born with anal malformations (Hakelius et al., 1980). The first group consists of 38 patients, 33 females and 5 males, aged 23–72 years (average 48.4 yr) at surgery. The aetiology of the incontinence was perineal tear at delivery in 15 cases, repair of anal fistula in 6, congenital imperforate anus in 6, surgery for haemorrhoids in 5, pull-through operation for rectal cancer in 1, and unknown cause in 5 cases. The duration of incontinence before surgery was at least 2 yr and in most of the cases the period of incontinence was much longer, up to 50 yr in one case. All the patients had pronounced incontinence, which means that they were unable to hold formed stools at will, and they all used pads in their underwear. Thus, all patients were severely socially disabled. In 29 of these cases, the palmaris longus muscle was used as transplant and in 9 the sartorius. The results of the operations have been judged through palpation of the transplant, X-ray examinations (*Figure 12.35*) and the patients' estimation.

The only postoperative complications were infection in the perineal wounds in 6 cases. In one of these, a relatively big abscess was drained. This patient also had signs of septicaemia. In the remaining 5 cases, the infection was superficial and did not threaten the grafts.

The usual course in the postoperative period has been that during the first 3 months after transplantation there was no improvement. The transplants were palpable, but they had no contractile function. This delay in function depends on the long time required for reinnervation of the graft to occur. Between the third and the sixth month an improvement was noted. As the first sign, the patients reported that they could feel the presence of faeces in the rectum, but they could not retain the stools. Later, the ability to retain the stools increased and this improvement continued up to 1 yr postoperatively.

The follow-up time was 1–7 yr, with an average of 40 months. Sixteen of the patients were totally cured of their incontinence; 12 were markedly improved, needed no more pads in their underwear and could retain their stools for a minimum of 5 min. These 12 patients live a practically normal social life. In 10 cases the transplantation had no effect.

All the unsuccessful cases were women—one was the oldest and one the third oldest in the group. In these cases, no contraction of the transplants developed either by palpation or by X-ray examination. Both were operated at the beginning of the series. They had laxity of the pelvic floor and a tendency towards prolapse. One case had severe damage to her perineum after a tear at delivery, and probably should have been treated with a perineoplasty. She has since been offered such an operation. One patient was incontinent because of multiple fistulae that had been incised repeatedly. The operative field was very fibrotic, so that the conditions for a good take of the graft were poor. She now has a colostomy. In six cases there was no obvious cause of failure of the transplantation.

The paediatric material consists of 13 children with anal incontinence due to congenital malformations. There are 11 boys and 2 girls. The age at surgery was

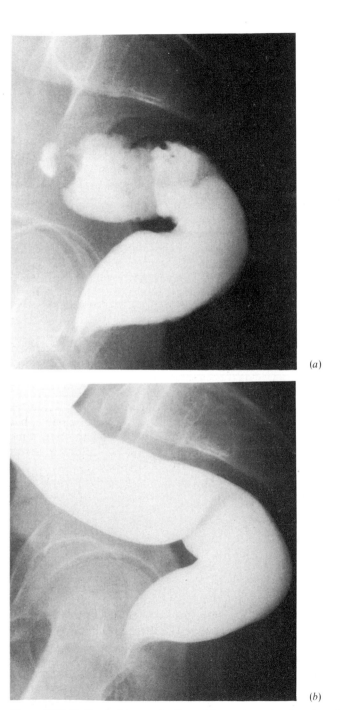

(a)

(b)

Figure 12.35. Radiographic examination of the anal canal and rectum. Lateral views. (a) Preoperative examination. Patient trying to retain the contrast. Note the obtuse anorectal angle and the diffuse and blunt lower boundary of the barium contrast, indicating incontinence. (b) Nine months postoperatively. The angulation between the rectum and anal canal is restored and the contrast ends at this level in a well-defined funnel-like tip

TABLE 12.5. The clinical Kelly score

	Points*		
	2	1	0
'Accidents'	Never	Sometimes	50 per cent
Soiling	Never	Sometimes	Always
Sphincter action	Strong	Partial or weak	Absent

* 0–2, 'poor'; 3–4, 'fair'; 5–6, 'good'.

8–15 years (average 11.5 yr). The primary diagnosis was anorectal agenesis in 11 cases, congenital megacolon in 1 case, and anorectal diaphragm in 1 case. All these cases had been operated on before. Preoperatively, all patients had severe incontinence and wore pads or diapers. Their degree of incontinence was estimated by means of the Kelly score (Kelly, 1969) (*Table 12.5*). The patients have been followed from 2 to 5 yr (mean 36 months) after surgery. All of them were Kelly 1.0 preoperatively and all except one have improved. Eleven have reached 3 points or more, which means that they have achieved social continence and no longer need pads or diapers.

Conclusions

Free autogenous muscle transplantation is a good method for curing anal incontinence due to a traumatized or congenitally lacking puborectalis muscle. The transplant forms a dynamic sling that becomes innervated from the muscles of the pelvic floor and is thus automatically incorporated in the anal reflex mechanism.

C. Treatment: (vi) Biofeedback

M. M. Schuster

Introduction

Biofeedback is a specific form of behavioural modification which is aimed at training for control over bodily functions. Since instruments are used to monitor and feed back to the subject information concerning these functions, biofeedback is sometimes called instrumental learning. Feedback is a basic ingredient of all learning, since it provides information concerning the degree of success and therefore permits improvement of performance. For example, a tennis serve can be improved by utilizing the visual feedback of the observed trajectory of the ball that has been served. This observation will permit the server to alter the toss-up or the racket-swing in order to improve and perfect the serve.

Biofeedback training differs from classical Pavlovian conditioning in that Pavlovian conditioning requires a specific, unconditioned stimulus (such as meat) to elicit and reinforce a specific response (e.g. salivation). By contrast, biofeedback can use any reward to reinforce any preceding event. It does not elicit the event, but instead, reinforces it.

Anal incontinence which results from organic neuromuscular impairment of sphincter function has been successfully treated with biofeedback techniques, utilizing pressure recordings or electromyographic recordings of sphincter function in order to learn or relearn sphincteric control. Biofeedback can successfully treat both sensory impairment, which is neurological, or motor impairment, which may be neurological or muscular.

Sphincteric incontinence

Neuromuscular sphincteric impairment most commonly results from either systemic or local disorders (Alva, Mendeloff and Schuster, 1967; Schuster, 1968; Cerulli, Nikoomanesh and Schuster, 1979). Among the systemic disorders which impair these functions are neuromuscular diseases such as myotonic dystrophy, collagen vascular disorders such as scleroderma which affects the smooth muscle function of the internal sphincter, or polymyositis which can affect the striated external sphincter. Cerebro-vascular accidents, birth injuries such as myelomeningocele and spina bifida, and spinal cord injuries, similarly can produce afferent or efferent nerve impairment, as can diabetes mellitus and alcoholism because of associated peripheral neuropathy. In addition, direct sphincter injury may follow anorectal surgery (haemorrhoidectomy or fissurectomy) or tears from delivery.

Mechanisms of continence

There are a number of colorectal mechanisms responsible for the maintenance of continence (Schuster, 1968). Compliant adaptation permits the colon to accommodate stool and therefore assists in storage. Structural changes such as fibrosis and functional influences such as spasm may interfere with compliance and with continence. The rectosigmoid flexures and sharp angulations further serve to impede the forward progress of stool by acting as valve-like impediments, which are more successful in retaining firm rather than liquid stool. The spiral valves of Houston act in a similar manner. Functional forces assist these mechanical factors. A reversed rectosigmoid gradient, which results from more frequent pressure waves in the lower rectum than in the higher rectum, acts to retard entry of stool into this area. The sharp angulation provided by the puborectalis sling is an even more powerful deterrent to the forward movement of stool. Sphincteric mechanisms become more significant after stool has entered the rectal ampulla.

Most instances of incontinence are due to sensorimotor dysfunction of the rectosphincteric segment. Impairment of sensory perception can result from resection of the rectosigmoid sensory organ, injury to afferent nerves, or spinal cord injury. Diabetic peripheral neuropathy, in particular, is known to impair the sensory perception of a defaecatory urge (Wald and Tunuguntla, 1984). It is obviously possible for sensory substitution to occur, since patients who have had low ileoproctostomies can relearn sensory awareness successfully enough to provide for effective continence. Motor nerve impairment can produce incontinence as a result of marked muscle weakness despite intact reflexes, or by neurological impairment of reflexes in the absence of muscle weakness.

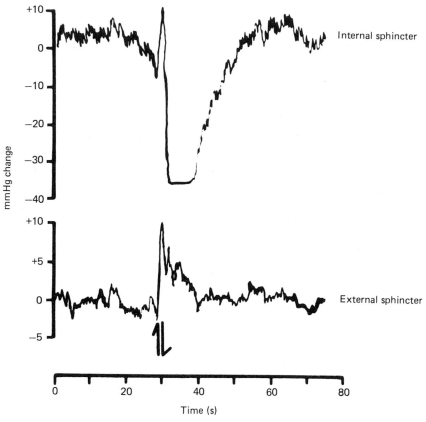

Figure 12.36. Normal rectosphincteric responses. Rectal distension (arrows over time axis) induces reflex relaxation of internal anal sphincter (top tracing) and simultaneous contraction of the external sphincter (lower tracing)

Motor control mechanisms

Balloon distension of the rectum or rectosigmoid mimics in a rough manner the arrival of stool in this area, initiates a cognitive awareness of a bolus within the rectum and also initiates motor responses. The latter consist of reflex inhibition (relaxation) of the autonomically innervated smooth muscle of the internal sphincter, with simultaneous active contraction of the somatically innervated striated muscle of the external sphincter (*Figure 12.36*). The internal sphincter inhibitory reflex is transmitted via afferent stretch receptors in the colonic muscle wall to the myenteric plexus and hence to the sphincter (Tobon *et al.*, 1968); it is therefore an intrinsic reflex. On the other hand, the external sphincter contractile response involves a spinal reflex arc. For this reason spinal cord injury, or transection of extraneous nerves, impairs the external sphincter response (often including its sensory component), whereas the intrinsically controlled internal sphincter reflex remains unaffected. For this reason also the internal sphincter inhibitory reflex can occur without sensory awareness after complete spinal cord transection or after general or spinal anaesthesia (Schuster, 1968).

The internal sphincter in its 'resting state' is in a condition of near maximal

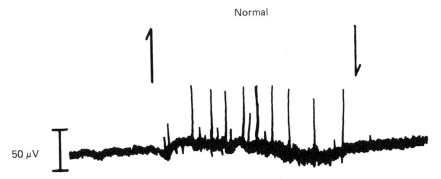

Normal

50 μV

Figure 12.37. Normal electromyogram (retouched) of external sphincter. Spike action potentials are induced by transient inflation of air into the rectal balloons and diminish when air is withdrawn

contraction and its normal reflex response is to relax. The external sphincter in its resting state emits only mild background noise on electromyography, indicating that it is in a minimal state of tonic contraction, but its normal automatic response is to contract phasically (*Figure 12.37*) (Schuster, 1968). It is believed that the tonically contracted internal sphincter provides continence under conditions when small amounts of material enter the rectum in quantities which do not cause sufficient distension to produce internal sphincter relaxation. This mechanism permits continence to be maintained without sensory awareness. However, larger quantities of material entering the rectum induce a sense of urgency and result in momentary contraction of the external sphincter, followed by further voluntary contraction if this is deemed necessary.

Sensory control mechanisms

A threshold for sensory perception of rectal distension can be established by progressively distending the rectum with smaller volumes of air until a level is reached at which distension is no longer appreciated; one might conversely proceed in the opposite direction using increments of distension until a perception is appreciated (*Figure 12.38*) (Schuster, 1977b; Whitehead, Engel and Schuster, 1980). Normally, subjects can sense volumes as small as 7.5 ml of distension. Lesions at L3 and above (Ihre, 1974; Whitehead, Engel and Schuster, 1980) result in elimination of rectal sensation, indicating that the sensory nerves involved in the afferent limb of rectosphincteric reflexes enter the spinal cord at this level. When sensation is impaired, as in diabetic peripheral neuropathy, a high sensory threshold results, manifested by requirements for a larger volume of air to be instilled into the rectum in order to be sensed. Sensory impairment may often be improved and sensory threshold lowered by biofeedback training.

If some slight sensation is present at the outset of biofeedback therapy, very large volumes of air which can be perceived by the patient are instilled, and gradually smaller and smaller quantities are inflated, with instructions to the patient to concentrate hard and to announce each distension as soon as it is perceived. If no sensory awareness is initially present, biofeedback may be employed announcing each distension, at first using large volumes, and then progressively lower volumes until awareness is achieved at each level, first with and then without the announced verbal feedback. If, using this biofeedback technique, the sensory level can be brought below 20 ml of distension, the

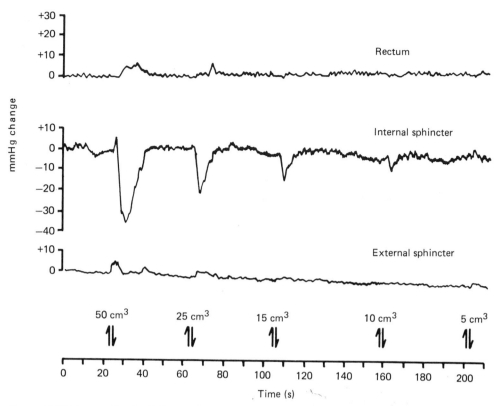

Figure 12.38. Sensory threshold. Decreasing volumes of air elicit decreasing relaxation in the internal sphincter and decreasing contraction in the external sphincter until a level is reached at which no further response is detected

patient has a chance to achieve continence by relearning sphincteric control. If this impairment is strictly afferent, this may be sufficient to return the patient to a continent state. In our experience, little success is obtained if the threshold cannot be brought below 30 ml of distension.

A technique which can be used to overcome selection bias is that of forced choice technique (Whitehead, Engel and Schuster, 1980). This method requires the patient to make a choice as to which of two distensions is 'real'. One distension is a 'false' distension (with the therapist instilling air through a syringe not connected to the rectal balloon), and one distension is 'real' (with the air being distended into the balloon). False and real distensions are alternated in a random fashion and the patient is asked to report which 'distension' is perceived.

Motor dysfunction and biofeedback treatment

Faecal incontinence in adults is most commonly due to neuromuscular impairment of external anal sphincter function (Schuster, 1966; Alva, Mendeloff and Schuster, 1967). Biofeedback is the treatment of choice for this type of incontinence (Engel, Nikoomanesh and Schuster, 1974; Cerulli, Nikoomanesh and Schuster, 1979;

Whitehead, Engel and Schuster, 1980). In our experience, 70 per cent of patients with organic neural or muscular impairment of sphincteric function regain continence completely or demonstrate 90 per cent improvement when treated by this technique (Cerulli, Nikoomanesh and Schuster, 1979), despite the fact that these patients had gross daily soiling which was unresponsive to other forms of treatment over periods of years. Patients whose incontinence results from direct muscle injury (usually operative) respond more favourably than those with spinal cord injuries or with generalized neuromuscular disorders (such as multiple sclerosis and myotonic dystrophy) or collagen vascular diseases (Cerulli, Nikoomanesh and Schuster, 1979).

The most commonly employed recording technique involves the use of a triple balloon system placed manually (without proctoscopic aid) so that the distending balloon lies in the rectum. The moulded double balloon straddles the anal canal, with the inner balloon surrounded by the internal anal sphincter and the outer balloon by the subcutaneous bundle of the external sphincter (*Figure 12.39*) (Schuster *et al.*, 1965;

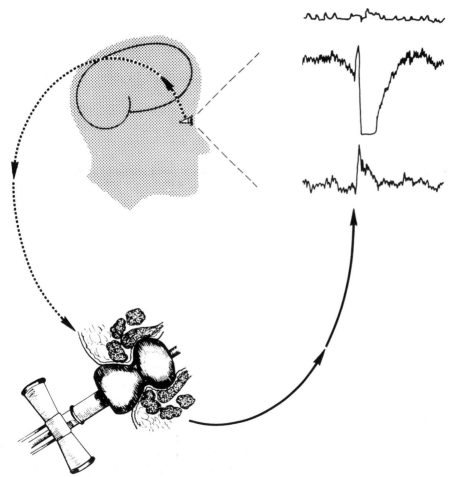

Figure 12.39. Biofeedback technique. The patient watches the tracing as it is being recorded and is instructed as to the appropriate sphincteric response

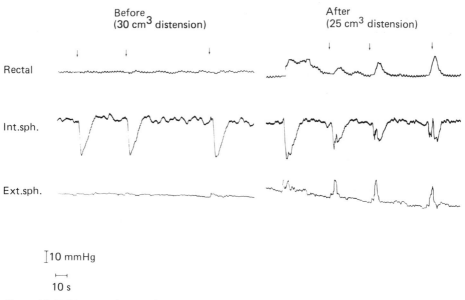

Figure 12.40. Manometric recording in an incontinent subject before and after biofeedback training. Before training no external sphincter is present. Good responses are obtained after training

Engel, Nikoomanesh and Schuster, 1974). The rectal balloon is composed of a condom tied around a catheter in such a manner that, when distended with 50 cm^3 of air, it is filled but not stretched. The other two balloons are filled with 10 cm^3 of air, which both positions them appropriately within the anal canal and also holds them in place unless extreme sphincter laxity permits them to slip, in which case the apparatus is fixed in place by taping it to the buttocks. Thresholds for internal sphincter reflex relaxation and for external sphincter contraction are established in a manner similar to sensory testing described above, using 10 ml increments of distension, until a point is reached at which responses from each of the two sphincters no longer occurs. The threshold for the sphincteric response is different for each of the two sphincters. Patients with sphincteric incontinence show no external sphincter contraction or a very weak contraction.

Biofeedback is provided by elevating the table upon which the patient lies or by elevating the patient's head with a pillow so that the patient can see the manometric tracing as it is being recorded. The patient is instructed to contract the external sphincter in synchrony with internal sphincter relaxation each time rectal distension is sensed (*Figure 12.40*). It is sometimes necessary to show the patient a normal record or to draw the normal pattern of response so that he or she will comprehend the task. After the appropriate response has been learned for one level of distension, attempts are made to lower the threshold by encouraging the patient to develop similar responses to lower volumes of distension until the lowest volume is reached to which a successful response is obtained. The goal is to shape the external sphincter contraction so that it is of normal amplitude (10 mmHg or greater) and of sufficient duration (2–3 s); and it must coincide with internal sphincter relaxation. This learning process takes anywhere from 15 min to half an hour and during this time the patient should learn to perform the task, first with visual feedback and then without visual feedback (*Figure 12.41*). Visual feedback is withheld quite simply by holding a paper between the patient's angle of

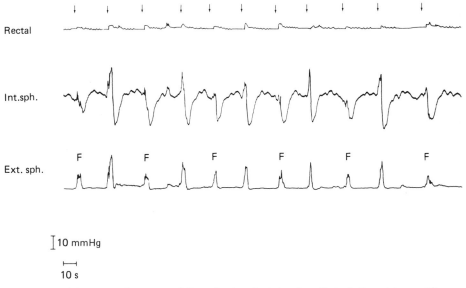

Rectal

Int.sph.

Ext. sph.

I 10 mmHg

⊢⊣
10 s

Figure 12.41. Manometry in a successfully trained patient showing effect of alternately providing feedback (F) and withholding feedback. External sphincter responds with contractions that are higher when feedback is withheld than when it is provided

vision and the recording paper during distension, so that the recording is visible to the therapist but not to the patient.

After the initial session, the patient is instructed to reinforce this automatic response by concentrating over the next 2 weeks on any rectal sensations which are remotely similar to the balloon distension or similar to a sensation of material entering the rectum. The instructions are to contract the sphincter to the count of 3 (in a manner similar to that learned during the biofeedback session) as soon as there is any hint of rectal distension. The patient should not wait until he or she is certain of the sensation, but should respond at the first hint of a sensation. At the end of 2 weeks it is assumed that this response will have become automatic and no further special attention need be paid to it.

In addition to retraining for automatic external sphincter contraction as described above, the patient is instructed to carry out sphincter strengthening exercises by contracting the external sphincter to the count of 3, then relaxing and immediately repeating the exercise, producing 5–10 such transient squeezes 5 times a day, and gradually increasing the number of squeezes over a period of weeks until a total of 40 squeezes are made 5 times a day. This exercise is continued until normal sphincter strength is achieved or incontinence is completely controlled.

The return visit is usually scheduled 6–8 weeks after the initial biofeedback session in order to re-evaluate the new baseline sphincter responses, to more finely tune and shape these responses, to correct any false impressions that the patient may have, and to reinforce the correct responses. In almost all instances only two sessions are required, as long as neuromuscular function remains stable. Patients with progressive neuromuscular disorders such as multiple sclerosis may benefit from further biofeedback sessions as neuromuscular function continues to deteriorate.

Biofeedback training is usually successful when innervation is not completely disrupted and when some muscle response can be recruited. It is unsuccessful when there is complete spinal cord transection or complete denervation. Experience with patients who have sensory nerve damage suggests that utilization of alternative nerve pathways may be the mechanism for successful relearning of control. Patients who regain appreciation of distension as a cue for continence often report that the sensation which they perceive during biofeedback training for sensory awareness is different from the sensation which they appreciated before the nerve injury, implying that the signals are being transmitted through different nerve pathways. It is quite possible that motor control is relearned in a similar fashion.

Conclusions

In addition to providing a conceptual model for investigating mechanisms for successful rehabilitation of impaired neuromuscular function, biofeedback is also a useful form of treatment for a socially and psychologically disabling and chronic condition—faecal incontinence. When successful, it is more rapidly effective than any other technique, and it has the major advantage that it carries no risk of morbidity or mortality.

References

ADEYEMI, S. D. and DA ROCHA-AFODU, J. T. (1982). Management of imperforate anus at the Lagos University Teaching Hospital, Nigeria: a review of ten years' experience. *Progress in Paediatric Surgery*, 15, 187–194

ALVA, J., MENDELOFF, A. I. and SCHUSTER, M. M. (1967). Reflex and electromyographic abnormalities associated with fecal incontinence. *Gastroenerology*, 53, 101

AMANO, S. (1980). Rectoanal pressures and rectal compliance in constipated infants and children. *Journal of the Japanese Society of Pediatric Surgeons*, 16, 715–730

ANDERSON, R. S. (1984). A neurogenic element to urinary genuine stress incontinence. *British Journal of Obstetrics and Gynaecology*, 91, 41–45

BARTOLO, D. C. C., JARRATT, J. A. and READ, N. W. (1983). The use of conventional EMG to assess external sphincter neuropathy in man. *Journal of Neurology, Neurosurgery and Psychiatry*, 46, 1115–1118

BEERSIEK, F., PARKS, A. G. and SWASH, M. (1979). Pathogenesis of anorectal incontinence: a histometric study of the anal musculature. *Journal of the Neurological Sciences*, 42, 111–127

BILL, A. H. JR and JOHNSON, R. J. (1958). Failure of migration of the rectal opening as the cause for most cases of imperforate anus. *Surgery, Gynecology and Obstetrics*, 106, 643–644

BLACK, C. T., POKORNY, W. J., McGILL, C. W. and HARBERG, F. J. (1982). Anorectal trauma in children. *Journal of Pediatric Surgery*, 17, 501–504

BLAISDELL, P. C. (1940). Repair of the incontinent sphincter ani. *Surgery, Gynecology and Obstetrics*, 70, 692–697

BRANDESKY, G., GELEY, L. and JANOUT, D. (1984). Results of the modified Hartl gracilis plasty. *Progress in Pediatric Surgery*, 17, 115–122

BRENT, L. and STEPHENS, F. D. (1976). Primary rectal ectasia: a qualitative study of smooth muscle cells in normal and hypertrophied human bowel. *Progress in Pediatric Surgery*, 9, 41–63

BRINDLEY, G. S. (1981). Electroejaculation: its technique, neurological implications and uses. *Journal of Neurology, Neurosurgery and Psychiatry*, 44, 9–18

BROCKLEHURST, J. C. (1972). Bowel management in the neurologically disabled. The problems of old age. *Proceedings of the Royal Society of Medicine*, 65, 66–69

BROCKLEHURST, J. C. (1975). Management of anal incontinence. *Clinics in Gastroenterology*, 4, 479–487

BROWNE, D. (1951). Some congenital deformities of the rectum, anus, vagina and urethra. *Annals of the Royal College of Surgeons of England*, 8, 173–177

BROWNING, G. G. P. and MOTSON, R. W. (1983). Results of Parks' operation for faecal incontinence after anal injury. *British Medical Journal*, 286, 1873–1875

BROWNING, G. G. P. and PARKS, A. G. (1983). Postanal repair for neuropathic faecal incontinence: correlation of clinical result and anal canal pressures. *British Journal of Surgery*, 70, 101–104

BROWNING. G. G. P., RUTTER, K. R. P., MOTSON, R. W. and NEILL, M. E. (1984). Postanal repair for idiopathic faecal incontinence. *Annals of the Royal College of Surgeons of England*, Supplement, 30–33

BRYNDORF, J. and MADSEN, C. M. (1960). Ectopic anus in the female. *Acta Chirurgica Scandinavica*, 118, 466–468

BUCHMANN, P. and KEIGHLEY, M. R. (1982). Darmprolaps und/oder Stuhlinkontinenz. *Schweiz Medizinische Wochenschrift*, 112, 648–652

BUENO, F., CERULLI, M. and SCHUSTER, M. M. (1976). Operant conditioning of colonic motility in irritable bowel syndrome. *Gastroenterology*, 70, 867

BUTLER, E. C. B. (1954). Complete rectal prolapse following removal of tumours of the cauda equina. *Proceedings of the Royal Society of Medicine*, 47, 521–522

CALDWELL, K. P. S. (1963). The electrical control of sphincter incompetence. *Lancet*, ii, 174–175

CAMPBELL, R. E. (1941). A report on a series of complete tears of the perineum with extension up the posterior vaginal wall repaired by the vaginal flap method. *American Journal of Obstetrics and Gynecology*, 41, 403–411

CARLSSON, B. M. and GUTMANN, E. (1975). Regeneration in free grafts of normal and denervated muscles in the rat: morphology and histochemistry. *The Anatomical Record*, 183, 47–61

CERULLI, M. A., NIKOOMANESH, P. and SCHUSTER, M. M. (1979). Progress in biofeedback conditioning for fecal incontinence. *Gastroenterology*, 76, 742–746

CLARKE, N., HUGHES, A. O., DODD, K. J., PALMER, R. L., BRANDON, S., HOLDEN, A. N. and PEARCE, D. (1979). The elderly in residential care: patterns of disability. *Health Trends*, 11, 17

CONSTANTINIDES, C. G. and CYWES, S. (1983). Fecal incontinence: a simple pneumatic device for home biofeedback training. *Journal of Pediatric Surgery*, 18, 276–277

COOK, R. C. M. (1978). Anorectal malformations, in *Neonatal Surgery*, pp. 436–481 (P. P. Rickham, J. Lister and I. Irving, Eds). London; Butterworths

COOK, R. C. M. (1983). Anorectal malformations, in *Rob and Smith's Operative Surgery*, 4th edn, vol. 3, *Colon, Rectum and Anus*, pp. 602–616 (I. P. Todd and L. P. Fielding, Eds). London; Butterworths

CORMAN, M. L. (1978). Gracilis muscle transposition. *Contemporary Surgery*, 13, 9–16

CORMAN, M. L. (1980). Follow-up evaluation of gracilis muscle transposition for fecal incontinence. *Diseases of the Colon and Rectum*, 23, 552–555

CORMAN, M. L. (1983). Management of anal incontinence. *Surgical Clinics of North America*, 63, 177–192

CORMAN, M. L. (1984). *Colon and Rectal Surgery*, pp. 129–134. Philadelphia; Lippincott

CYWES, S., CREMIN, B. J. and LOUW, J. H. (1971). Assessment of continence after treatment for anorectal agenesis: a clinical and radiological correlation. *Journal of Pediatric Surgery*, 6, 132–136

DEWHURST, C. J. (1963). *Gynaecological Disorders of Infants and Children*. London; Cassell

DIAS, R. G., SANTIAGO, A. de P. G. and FERREIRA, M. C. (1982). Rectal atresia: treatment through a single sacral approach. *Journal of Pediatric Surgery*, 17, 424–425

DUTHIE, H. L. (1971). Progress report—anal continence. *Gut*, 12, 844–852

ENGEL, B. T., NIKOOMANESH, P. and SCHUSTER, M. M. (1974). Operant conditioning of rectosphincteric responses in the treatment of fecal incontinence. *New England Journal of Medicine*, 290, 646–649

FAULKNER, J. A., MAXWELL, L. C., MUFTI, S. A. and CARLSSON, B. M. (1976). Skeletal muscle fiber regeneration following heterotopic autotransplantation in cats. *Life Sciences*, 19, 289–296

FREEMAN, N. V., BURGE, D. M., SOAR, J. and SEDGWICK, E. M. (1980). Anal evoked potentials. *Zeitschrift für Kinderchirurgie*, 31, 22–30

FRITZ, G. K. and ARMBRUST, J. (1982). Enuresis and encopresis. *Psychiatric Clinics of North America*, 5, 283–296

GILLEARD, C. J. (1980). Prevalence of incontinence in local authority homes for the elderly. *Health Bulletin*, 38(6), 236–238

GOLDENBERG, D. A., HODGES, K., HERSH, T. and JINICH, H. (1980). Biofeedback therapy for fecal incontinence. *American Journal of Gastroenterology*, 74, 342–345

GOLIGHER, J. C. (1967). *Surgery of the Anus, Rectum and Colon*, 2nd edn. London; Baillière, Tindall and Cassell

HABEEB, M. C. and KALLSTROM, M. D. (1976). Bowel program for institutionalized adults. *American Journal of Nursing*, 76(4), 606–608

HAKELIUS, L. (1975). Free autogenous muscle transplantation in two cases of total anal incontinence. *Acta Chirurgica Scandinavica*, 141, 69–75

HAKELIUS, L. (1979). Reconstruction of the perineal body as treatment for anal incontinence. *British Journal of Plastic Surgery*, 32, 245–252

HAKELIUS, L. (1981). Treatment of anal and urinary incontinence with free muscle transplants, in *Muscle Transplantation*, pp. 237–241 (G. Freilinger, J. Holle and B. M. Carlsson, Eds). Vienna and New York; Springer Verlag

HAKELIUS, L., GIERUP, J., GROTTE, G. and JORULF, H. (1980). Further experience with free autogenous muscle transplantation in children with anal incontinence. *Zeitschrift für Kinderchirurgie*, 31, 141–147

HAKELIUS, L. and NYSTRÖM, B. (1975a). Blood vessels and connective tissue in autotransplanted free muscle grafts of the cat. *Scandinavian Journal of Plastic and Reconstructive Surgery*, 9, 87–91

HAKELIUS, L. and NYSTRÖM, B. (1975b). Histochemical studies of end-plate formation in free autologous muscle transplants in cats. *Scandinavian Journal of Plastic and Reconstructive Surgery*, **9**, 9–14

HAKELIUS, L., NYSTRÖM, B. and STÅLBERG, E. (1975). Histochemical and neurophysiological studies of autotransplanted cat muscle. *Scandinavian Journal of Plastic and Reconstructive Surgery*, **9**, 15–24

HECKER, W. Ch., HOLSCHNEIDER, A. M. and KRAEFT, H. (1980). Complications, deaths and long term results after surgery of anorectal atresia. *Zeitschrift für Kinderchirurgie*, **29**, 238–244

HENRY, M. M., PARKS, A. G. and SWASH, M. (1982). The pelvic floor musculature in the descending perineum syndrome. *British Journal of Surgery*, **69**, 470–472

HENTZ, V. R. (1982). Construction of a rectal sphincter using the origin of the gluteus maximus muscle. *Plastic and Reconstructive Surgery*, **70**, 82–85

HERTZ, A. F. (1909). *Constipation and Allied Disorders*. London; Oxford University Press

HOLLE, J. and FREILINGER, G. (1984). Improvement of continence by myoplasty of the pelvic floor. *Progress in Pediatric Surgery*, **17**, 123–130

HOLSCHNEIDER, A. M. (1983). Treatment and functional results of anorectal continence in children with imperforate anus. *Acta Chirurgica Belgica*, **3**, 191–204

HOLSCHNEIDER, A. M. and HECKER, W. Ch. (1981a). Flapped and free muscle transplantation in the treatment of anal incontinence. *Zeitschrift für Kinderchirurgie*, **32**, 244–258

HOLSCHNEIDER, A. M. and HECKER, W. Ch. (1981b). Reverse smooth muscle plasty: a new method of treating anorectal incontinence in infants with high anal and rectal atresia. *Journal of Pediatric Surgery*, **16**, 917–920

HOLSCHNEIDER, A. M., POSCHL, U. and KRAEFT, H. (1979). Pickrell's gracilis muscle transplantation and its effects on anorectal continence: a 5 year prospective study. *Zeitschrift für Kinderchirurgie*, **27**, 135–143

HOPKINSON, B. R. and LIGHTWOOD, R. (1966). Electrical treatment of anal incontinence. *Lancet*, **i**, 344–351

HYAMS, D. E. (1974). Gastrointestinal problems in the old. *British Medical Journal*, **1**, 107–110

IHRE, T. (1974). Studies on anal function in continent and incontinent patients. *Scandinavian Journal of Gastroenterology*, **9**, Supplement 25

ITO, Y., YOKOYAMA, J., NAMBA, S., MORIKAWA, Y. and KATSUMATA, K. (1981). Reappraisal of endorectal pull-through procedure. II. Animal experiment. *Journal of Pediatric Surgery*, **16**, 655–659

KEIGHLEY, M. R. (1984). Postanal repair for faecal incontinence. *Journal of the Royal Society of Medicine*, **77**, 285–288

KELLY, J. H. (1969). Cineradiography in anorectal malformations. *Journal of Pediatric Surgery*, **4**, 538–546

KELLY, J. H. (1972). The clinical and radiological assessment of anal continence in childhood. *Australian and New Zealand Journal of Surgery*, **42**, 62–63

KIESEWETTER, W. B. (1967). Imperforate anus. II. The rationale and technique of the sacro-abdomino-perineal operation. *Journal of Pediatric Surgery*, **2**, 106–111

KIESEWETTER, W. B. and JEFFERIES, M. R. (1981). Secondary anorectal surgery for the missed puborectalis muscle. *Journal of Pediatric Surgery*, **16**, 921–927

KIESEWETTER, W. B. and NIXON, H. H. (1967). Imperforate anus. I. Its surgical anatomy. *Journal of Pediatric Surgery*, **2**, 60–68

KIFF, E. S. and SWASH, M. (1984a). Slowed conduction in the pudendal nerves in idiopathic (neurogenic) faecal incontinence. *British Journal of Surgery*, **71**, 614–616

KIFF, E. S. and SWASH, M. (1984b). Normal proximal and delayed distal conduction in the pudendal nerves of patients with idiopathic (neurogenic) faecal incontinence. *Journal of Neurology, Neurosurgery and Psychiatry*, **47**, 820–823

KING'S FUND CENTRE (1983). Action on incontinence—report of a working group. Project Paper 43, pp. 1–47

KOTTMEIER, P. K. and DZIADIW, R. (1967). The complete release of the levator sling in fecal incontinence. *Journal of Pediatric Surgery*, **2**, 111–117

KUGELBERG, E., EDSTRÖM, L. and ABBRUZZESE, M. (1970). Mapping of motor units and experimentally reinnervated rat muscle. *Journal of Neurology, Neurosurgery and Psychiatry*, **33**, 319–329

LABERGE, J. M., BOSC, O., YAZBECK, S., YOUSSEF, S., DUCHARME, J. C., GUTTMAN, F. M. and N'GUYEN, L. T. (1983). The anterior perineal approach for pull-through operations in high imperforate anus. *Journal of Pediatric Surgery*, **18**, 774–778

LEIGH, R. J. and TURNBERG, L. A. (1982). Faecal incontinence: the unvoiced symptom. *Lancet*, **i**, 1349–1351

LEVINE, M. D. (1982). Encopresis: its potentiation, evaluation and alleviation. *Pediatric Clinics of North America*, **29**, 315–330

LOENING-BAUCKE, V. A. and YOUNOSZAI, M. K. (1982). Abnormal anal sphincter response in chronically constipated children. *Journal of Pediatrics*, **100**, 213–218

LOUW, J. H. (1962). Some observations on the musculature of the pelvic floor, the anal sphincters, and rectal continence. *South African Journal of Clinical Medicine*, **8**, 54–58

MAGNUS, R. V. (1972). Congenital rectovesical fistula and its associated anomalies. *Australian and New Zealand Journal of Surgery*, **42**, 197–200

MAGNUS, R. V. (1974). Urinary abnormalities in children with congenital recto-vesical fistulae. *Australian Paediatric Journal*, **10**, 82–85

MARTIUS, H. (1954). *Die Gynäkologischen Operationen*. Stuttgart; Georg Thieme Verlag

McLAREN, S. M., McPHERSON, F. M., SINCLAIR, F. and BALLINGER, B. R. (1981). Prevalence and severity of incontinence among hospitalised female psychogeriatric patients. *Health Bulletin*, **39**(3), 157–161

MIKKELSEN, E. J., BROWN, G. L., MINICHIELLO, M. D., MULLICAN, F. K. and RAPOPORT, J. L. (1982). Neurologic status in hyperactive, enuretic, encopretic and normal boys. *Journal of the American Academy of Child Psychiatry*, **21**, 75–81

MILLER, N. F. and BROWN, W. (1937). The surgical treatment of complete perineal tears in the female. *American Journal of Obstetrics and Gynecology*, **34**, 196–209

MOLANDER, M. L. and FRENCKNER, B. (1983). Electrical activity of the external anal sphincter at different ages in childhood. *Gut*, **24**, 218–221

MUNN, J. (1972). Bowel management in the neurologically disabled: the patient's viewpoint. *Proceedings of the Royal Society of Medicine*, **65**, 65

NAGASAKI, A., IKEDA, K. and HAYASHIDA, Y. (1984). Assessment of bowel control with anorectal manometry after surgery for anorectal malformation. *Japanese Journal of Surgery*, **14**, 229–234

NEILL, M. E., PARKS, A. G. and SWASH, M. (1981). Physiological studies of the pelvic floor in idiopathic faecal incontinence and rectal prolapse. *British Journal of Surgery*, **68**, 531–536

NEILL, M. E. and SWASH, M. (1980). Increased motor unit fibre density in the external anal sphincter muscle in anorectal incontinence: a single fibre EMG study. *Journal of Neurology, Neurosurgery and Psychiatry*, **43**, 343–347

NIXON, H. H. (1984). Possibilities and results of management of bowel incontinence in children. *Progress in Pediatric Surgery*, **17**, 105–113

PALKEN, M., JOHNSON, R. J., DERRICK, W. and BILL, A. H. JR. (1972). Clinical aspects of female patients with high ano-rectal agenesis. *Surgery, Gynecology and Obstetrics*, **135**, 411–414

PARKS, A. G. (1975). Anorectal incontinence. *Proceedings of the Royal Society of Medicine*, **68**, 681–690

PARKS, A. G. and McPARTLIN, J. F. (1971). Late repair of injuries of the anal sphincter. *Proceedings of the Royal Society of Medicine*, **64**, 1187–1189

PARKS, A. G. and McPARTLIN, J. F. (1983). Surgical repair of anal sphincters following injury, in *Rob and Smith's Operative Surgery—Alimentary Tract and Abdominal Wall*, vol. 3, *Colon, Rectum and Anus*, pp. 440–442 (I. P. Todd and L. P. Fielding, Eds). London; Butterworths

PARKS, A. G. and PERCY, J. (1983). Postanal pelvic floor repair for anorectal incontinence, in *Rob and Smith's Operative Surgery—Alimentary Tract and Abdominal Wall*, vol. 3, *Colon, Rectum and Anus*, pp. 433–438 (I. P. Todd and L. P. Fielding, Eds). London; Butterworths

PARKS, A. G., SWASH, M. and URICH, H. (1977). Sphincter denervation in anorectal incontinence and rectal prolapse. *Gut*, **18**, 656–665

PENFOLD, J. C. B. and HAWLEY, P. R. (1972). Experiences of Ivalon sponge implant for complete rectal prolapse at St Mark's Hospital, 1960–1970. *British Journal of Surgery*, **59**, 846–848

PERCY, J., NEILL, M. E., KANDIAH, T. K. and SWASH, M. (1982). A neurogenic factor in faecal incontinence in the elderly. *Age and Ageing*, **11**, 175–179

PERCY, J. P., NEILL, M. E., SWASH, M. and PARKS, A. G. (1981). Electrophysiological study of motor nerve supply of pelvic floor. *Lancet*, **i**, 16–17

PHANEUF, L. E. (1938). Complete laceration of the perineum and rectovaginal fistula. *American Journal of Obstetrics and Gynecology*, **36**, 899–907

PHANEUF, L. E. (1950). Vaginal plastic surgery in the treatment of lacerations and displacements of the female genital tract. *American Journal of Obstetrics and Gynecology*, **60**, 1068–1087

PICKRELL, K. L. (1952). Construction of a rectal sphincter in restoration of anal continence by transplanting the gracilis muscle. *Annals of Surgery*, **135**, 853–859

PICKRELL, K. L., BROADBENT, T. R., MASTERS, F. W. and METZGER, J. (1952). Construction of a rectal sphincter and restoration of anal continence by transplanting gracilis muscle: report of four cases in children. *Annals of Surgery*, **135**, 853–862

PICKRELL, K., MASTERS, F., GEORGIADE, N. and HORTON, C. (1954). Rectal sphincter reconstruction using gracilis muscle transplant. *Plastic and Reconstructive Surgery*, **13**, 46–55

POTTS, W. J. (1959). *The Surgeon and the Child*. Philadelphia; Saunders

PRESTON, D. M., LENNARD-JONES, J. E. and THOMAS, B. M. (1984). The balloon proctogram. *British Journal of Surgery*, **71**, 29–32

PROCHIANTZ, A. and GROSS, P. (1982). Gluteal myoplasty for sphincter replacement: principles, results and prospects. *Journal of Pediatric Surgery*, **17**, 25–30

PURI, P. and NIXON, H. H. (1976). Levatorplasty: a secondary operation for fecal incontinence following primary operations for anorectal agenesis. *Journal of Pediatric Surgery*, **11**, 77–82

PURI, P. and NIXON, H. H. (1977). The results of treatment of anorectal anomalies: a 13–20 year follow-up. *Journal of Pediatric Surgery*, **12**, 27–32

RAFFENSPERGER, J. G. (1980). *Swenson's Pediatric Surgery*, 4th edn, pp. 577–561. New York; Appleton-Century-Crofts

RAPPERT, E. (1952). Plastischer Ersatz des Musculus sphincter ani. *Zentralblatt für Chirurgie*, **77**, 579–581

REFSUM, S. and KNUTRUD, O. (1980). Free autogenous muscle transplantation in children with anal incontinence. *Zeitschrift für Kinderchirurgie*, **31**, 30–35

REHBEIN, F. (1959). Operation for anal and rectal atresia with recto-urethral fistula. *Chirurgie*, **30**, 417–419

REVILLON, Y., JEHANNIN, B. and ARHAN, P. (1979). Constipation in the child. *Chirurgie Pédiatrique*, **20**, 181–184

RUSSELL, W. (1932). *Colonic Irrigation*. Edinburgh; Churchill Livingstone

SAKANIWA, M., TAKAHASHI, H. and MAIE, M. (1981). Anorectal manometry in myelomeningocele. *Journal of the Japanese Society of Pediatric Surgeons*, **17**, 635–642

SANTULLI, T. V., KIESEWETTER, W. B. and BILL, A. H. JR. (1970). Anorectal anomalies: a suggested international classification. *Journal of Pediatric Surgery*, **5**, 281

SARAHAN, T., WEINTRAUB, W. H., CORAN, A. G. and WESLEY, J. R. (1982). The successful management of chronic constipation in infants and children. *Journal of Pediatric Surgery*, **17**, 171–174

SAXENA, N., BHATTACHARYYA, N. C., KATARIYA, S., MITRA, S. K. and PATHAK, I. C. (1981). Perineal anal transplant in low anorectal anomalies. *Surgery*, **90**, 464–467

SCHARLI, A. F. (1984). Analysis of anal incontinence. *Progress in Pediatric Surgery*, **17**, 93–104

SCHARLI, A. F. and KIESEWETTER, W. B. (1970). Defecation and continence: some new concepts. *Diseases of the Colon and Rectum*, **13**, 81–107

SCHMIDT, E. (1978). Die chirurgische Behandlung der analen Incontinenz mittels frei transplantierter autologer körpereigener Darmmuskulatur. *Chirurgie*, **49**, 320–321

SCHREIBER, H. (1964). Unsere Erfahrung mit der Sphinkter-Damm-Plastik bei alten Dammrissen III. Grades. *Zentralblatt für Gynäkologie*, **86**, 1565–1568

SCHUSTER, M. M. (1966). Clinical significance of motor disturbances of the enterocolonic segment. *American Journal of Digestive Diseases*, **2**, 320

SCHUSTER, M. M. (1968). Motor action of the rectum and anal sphincters in continence, in *Handbook of Physiology* (C. Code and C. Ladd Prosser, Eds). Baltimore, Maryland; American Physiological Society/Williams and Wilkins

SCHUSTER, M. M. (1977a). Biofeedback for fecal incontinence. *Journal of the American Medical Association*, **238**, 2595–2596

SCHUSTER, M. M. (1977b). Biofeedback treatment of gastrointestinal disorders. *Medical Clinics of North America*, **61**, 907–912

SCHUSTER, M. M., HOOKMAN, P., HENDRIX, T. R. and MENDELOFF, A. I. (1965). Simultaneous manometric recording of internal and external anal sphincter reflexes. *Bulletin of the Johns Hopkins Hospital*, **116**, 79

SCIAFFINO, S., SJÖSTRÖM, M., THORNELL, L. E., NYSTRÖM, B. and HAKELIUS, L. (1975). The process of survival of denervated and freely autotransplanted skeletal muscle. *Separatum Experientia*, **31**, 1328–1330

SCOTT, J. E. S. (1966). The microscopic anatomy of the terminal intestinal canal in ectopic vulval anus. *Journal of Pediatric Surgery*, **1**, 441–443.

SHAFIK, A. (1975). A new concept of the anatomy of the anal sphincter mechanism and the physiology of defecation. *Investigative Urology*, **13**, 175–182

SKEF, Z., RADHAKRISHNAN, J. and REYES, H. M. (1983). Anorectal continence following sphincter reconstruction utilizing the gluteus maximus muscle: a case report. *Journal of Pediatric Surgery*, **18**, 779–781

SMITH, G. and LINTON, J. R. (1929). Complete laceration of the perineum. *Surgery, Gynecology and Obstetrics*, **49**, 702–705

SNOOKS, S. J., BARNES, R. P. H. and SWASH, M. (1984). Damage to the innervation of the voluntary anal and periurethral striated sphincter musculature in incontinence; an electrophysiological study. *Journal of Neurology, Neurosurgery and Psychiatry*, **47**, 1269–1273

SNOOKS, S. J., HENRY, M. M. and SWASH, M. (1984). Anorectal incontinence and rectal prolapse: differential assessment of the innervation to puborectalis and external anal sphincter muscles. *Gut* (in press)

SNOOKS, S. J., SETCHELL, M., SWASH, M. and HENRY, M. M. (1984). Injury to innervation of pelvic floor sphincter musculature in childbirth. *Lancet*, **ii**, 546–550

SNOOKS, S. J. and SWASH, M. (1984a). Abnormalities of the innervation of the urethral striated sphincter musculature in incontinence. *British Journal of Urology*, **56**, 401–405

SNOOKS, S. J. and SWASH, M. (1984b). Perineal nerve and transcutaneous spinal stimulation; new methods for investigation of the urethral striated sphincter musculature. *British Journal of Urology*, **56**, 406–409

✗ SNOOKS, S. J., SWASH, M., SETCHELL, M. and HENRY, M. M. (1984). Injury to innervation of pelvic floor sphincter musculature in childbirth. *Lancet*, **ii**, 546–550

STEPHENS, F. D. (1953a). Imperforate anus: a new surgical technique. *Medical Journal of Australia*, **2**, 202–204

STEPHENS, F. D. (1953b). Congenital imperforate rectum, recto-urethral and recto-vaginal fistulae. *The Australian and New Zealand Journal of Surgery*, **22**, 161–172

STEPHENS, F. D. (1963). *Congenital Malformations of the Rectum, Anus and Genito-Urinary Tracts*. Edinburgh; Livingstone.

STEPHENS, F. D. and SMITH, E. D. (1971). *Anorectal Malformations in Children*. Chicago; Year Book Medical Publishers

STEPHENS, F. D. and SMITH, E. D. (1984). *Anorectal Anomalies*. Report of a workshop meeting at 'Wingspread' Convention Center, Racine, Wisconsin, USA

STEWART, M. (1971). Constipation and faecal incontinence in the elderly. *Journal of Medical Women's Federation*, **53**, 25–29

STONE, H. B. (1929). Plastic operation for anal incontinence. *Archives of Surgery*, Chicago, **18**, 845–851

STUDITSKY, A. N. (1964). Dynamics of the development of myogenic tissue under conditions of explantation and transplantation, in *Cinemicrography in Cell Biology*, pp. 171–200 (G. G. Rose, Ed.). New York; Academic Press

SWASH, M. (1982). The neuropathology of idiopathic faecal incontinence, in *Recent Advances in Neuropathology*, pp. 242–271 (W. Thomas Smith and J. B. Cavanagh, Eds). Edinburgh; Churchill Livingstone

SWENSON, O. and DONNELLAN, W. L. (1967). Preservation of the puborectalis sling in imperforate anus. *Surgical Clinics of North America*, **47**, 173

TALALAY, P., Ed. (1964). *Drugs in Our Society*, pp. 1–16. London; Oxford University Press

THIERSCH, K. (1891). Quoted by Goligher (1967)

THOMAS, T. M. (1984). Community medicine (in press)

THOMAS, T. M., PLYMAT, K. R., BLANNIN, J. and MEADE, T. W. (1980). Prevalence of urinary incontinence. *British Medical Journal*, **281**, 1243–1245

THOMPSON, N. (1971a). Investigation of autogenous skeletal muscle grafts in the dog. *Transplantation*, **12**, 353–363

THOMPSON, N. (1971b). Autogenous free grafts of skeletal muscle. *Plastic and Reconstructive Surgery*, **48**, 11–27

TOBON, F., REID, N. C. R. W., TALBERT, J. L. and SCHUSTER, M. M. (1968). A non-surgical diagnostic test for Hirschsprung's disease. *New England Journal of Medicine*, **278**, 188

de VRIES, P. A. and PEÑA, A. (1982). Posterior sagittal anorectoplasty. *Journal of Pediatric Surgery*, **17**, 638–643

WALD, A. and TUNUGUNTLA, A. K. (1984). Anorectal sensorimotor dysfunction in fecal incontinence and diabetes mellitus. *New England Journal of Medicine*, **310**, 1282–1287

WARREN, J. C. (1882). A new method of operation for the relief of rupture of the perineum through the sphincter and rectum. *Transactions of American Gynecologic Society*, **72**, 322–330

WEISENBERG, S. (1926). Encopresis. *Zeitschrift für Kinderheilk*, **40**, 674–677

WHITEHEAD, W. E., ENGEL, B. T. and SCHUSTER, M. M. (1980). Irritable bowel syndrome: physiological and psychological differences between diarrhea-predominant and constipation-predominant patients. *Digestive Diseases and Sciences*, **5**, 404

WHITING, J. and CHILD, I. L. (1953). *Child Training and Personality*. New Haven; Yale University Press.

WREDEN, R. R. (1929). A method of reconstructing a voluntary sphincter ani. *Archives of Surgery*, Chicago, **18**, 841–844

WRIGHT, L. (1974). Bowel function in hospital patients. Nursing Care Project Reports, Series 1, no. 4. London; Royal College of Nursing

Chapter 13

Solitary ulcer syndrome of the rectum: its relation to mucosal prolapse

K. R. P. Rutter

Introduction

Solitary rectal ulcer syndrome (SRUS) is a chronic, benign condition principally affecting young adults, characterized by the passage of blood and mucus per rectum, disordered defaecation and anal pain. It has a well-defined histological appearance which should allow a confident diagnosis on biopsy. In its classical form of a solitary rectal ulcer, it is undoubtedly rare. However, there is increasing awareness of a non-ulcerated form showing the same symptomatology and pathology which is not at all unusual and which should be considered in any patient with atypical rectal disease.

The syndrome never goes on to malignancy and major excisional surgery is virtually never required. Yet in a recent survey of 31 patients with the condition (Misumi et al., 1981), 8 patients were treated by abdominoperineal excision of the rectum (one a 19 year old), 2 had anterior resections (both 13 year olds), 2 had colostomies and 1 had a sigmoidectomy. There is clearly an urgent need for greater understanding of the condition by surgeons and pathologists alike.

The first description of the condition is generally credited to Cruveilhier (1870) and there were several other reports towards the end of the nineteenth century, but it is difficult to be sure, in retrospect, whether this was the condition we now recognize. The term solitary rectal ulcer was first used by Lloyd-Davis at St Mark's Hospital in 1937 (personal communication) and the condition has been well recognized there since that time. The first well-documented case was described by Madigan (1964) and a further four cases were reported by Haskell and Rovner (1965). Madigan and Morson (1969) reviewed a total of 68 patients seen at St Mark's Hospital and, in a clear exposition, laid down the histological criteria required for a biopsy diagnosis. Rutter and Riddell (1975) stressed the strong association with rectal prolapse and suggested that the histological changes seen in the condition might be produced by a combination of mucosal prolapse, tissue ischaemia and trauma all brought about by excessive straining at stool. Several subsequent studies (Schweiger and Alexander-Williams, 1977; Martin, Parks and Biggart, 1981) have again confirmed the association with rectal prolapse and there is broad agreement that there is a close relationship between the two conditions. However, the precise aetiology has yet to be proved and occasional patients are seen with a firm histological diagnosis of solitary rectal ulcer syndrome in whom no prolapse can be demonstrated. It is likely that there are a number of different factors involved.

Presentation

The SRUS is remarkable for the wide variety of ways in which it may present and for the number of other diseases it can mimic. It should always be considered in the differential diagnosis of any atypical lesion affecting the anorectal region. It is easily mistaken for prolapsed haemorrhoids, non-specific proctitis, ischaemic proctitis, rectal Crohn's disease, pseudomembranous colitis, villous adenoma of the rectum or even carcinoma, and the situation is further complicated by the close association between SRUS and all forms of rectal prolapse.

Symptoms

Bleeding is almost invariably present in these patients, but there is no particular pattern to suggest the diagnosis of SRUS. The blood is usually fresh and separate from the stool, but equally can be dark and mixed in; it is unusual for it to be heavy, although occasionally it can be sufficient to require transfusion and, on occasions, emergency surgery has been needed. The passage of mucus is also very common and is sometimes profuse. Patients frequently describe a feeling of tenesmus, relieved by the passage of small quantities of mucus.

Pain is another common symptom, but again there are no consistent features to it. It may be suprapubic, lumbar, rectal or anal. It may be present all the time or intermittently, is occasionally postural or related to exercise; sometimes it only becomes noticeable on defaecation.

The symptom that causes most confusion, is frequently overlooked and yet may be almost diagnostic of the condition, is the disorder of defaecation that almost invariably occurs. It is variously described as constipation or as diarrhoea, as a need to strain excessively at stool or as a sensation of anal blockage. Understandably, many patients are embarrassed and have difficulties in explaining the symptoms. This is compounded by the fact that we have no acceptable definition of a normal defaecation pattern. On close questioning, patients admit to frequent visits to the lavatory, resulting in the passage of small quantities of mucus without resolution of the urge to defaecate. Others describe the same habit as constipation, sitting on the lavatory for long periods, frequently straining a great deal, often without success. Yet other patients describe a peculiar difficulty in defaecation when they are aware of the presence of a stool in the rectum, and a strong urge to defaecate but feel something is 'blocking' the way out. A proportion of these patients discover that passing a finger into the anal canal relieves the feeling of obstruction, allowing defaecation to proceed, although they may need to repeat the process to achieve complete evacuation. There is good evidence that the obstruction in these patients is due to an anterior rectal mucosal prolapse occluding the anal canal.

Thus, there is no absolutely consistent pattern of symptoms on which one can base a diagnosis of SRUS. However, one aspect of the history is common and should alert one to the diagnosis. This is the history some patients give of rectal bleeding with the passage of mucus, together with a bowel habit that involves repeated visits to the lavatory, as many as six or seven times a day, where they sit straining forcibly for long

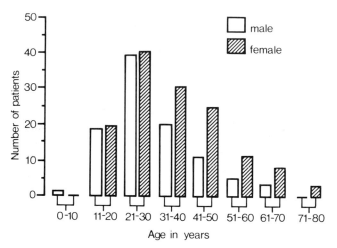

Figure 13.1. Age and sex distribution of patients with solitary rectal ulcer syndrome

periods, frequently for up to an hour or more. Notwithstanding these efforts, they may be quite unable to pass a stool. Not surprisingly, in view of the long periods of time involved, these patients must organize their whole life-style around their disordered bowel habit and many of these patients are thought of as odd, deviant or fetishist, although these labels would seem to be quite unfair and unjustified.

Age and sex presentation

Figure 13.1 shows the age distribution of patients with the syndrome and it can be seen that it is rare in children, is commonest in the second, third and fourth decades, with a peak in the thirties, and then becomes progressively less common in older age groups. It is principally a condition affecting healthy, young adults. Overall, it is commoner in women than men, although it is only after the third decade that the female preponderance becomes obvious. This may be due to the fact that rectal prolapse is commoner in middle-aged and elderly women.

Clinical signs

General examination is usually normal (apart from occasional tenderness in the left iliac fossa) and abnormalities are only found on rectal examination. An obvious finding is the presence of an easily palpable, thickened but mobile area of mucosa on the low anterior rectal wall, just above the anorectal junction. Sometimes, the induration is nodular or villous in character and might suggest a polyp or even carcinoma. Occasionally, it is possible to feel a ring of thickened tissue encircling the lower rectum.

Sigmoidoscopy

The solitary ulcer has a very characteristic appearance; it is usually shallow and 'punched out' with a greyish-white, sloughy base. Surrounding it is a hyperaemic halo extending for a few millimetres before merging into relatively normal mucosa. Sometimes, there can be quite a wide area of rather inflamed granular mucosa surrounding the ulcer. The ulcers tend to occur adjacent to rectal valves and not infrequently lie astride them. There is wide variation in the morphology of the ulcers: they vary from a few millimetres to several centimetres in diameter and, although generally round or oval, linear and serpiginous forms are not infrequently seen. Sometimes, large circumferential ulcers occur, although these are rare. Despite the name of the syndrome, it is not unusual to see multiple ulcers, sometimes small and aphthoid in appearance and sometimes quite large. In the absence of ulceration, a localized area of inflamed mucosa may be seen and this may have many of the typical features of non-specific proctitis with granularity, friability and contact bleeding. Sometimes there is an overlying area of greyish-white slough which may be punctate or diffuse and, on occasions, can be so extreme as to suggest a diagnosis of pseudo-membranous colitis. The mucosa may be heaped up or nodular and sometimes has a polypoid appearance.

Thus, there is a wide variation in the naked eye appearance of the mucosa and the clue to the diagnosis lies in the location of the mucosal changes. These changes, whether involving ulceration or not, are almost invariably seen between 4 and 12 cm from the anal verge, and a peculiarity of the condition is the remarkable frequency with which the changes occur on the low anterior rectal wall immediately above the anorectal junction. If the patient is asked to strain with a proctoscope in position, the affected area may enter the end of the instrument and obstruct the view.

There are thus two distinct forms of the syndrome, one ulcerated and the other non-ulcerated, with a large degree of overlap between them. The term solitary rectal ulcer syndrome is clearly unsatisfactory since, in many cases, no true ulceration is seen and when ulcers are present they are frequently not solitary. Furthermore, a number of other terms such as hamartomatous inverted polyps of the rectum (Allen, 1966), colitis cystica profunda (Wayte and Helwig, 1967), enterogenous cyst of the rectum (Talerman, 1971) and inflammatory cloacogenic polyp (Lobert and Appleman, 1981) have been used to describe what are probably variants or complications of the condition. Du Boulay, Fairbrother and Isaacson (1983), in a recent study, have again stressed the association of SRUS with mucosal prolapse and have proposed that a common clinicopathological term, mucosal prolapse syndrome, should be used to cover all the variations of the condition. This proposal has much to commend it and should be adopted.

Evolution of the syndrome

The outcome of untreated SRUS is unpredictable, although resolution is unusual. Madigan and Morson (1969) reported 52 patients observed over an average duration of 8 years and found that ulcers showed remarkably little change over this period. They described one male patient with a persistent ulcer that remained virtually unchanged over a period of 34 years. Others, including the author, have observed a more dynamic situation where ulcerated and non-ulcerated forms undergo considerable changes of morphology, with ulcers occasionally healing spontaneously or changing to a non-ulcerated form and vice versa. Franzin et al. (1982) studied 27 patients over a 4-year period and found that although symptoms changed little over this time, there were marked but unpredictable naked eye and histological changes.

Complications

Serious complications are rarely seen in patients with this syndrome, and the only life-threatening complication is massive blood loss requiring transfusion. Martin, Parks and Biggart (1981) described 3 cases out of 51 requiring transfusion, and Madigan and Morson (1969) described 4 out of 68. In neither of these studies did any patients die.

In view of the marked fibrosis that is such a feature of the condition, it would be expected that rectal stenosis might be a problem. A number of investigators (Lewis, Mahoney and Heffernan, 1977; Chapa, Smith and Dickinson, 1981) have described rectal stenosis on barium enemas in these patients, but symptomatic rectal stenosis is rare.

Fistulation would not be expected because, in contradistinction to Crohn's disease where the inflammation is transmural, the ulceration in patients with SRUS is always superficial. There has been a single report of fistulation to the bladder producing a pseudocloaca (Eisenstat and Herbst, 1979).

Histology

A number of specific histological features may be seen which permit a confident diagnosis of SRUS to be made. These changes are best seen in the mucosa adjacent to an ulcer or in the pre-ulcerative or non-ulcerated form of the condition. The most characteristic changes consist of the replacement of the normal lamina propria by fibroblasts and smooth muscle cells derived from the muscularis mucosae which pass up between the crypts towards the luminal surface (*Figure 13.2*). The proportion of muscle fibres to fibroblasts is variable. Sometimes, fibroblasts and collagen

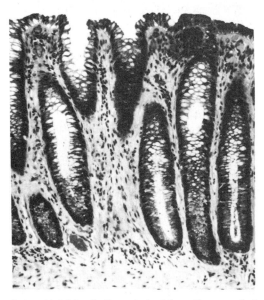

Figure 13.2. Muscle fibres derived from the muscularis mucosae passing up between the tubules (Haematoxylin and eosin, × 16)

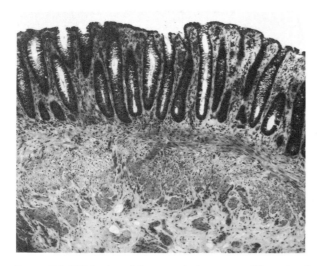

Figure 13.3. Thickening of the muscularis mucosae (Haematoxylin and eosin, × 16)

predominate while, on other occasions, particularly in more severe disease, the excess of smooth muscle fibres may be so pronounced that they form thick fascicles arising from a greatly thickened muscularis mucosae (*Figure 13.3*) and filling the space between the epithelial tubules. These changes may be so extreme that they simulate a smooth muscle tumour and mistakes in diagnosis have been made on this basis.

The crypts show regenerative features, with branching, distortion and shortening, although this latter feature may be difficult to identify due to the alteration in the architecture of the muscularis mucosae. The epithelium itself shows hyperplasia with increased mitoses, pseudostratification and a variable amount of mucin depletion. Studies of mucin histochemistry in these patients have shown a loss of the normal mucin pattern, with sialomucins predominating throughout the crypt length (Du Boulay, Fairbrother and Isaacson, 1983). The mucosa is usually thickened, occasionally becoming markedly villous, and it is on these villous processes that superficial ulceration first occurs. This is accompanied by a marked fibrinous and polymorph exudate which eventually produces the white floor so characteristic of the true solitary ulcer. This may be so florid as to suggest a diagnosis of pseudo-membranous colitis. Ulceration is always superficial and never penetrates deeply into the submucosa. Even in quite marked ulceration there may be surprisingly little inflammatory reaction. Associated with the ulceration, dilatation and congestion of the capillary channels beneath the surface epithelium are often seen and, in some cases, abnormalities may be apparent in the arterial wall, with thickening of the vascular media and fibrinoid necrosis.

An unusual complication of the condition, best known as localized colitis cystica profunda, occurs when misplaced glands are seen in the submucosa (*Figure 13.4*), the glands being filled with mucus and lined by normal colonic epithelium. These cysts are often surrounded by haemosiderin and occasionally by foreign body giant cells or foci of calcification. It is this appearance that can sometimes suggest a focus of carcinoma, although close inspection should show that the epithelium is not neoplastic. Other features which may only be seen in particularly deep biopsies or resection specimens are marked submucosal fibrosis and gross thickening of the muscularis propria. This

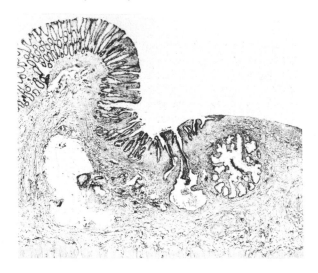

Figure 13.4. Localized colitis cystica profunda (Haematoxylin and eosin, ×6)

thickening may extend to a considerable distance beyond the area of mucosal change. The biopsy diagnosis of SRUS is made more difficult when sections have been cut tangentially across the base of hyperplastic crypts. This can give a false impression of invasive carcinoma surrounded by collagen and smooth muscle cells.

Pathogenesis

A number of different explanations, described below, have been advanced to account for the mucosal changes seen in the syndrome.

Inflammatory bowel disease

The naked eye appearance of the mucosa can be indistinguishable from non-specific proctitis and not surprisingly it has been suggested (Jalan *et al.*, 1970) that SRUS, particularly when no ulcer is present, is a localized form of inflammatory bowel disease. However, there are several reasons why this seems unlikely. The histological appearances are dissimilar and studies of mucin secretion show an excess of sialomucins compared with the normal mucin pattern, suggesting that the two conditions are different (Ehsamullah, Filipe and Gazzard, 1982). Furthermore, patients with SRUS never respond to treatment with sulphasalazine and steroids and no patient has ever been described going on to develop total ulcerative colitis.

Congenital duplication

Madigan and Morson (1969), in putting forward several possibilities, speculated that solitary ulcers might be areas of localized heterotopia or congenital duplication of the rectal wall undergoing cystic change due to retention of mucin. It was postulated that ulceration might occur when these cysts burst into the lumen. Over the past 15 years, there has been no supplementary evidence to support the theory and it would seem to be unlikely.

Trauma

It has been suggested that these ulcers might be the result of trauma, either self-inflicted or homosexual; indeed, as described above, there is no doubt that a significant proportion of these patients, perhaps as many as 50 per cent (Martin, Parks and Biggart, 1981), will admit, on close questioning, to self-digitation and it is possible that this may have a minor aetiological role. However, it is difficult to believe that this is an important factor. The histological appearances are not what one would expect from simple trauma and many of the areas of abnormal mucosa are well out of the range of the patient's finger. Furthermore, large numbers of patients with SRUS denied that they could traumatize themselves digitally and there is no reason to doubt this. In an investigation into the rectal mucosal changes in a group of homosexuals (Sohn and Robilotti, 1977), 31 patients were observed with non-specific inflammatory changes and none of these showed the histological features of SRUS. In a total of 260 patients, only 6 were seen with a solitary ulcer in the rectum and only 1 of these showed changes compatible with a diagnosis of SRUS.

Infection

Rectal ulceration and inflammation can occur as a result of a wide range of infective conditions such as syphilis, gonorrhoea, amoebiasis, shigellosis and lymphogranuloma venereum. However, none of these produce the typical histological picture of SRUS, nor have patients with the syndrome ever been shown to have any of these specific infections, despite careful investigation.

Ischaemia

Devroede *et al.* (1973) presented a patient with a solitary rectal ulcer apparently caused by stenosis of the inferior mesenteric artery. The ulceration healed following surgical relief of the stenosis. There is no evidence to suggest that large vessel ischaemia is involved in the aetiology of SRUS.

Prolapse

The histological features of SRUS, although easily recognized, are by no means specific and can be seen in a wide range of other clinical situations (B. Morson, personal communication), for example:

1. Prolapsed haemorrhoids.
2. Rectal mucosal prolapse.
3. Full thickness rectal prolapse.
4. Prolapsing anorectal adenomatous polyps.
5. Ileostomies.
6. Colostomies.
7. Gastric mucosa prolapsing into the duodenum.

The one constant and striking factor in all these situations is the occurrence of mucosal prolapse with movement of the mucosa over the submucosa, and the conclusion that prolapse is in some way involved in the pathogenesis of SRUS would seem irresistible.

Another curious feature of the condition is the marked predilection of the mucosal abnormality for the low anterior rectal wall. Taking into account the large number of

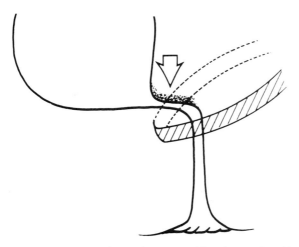

Figure 13.5. 'Flap' valve at the anorectal junction produced by the pull of the puborectalis muscle

patients with SRUS who admit to powerful and prolonged straining efforts at stool, it would seem more than coincidence that the mucosal damage is found so commonly on the low anterior rectal wall which is the area intimately involved in the maintenance of continence.

Although many theories have been advanced to account for the maintenance of faecal continence, it is now wisely accepted that the 'flap' valve theory of Parks (Parks, Porter and Hardcastle, 1966; Parks, 1975) is the most plausible. The low rectum swings forward almost horizontally along the pelvic floor to meet the anal canal at an angle of about 90° and this angulation is maintained by the pull of the puborectalis muscle (*Figure 13.5*). This muscle is unusual in that unlike most other muscles in the body it is in a state of continuous tonic activity, even during sleep (Floyd and Walls, 1953). As a result of this angulation, the low anterior rectal wall comes to lie over the upper end of the anal canal occluding it. Any increase in intra-abdominal pressure threatening continence results in an increase in activity in the puborectalis, pulling the anorectal angle forwards and upwards, exaggerating the angle and rendering the closure even more secure. For defaecation to occur, the anorectal angle must be 'unlocked' and this takes place by lengthening of the puborectalis.

Electromyographic studies have shown that in most people this takes place by reflex inhibition in the muscle (Porter, 1961), although it has also been shown (Kerremans, 1969; Rutter, 1974) that, in some normal individuals, inhibition does not occur and lengthening only results as a consequence of passive stretching brought about as the result of a straining effort. Indeed, it has been suggested that there are two broad types of defaecation habit: people with easy puborectalis inhibition are able to defaecate rapidly without straining, whereas those in whom inhibition does not occur so easily are the group who strain. Studies of intra-abdominal pressures, using a radiotelemetry pill, give some support to this contention (unpublished observations).

Electromyography in patients with SRUS (Lane, 1974; Rutter, 1974) has shown that some of them have a gross disturbance in the behaviour of the puborectalis muscle. During a bearing-down effort, far from achieving inhibition, the puborectalis muscle goes into a state of extreme overactivity, which persists as long as the bearing-down effort is maintained. The effect of this failure of inhibition is that these patients must strain at stool and can only defaecate through an unrelaxed pelvic floor. Since the low

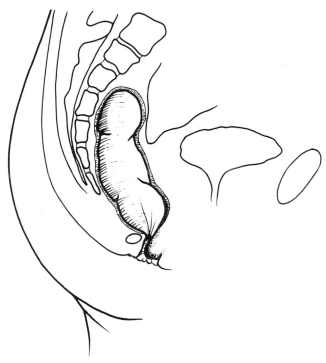

Figure 13.6. Anterior rectal mucosal prolapse filling anal canal

anterior rectal wall forms the 'flap' of the flap valve, it is this area in particular which is affected by prolonged straining efforts during defaecation.

The end result of persistent straining efforts over the years, whatever the explanation of the need to strain, is that eventually the anterior rectal wall begins to slide down the anal canal. As time goes by, a significant anterior wall prolapse develops and eventually this reaches the outside. In some patients, this anterior wall prolapse becomes so large that it forms a bolus obstructing the anal canal (*Figure 13.6*) and it is this obstructing prolapse that causes problems with defaecation and which may force the patient to practice self-digitation. Only in this way can he or she clear the lumen and allow defaecation to occur.

Thus, there are several ways in which damage can occur to the anterior rectal wall as a result of straining efforts.

Ischaemia

Ischaemia could be due to the following:

1. Pressure necrosis when the anterior rectal wall is forced into the upper end of the anal canal and pinched by an actively contracting external sphincter. Many of these patients are young with healthy musculature.
2. Fibrous and muscular tissue in the lamina propria obliterating the submucosal capillaries.
3. Stretching and rupture of submucosal vessels occurring as a result of shearing movements between the mucosa and submucosa.

This concept of ischaemia causing mucosal damage is supported by the fact that ulceration tends to occur at a position most remote from the blood supply, i.e. on the apex of a prolapse.

Trauma

Trauma may be brought about by the following:

1. Direct trauma caused by self-digitation.
2. Abrasion by clothing of exteriorized rectal mucosa.

Some of the other histological features seen in the syndrome may also be due to the prolapse. The striking thickening of the muscularis mucosae, and the change in polarity of the fibres derived from it, may represent an attempt by the tissues to resist the shearing forces between the mucosa and submucosa.

The misplaced glands seen in the submucosa in cases with localized colitis cystica profunda may be explained by 'pinching off' of the base of a crypt by the actively squeezing sphincter. Alternatively, the primary lesion may be submucosal haemorrhage brought about by trauma, resulting in rupture of blood vessels. The haemorrhage may organize and, if it makes contact with the base of the crypt, the epithelium may proliferate and cover the lining of the cavity, as if it were a superficial ulcer.

Similar mechanisms may explain the relationship between SRUS and complete rectal prolapse. The Moschcowitz (1912) theory, that complete rectal prolapse is a direct sliding hernia of the rectum, is no longer tenable and the current opinion is that full thickness rectal prolapse begins as a mid-rectal intussusception which progressively advances until it reaches the exterior (Ripstein and Lanter, 1963; Broden and Snellman, 1968; Ihre, 1972) (*Figure 13.7*). The concept of mid-rectal intussusception, internal procidentia or occult rectal prolapse is now accepted and the association with solitary rectal ulcer syndrome is acknowledged (Rutter and Riddell, 1975; Schweiger and Alexander-Williams, 1977; Biehl, Ray and Gathright, 1978; White, Findlay and Price, 1980). The same mechanisms that bring about the changes of SRUS in cases with mucosal prolapse can be invoked with complete rectal prolapse, even when the prolapse has not reached the outside. As the intussusception develops and prolapses down the rectum towards the anal canal, ischaemia may occur as a result of any of the mechanisms described above. Eventually, the prolapse enters the anal canal and descends to reach the exterior where direct trauma may occur.

The relationship between 'high' prolapse beginning as intussusception and 'low' prolapse has yet to be defined. Although there is a large degree of overlap between them, both forms usually exist independently and there is no obvious evidence that the one develops into the other. It may be that both represent different defects in rectal supporting tissues. The author has seen a patient with SRUS in association with a high prolapse whose ulcer healed following treatment by rectopexy, only to develop another ulcer in a new location immediately above the anorectal angle at a later date. Schweiger and Alexander-Williams (1977) describe a similar patient. There is, as yet, no consensus as to which is the commoner form of prolapse to be found with SRUS. Schweiger and Alexander-Williams (1977) and Martin, Parks and Biggart (1981) describe a large preponderance of cases with high prolapse, whereas others, including the author, have found the majority to be associated with the low form with no evidence of intussusception. This discrepancy is probably accounted for by the enthusiasm with which low rectal biopsies are taken in patients with symptoms suggestive of SRUS.

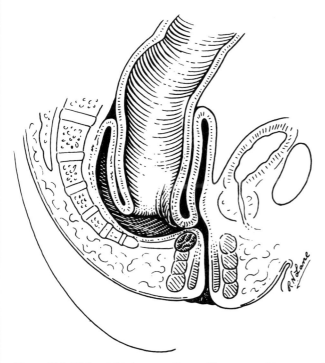

Figure 13.7. Mid-rectal intussusception, with apex reaching anorectal angle

Most patients with mucosal prolapse will show the histological changes of SRUS, even though they may not warrant such a diagnosis on the history alone.

Several authors have pointed out (Kennedy, Hughes and Masterton, 1977; Martin, Parks and Biggart, 1981; Du Boulay, Fairbrother and Isaacson, 1983) that this discussion concerns a spectrum of conditions, all aetiologically related, sharing a similar histological picture. The stress on the ulcerative form of this group of conditions brought about by the current nomenclature has perhaps been responsible for the failure of the condition to be more widely recognized and, for this reason, it would seem sensible for the old term to be discarded and the name 'mucosal prolapse syndrome' to be adopted in its place.

Treatment

There is often a long delay between the onset of symptoms and referral for specialist treatment, partly because the symptoms may be so bizarre and unexpected that they are not taken seriously and partly because the diagnosis can only be made following a sigmoidoscopy. Many general practitioners have neither the equipment nor the expertise to carry out the examination. As a result, many of these patients remain undiagnosed for a long time and become disenchanted with the medical profession. Hence, they require particularly sympathetic and sensitive handling. However, finding a doctor who will accept their symptoms as genuine and will examine them and find something to account for their problems, may in itself be therapeutic. Indeed, explanation and reassurance may be the only treatment required by these patients.

BRODEN, B. and SNELLMAN, B. (1968). Procidentia of the rectum studied with cine radiography: a contribution to the discussion of causative mechanism. *Diseases of the Colon and Rectum*, **11**, 330

CHAPA, H. J., SMITH, H. J. and DICKINSON, T. A. (1981). Benign (solitary) ulcer of the rectum: another cause for rectal stricture. *Gastro-intestinal Radiology*, **6**, 85–88

CRUVEILHEIR, J. (1870). Ulcère chronique du rectum, in *Anatomie Pathologique du Corps Humain*, vol. 2, no. 25, *Maladies du Rectum*, p. 4. Paris; J. B. Balliere

DEVROEDE, G., BEAUDRY, R., HADDAD, H. and ENRIQUEZ, P. (1973). Discrete ulcerations of the rectum and sigmoid. *Digestive Diseases*, **18**, 695–702

DU BOULAY, C. E., FAIRBROTHER, J. and ISAACSON, P. G. (1983). Mucosal prolapse syndrome—a unifying concept for solitary ulcer syndrome and related disorders. *Journal of Clinical Pathology*, **36**(11), 1264–1268

EHSANULLAH, M., FILIPE, M. I. and GAZZARD, B. (1982). Morphological and mucus secretion criteria for differential diagnosis of solitary ulcer syndrome and non-specific proctitis. *Journal of Clinical Pathology*, **35**(1), 26–30

EISENSTAT, T. E. and HERBST, J. (1979). Solitary rectal ulcer progressing to pseudo-cloaca: a case report. *American Journal of Surgery*, **45**, 57–59

FLOYD, W. F. and WALLS, E. W. (1953). Electromyography of the sphincter ani externus in man. *Journal of Physiology*, **122**, 599–609

FRANZIN, G., DINA, R., SCARPA, A. and FRATTON, A. (1982). The evolution of the solitary ulcer of the rectum; an endoscopic and histopathological study. *Endoscopy*, **14**(4), 131–134

HASKELL, B. and ROVNER, H. (1965). Solitary ulcer of the rectum. *Diseases of the Colon and Rectum*, **8**, 333–336

IHRE, T. (1972). Internal procidentia of the rectum—treatment and results. *Scandinavian Journal of Gastroenterology*, **7**, 643–646

JALAN, K. N., BRUNT, P. W., MACLEAN, N. and SIRCUS, W. (1970). Benign solitary ulcer of the rectum—a report of 5 cases. *Scandinavian Journal of Gastroenterology*, **5**, 143–147

KENNEDY, D. K., HUGHES, E. S. R. and MASTERTON, J. P. (1977). The natural history of benign ulcer of the rectum. *Surgery, Gynecology and Obstetrics*, **144**, 718–720

KERREMANS, R. (1969). In *Morphological and Physiological Aspects of Anal Continence and Defaecation*. Brussels; Editions Arscia

LANE, R. H. (1974). Clinical application of anorectal physiology. *Proceedings of the Royal Society of Medicine*, **68**, 28–30

LEWIS, F. W., MAHONEY, M. P. and HEFFERNAN, C. K. (1977). The solitary ulcer syndrome of the rectum: radiological features. *British Journal of Radiology*, **50**(591), 227–228

LOBERT, P. F. and APPLEMAN, H. D. (1981). Inflammatory cloacogenic polyps. *American Journal of Surgical Pathology*, **5**, 761–766

MADIGAN, M. R. (1964). Solitary ulcer of the rectum. *Proceedings of the Royal Society of Medicine*, **57**, 403

MADIGAN, M. R. and MORSON, B. C. (1969). Solitary ulcer of the rectum. *Gut*, **10**, 871–881

MARTIN, C. J., PARKS, T. G. and BIGGART, J. D. (1981). Solitary rectal ulcer syndrome in Northern Ireland, 1971–1980. *British Journal of Surgery*, **68**(10), 744–747

MISUMI, A., HERA, Y., MATSUDA, M., INAMORI, Y., KAWANO, H., TAKANO, S., MURAKAMI, A. and AKAGI, M. (1981). Solitary ulcer of the rectum: report of a case and review of the literature. *Gastroenterologia Japonica*, **16**(3), 286–294

MOSCHCOWITZ, A. V. (1912). The pathogenesis, anatomy and cure of prolapse of the rectum. *Surgery, Gynecology and Obstetrics*, **15**, 7

PARKS, A. G. (1975). Anorectal incontinence. *Proceedings of the Royal Society of Medicine*, **68**, 681–690

PARKS, A. G., PORTER, N. H. and HARDCASTLE, J. (1966). The syndrome of the descending perineum. *Proceedings of the Royal Society of Medicine*, **59**, 477–482

RIPSTEIN, C. B. (1965). Surgical care of massive rectal prolapse. *Diseases of the Colon and Rectum*, **8**, 34–38

RIPSTEIN, C. B. and LANTER, B. (1963). Etiology and surgical therapy of massive prolapse of the rectum. *Annals of Surgery*, **157**, 259

RUTTER, K. R. P. (1974). Electromyographic changes in certain pelvic floor abnormalities. *Proceedings of the Royal Society of Medicine*, **67**, 53–56

RUTTER, K. R. P. and RIDDELL, R. H. (1975). Solitary ulcer syndrome of the rectum. *Clinics in Gastroenterology*, **4**, 505–530.

SCHWEIGER, M. and ALEXANDER-WILLIAMS, J. (1977). Solitary ulcer syndrome of the rectum: its association with occult rectal prolapse. *Lancet*, **1**, 170–171

SOHN, N. and ROBILOTTI, J. G. (1977). The gay bowel syndrome. *American Journal of Gastroenterology*, **67**, 478–484

TALERMAN, A. (1971). Enterogenous cysts of the rectum. *British Journal of Surgery*, **58**, 643–647

WAYTE, D. M. and HELWIG, E. B. (1967). Colitis cystica profunda. *American Journal of Clinical Pathology*, **48**, 159–169

WELLS, C. (1959). New operation for rectal prolapse. *Proceedings of the Royal Society of Medicine*, **52**, 602–603

WHITE, C. M., FINDLAY, J. M. and PRICE, J. J. (1980). The occult rectal prolapse syndrome. *British Journal of Surgery*, **67**, 528–530

Chapter 14

Descending perineum syndrome

M. M. Henry

Introduction

The descending perineum syndrome is a pelvic floor disorder which was first recognized by Parks and his colleagues in 1966, during their investigations of patients with rectal prolapse. Although considered here in isolation, this disorder is frequently a recognizable part of the whole range of clinical disorders dealt with in this section of the book. In the author's experience, the disorder is relatively common and mostly occurs in women.

Definition

The syndrome was initially defined quantitatively in terms of the relationship of the anorectal angle to the pubococcygeal line, as demonstrated by lateral radiographs of the pelvis in which the anal canal and rectum were outlined by strips of barium-impregnated Ivalon sponge (Hardcastle and Parks, 1970). Using this technique, Hardcastle and Parks demonstrated that the pelvic floor occupied a lower position with reference to the bony plane in patients with faecal incontinence than in normal controls. In the clinical context, the syndrome is recognized when on examining the patient in the left lateral position the perineum balloons downwards during a straining effort. Using a simple clinical device (Henry, Parks and Swash, 1982) it was found that the syndrome can be simply defined as being present when the plane of the perineum extends beyond that of the ischial tuberosities during a straining effort.

Clinical features

Straining

The most prominent and persistent feature is a pronounced difficulty with defaecation, which results in long periods of fruitless straining and a sense of incomplete evacuation at the completion of such efforts. Pelvic floor descent leads to destruction of the anorectal angle and the 'flap' valve mechanism (see Chapter 3). As a consequence, prolapse of the anterior rectal wall into the lumen of the anal canal is encouraged, particularly during a straining effort. The prolapsing mucosa can act as a plug to block the free passage of faeces through the anal canal during defaecation. Such patients may need to insert a finger into the anal canal to deflect the mucosa, in order to achieve satisfactory defaecation. If the prolapsed mucosa fails to retract at the completion of defaecation, it may lie in constant contact with the sensory rich zone of epithelium at and below the dentate line. The sensation of a full rectum may ensue, with the result that repeated and futile attempts at defaecation may occur (*Figures 14.1–14.3*).

Rectal bleeding and mucus discharge

In a similar fashion to haemorrhoidal prolapse, prolapse of the anterior rectal mucosa may be responsible for mucus discharge and, if traumatized, rectal bleeding may develop.

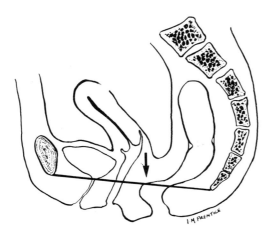

Figure 14.1. Normal resting state; the plane of the pelvic floor is close to that occupied by the pubococcygeal line

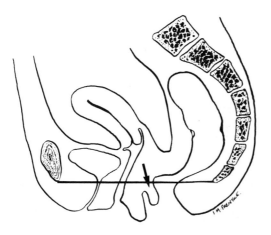

Figure 14.2. Straining is initiated and pelvic floor descent commences. The anorectal 'flap' valve is defective and prolapse of the anterior rectal wall into the lumen of the anal canal occurs

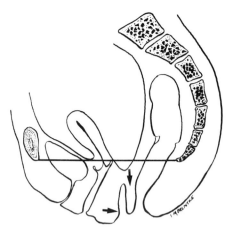

Figure 14.3. The end stage of a defaecatory effort. There has been marked descent of the pelvic floor in relation to the pubococcygeal line. The anterior rectal wall now lies in contact with sensory 'anoderm' at the dentate line, so eliciting the false impression of a full rectum and of incomplete evacuation

Perineal pain

Some patients describe a poorly localized deep perineal discomfort which is often precipitated by prolonged standing, and relieved by lying down or by sleep. There is usually no clear relation to defaecation, although sometimes the pain is precipitated by this act and the history suggests that a fissure may be present.

Urinary incontinence and vaginal prolapse

Some female patients develop functional abnormalities of urinary function, consisting mostly of stress incontinence. This may be accompanied by vaginal prolapse of varying severity.

Pathogenesis

The clinical relationship between faecal incontinence and perineal descent has been noted previously (Hardcastle and Parks, 1970). The possibility of perineal descent being an aetiological factor in faecal incontinence has arisen from the observation that denervation changes occur in the pelvic floor and external sphincter muscles of patients with idiopathic faecal incontinence (see Chapter 12). Some patients with perineal descent have the same histological and electrophysiological abnormalities that are recorded in patients with faecal incontinence (Henry, Parks and Swash, 1982). In this syndrome, abnormal descent of the pelvic floor of the order of 2–3 cm occurs. The terminal portion of the pudendal nerve in the adult is approximately 9 cm; thereby a stretching force to this segment of the nerve of the order of 20–30 per cent is exerted in patients with perineal descent. Since irreversible nerve damage develops when nerves are stretched by as little as 12 per cent (Sunderland, 1978), it is possible that stretching of the nerves leads to secondary neuropathic damage to these muscles.

Parks's original belief was that an abnormal pattern of defaecation resulted in a reduction of 'tone' of the pelvic floor muscles over a number of years. The neuropathy then occurred secondarily. However, it is equally possible that the neurological damage is a primary event (see Chapter 8) which is compounded by a further stretch injury. There is no possible means, at this stage, of determining which is cause and effect.

Treatment

Since there appears to be an important relationship between the syndrome and straining, common sense dictates that the primary aim is to correct this wherever possible. Bulking agents supported by the use of an irritant suppository may prove effective. However, much more can be achieved if the purposelessness of excessive straining in order to evacuate the patient's own rectal mucosa is fully explained to the individual affected.

An attempt can be made to minimize the effects caused by the prolapsing anterior rectal wall mucosa by direct local measures. These can comprise injection sclerotherapy, application of Barron's band, cryotherapy or formal excision. In the author's experience there is a high recurrence rate, particularly if the patient continues to strain.

If the patient with perineal descent develops faecal incontinence, specialized surgery (see Chapter 12) may be indicated.

It has to be said that, on the whole, treatment can be fairly unsatisfactory for clinician and patient alike. Even if treatment is initially successful, symptoms seem to recur commonly and become refractory to further treatment. Perineal pain is particularly difficult to manage and as yet no satisfactory means of help is available for the majority of these unfortunate and unhappy patients.

Recognition of this syndrome is of key importance to the proctologist. Many patients with perineal descent have symptoms which mimic or co-exist with haemorrhoids. If the pelvic floor and external sphincter have been denervated, continence may be dependent on a normal internal sphincter. Treatment by manual dilatation of the anus may result in severe faecal incontinence and a supremely dissatisfied patient.

References

HARDCASTLE, J. D. and PARKS, A. G. (1970). A study of anal incontinence and some principles of surgical treatment. *Proceedings of the Royal Society of Medicine*, **63**, 116–118

HENRY, M. M., PARKS, A. G. and SWASH, M. (1982). The pelvic floor musculature in the descending perineum syndrome. *British Journal of Surgery*, **69**, 470–472

SUNDERLAND, S. (1978). *Nerves and Nerve Injuries*, 2nd edn, pp. 62–66. Edinburgh; Churchill Livingstone

Chapter 15

Rectal prolapse

A. Pathogenesis and clinical features

D. J. Schoetz, Jr and M. C. Veidenheimer

Introduction

Prolapse of the rectum has been defined as a protrusion of part or all layers of the rectum through the anal orifice. Most physicians differentiate mucosal prolapse, in which anal and distal rectal mucosa protrudes from the anus, from complete rectal prolapse, in which all layers of the rectum extrude. Complete rectal prolapse is also referred to as rectal procidentia. Rectal prolapse has been divided into four types: *partial*, meaning involvement of the mucous membrane only; *complete*, which includes the mucocutaneous junction as part of the prolapse, also known as *first degree* prolapse; complete prolapse without involvement of the mucocutaneous junction, also known as *second degree* prolapse; and *concealed* or internal prolapse, in which the rectum invaginates within itself but does not present through the anus, also known as *third degree* prolapse (Roseman, de Peyster and Gilchrist, 1975).

Aetiology

The aetiology of rectal prolapse is probably multifaceted. Two proposed causative mechanisms have enjoyed widespread popularity and have formed the basis of many operative procedures used to treat this disease process.

Moschcowitz (1912) advanced the theory that rectal prolapse is a form of sliding hernia resulting from an abnormally deep cul-de-sac of Douglas. As a result of increased intra-abdominal pressure, the anterior wall of the rectum evaginates; ultimately, the intra-abdominal contents overcome the resistance offered by the rectum itself and by the posterior supportive structures of the pelvis to herniate through the levator musculature. According to this view, complete protrusion through the anal orifice requires progressive laxity of the lateral and posterior attachments of the rectum and is a late stage of the pathological process. Moschcowitz based his theory on the clinical observation that the anterior portion of the prolapsed rectum frequently contains small bowel that can be palpated within the externalized prolapse.

Broden and Snellman (1968) have advocated the theory of intussusception as the primary pathological process of rectal prolapse, based on their cineradiographic observations. They studied cineproctograms of 54 patients obtained during straining and concluded that the lead point of the circumferential intussusception was 6–8 cm inside the rectum; in no instances did the rectosigmoid form the lead point. Twenty patients had internal prolapse, and 4 of these had an associated enterocele. Similarly, 11 of 28 patients with procidentia had an enterocele, but in almost all instances the enterocele did not form until after intussusception. These observations resulted in the conclusion that the enterocele, which corresponds to the sliding hernia of Moschcowitz (1912), is a late manifestation of chronic intussusception associated with defaecation and straining.

Altemeier *et al.* (1971) acknowledged the possibility that both the mechanisms suggested by Moschcowitz (1912) and by Broden and Snellman (1968) could produce rectal prolapse. They described three types of prolapse: type I, which they classified as false prolapse, was a mucosal prolapse extending for 1–3 cm that was usually due to haemorrhoid disease; type II was an intussusception of all layers of the rectum, beginning above the anus but without any associated sliding hernia of the cul-de-sac; and type III, which was described as true or complete, included a sliding hernia through a defect in the pelvic diaphragm that ultimately produced a circumferential intussusception. Altemeier *et al.* (1971) stated that most cases of rectal prolapse are type III.

All investigators have noted consistent anatomical abnormalities in rectal procidentia and have based their theories of pathophysiology on these observations. Diastasis of the levator muscles, a deep pouch of Douglas, a redundant rectosigmoid, and lax lateral and posterior attachments of the rectum to the sacrum, with an elongated mesorectum, are anatomical findings common to all patients with rectal prolapse (*Figure 15.1*). It is probable that the inadequate posterior fixation of the rectum allows straightening of the rectum during straining, thus permitting propulsive force to be transmitted toward the anus and predisposing to an intussusception beginning at the anterior peritoneal reflection of the rectum. This concept is supported by observation of the effect of the absence of a sacral curvature noted in early childhood; most cases of prolapse in children occur before the age of 3 years, and in

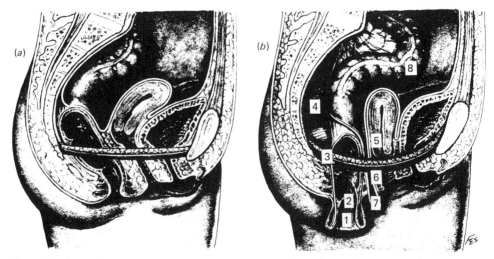

Figure 15.1. Anatomical pathology in rectal prolapse. (*a*) Normal. (*b*) Rectal prolapse, 1; patulous anus, 2; laxity and diastasis of levators, 3; increased retrorectal space and elongated mesorectum, 4; uterine prolapse, 5; rectocele, 6; deep cul-de-sac of Douglas, 7; redundant rectosigmoid, 8

many the condition will resolve spontaneously with skeletal maturation and resultant posterior fixation of the rectum.

Characteristically, the anus of a patient with rectal prolapse is patulous and gaping, and faecal incontinence is a frequent accompaniment of this condition. It is probable that the gaping anus with a compromised sphincter is an effect of the intruded prolapse rather than an important cause of the disease. However, damage to the sphincter from obstetrical trauma or extensive fistulotomy has been implicated as a contributory factor in some patients (Nigro, 1966).

The sliding hernia theory and the intussusception theory are not mutually exclusive. Rectal prolapse appears to represent a spectrum of anatomical characteristics resulting from some underlying abnormality that allows the process to occur. Recently, attention has been directed to the pelvic floor.

Electromyography of the pelvic floor muscles by Porter (1962a) suggested that straining efforts in patients with rectal prolapse resulted in complete and protracted reflex inhibition of the puborectalis and thus predisposed to progressive prolapse. Refinements in electromyographic (EMG) technique allowed the observation that in some individuals a paradoxical increase in puborectalis activity occurs during defaecation, resulting in pushing against an unyielding pelvic floor (Rutter, 1974). This paradoxical hyperactivity is seen in patients with solitary rectal ulcer and perineal descent syndrome. Parks, Swash and Urich (1977) observed the frequent association of descending perineum, faecal incontinence and rectal prolapse and proposed a unifying theory based on the histological demonstration of partial denervation of the puborectalis and external sphincter muscles in patients with these disorders. They suggested that repeated straining during defaecation results in stretching of the pudendal and inferior rectal nerves with progressive partial denervation of the pelvic floor musculature; the laxity of the puborectalis then allows increased intra-abdominal pressure to initiate the process of rectal prolapse.

The relationship between solitary rectal ulcer and rectal prolapse has also been discussed (Kennedy, Hughes and Masterton, 1977; Schweiger and Alexander-Williams, 1977). Some investigators believe that the ulcer is a precursor of rectal prolapse and that the characteristic histological changes in the rectal mucosa are the result of repetitive traumatic invagination of the pelvic peritoneum on the anterior rectal wall against the rigid puborectalis muscle, resulting in hyperaemia, oedema and ulceration. We have not been able to accept this theory, since we have seen essentially no ulcerations in any of the more than 150 patients with rectal prolapse we have treated surgically; the only ulcerations noted were those from surface irritation or ischaemia of the mucosa of the prolapsed rectum.

Clinical features

Rectal prolapse occurs predominantly in women, with an incidence varying from six to ten times that in men (Küpfer and Goligher, 1970; Theuerkauf, Beahrs and Hill, 1970; Altemeier et al., 1971; Jurgeleit et al., 1975; Parks, Swash and Urich, 1977; Lescher et al., 1979; Keighley and Matheson, 1981). Most patients are thin and elderly; the peak age incidence is in the sixth to seventh decade. The condition tends to develop at an earlier age in men, and the incidence in men does not increase after the age of 40 (Küpfer and Goligher, 1970). A higher incidence is seen in nulliparous women than in multiparous women (Goligher, 1984), an observation that minimizes the role of birth injury and stretching of the pelvic floor during labour as a primary causative factor.

Associated medical conditions may contribute to the development of prolapse. Psychiatric disorders were noted in 52 per cent of patients described by Altemeier *et al.* (1971) and in a sizable percentage of the series reported by Goligher (1984). The aetiological role of mental illness is unclear. Neurological diseases, such as multiple sclerosis, tabes dorsalis and cauda equina syndrome, have been a cause of prolapse in a small percentage (generally less than 5 per cent) of patients. Ageing, which results in diminished muscle tone of the pelvic floor, may play a role. Chronic constipation and long-standing abuse of laxatives are frequently seen (Parks, Swash and Urich, 1977). In addition, uterine prolapse is commonly coincident with rectal prolapse (Küpfer and Goligher, 1970).

The patient usually complains of a protrusion at the anal area, a feeling of incomplete evacuation after bowel movements, and sometimes of incontinence of stool. Early in the course, the protrusion may be present only when the patient is straining at stool or lifting heavy objects; in time, however, the prolapse may occur when assuming an erect posture or walking. Attempts by the patient to reduce the prolapse manually become increasingly futile until finally the rectum protrudes all the time. At this point, a continuous mucoid discharge and frequent bleeding from irritation of the exposed mucosa are present. During the development of this state the patient has usually become a homebound social recluse because of the problems associated with the prolapse.

Examination of the patient with suspected rectal prolapse should begin with the patient sitting on the toilet and straining. A prolapse will seldom protrude more than 13–15 cm. The surface is usually oedematous and hyperaemic, and superficial ulcerations may be seen. The thickness of the protruding intestine may be appreciated by the gloved examining fingers. Both walls of the bowel can be palpated in the prolapsed segment; thickening is more likely to be prominent anteriorly than posteriorly. In some instances small bowel can be felt anteriorly, corresponding to the hernia of the pouch of Douglas. Further inspection reveals the concentric rings of mucosa over the prolapsed rectum; the tip of the prolapse is usually placed posteriorly (*Figure 15.2*). Excoriation of the perineal skin resulting from faecal soiling and mucous discharge is common.

Reduction of the prolapse reveals a patulous anus with lax anal sphincters that easily admit three or four fingers painlessly. Anal pain is surprisingly absent from the clinical presentation of rectal prolapse; the presence of pain indicates incarceration with impending strangulation or some other painful condition not necessarily related to the prolapse.

Sigmoidoscopy should always be performed. Oedema and mucosal friability in the distal 6–8 cm of the rectum are characteristic of rectal prolapse. In rare instances a neoplasm may act as a lead point for the intussusception. Biopsy of suspicious lesions should be performed at this initial examination for adequate planning of treatment.

A barium enema study is also usually obtained as part of the complete evaluation of rectal prolapse. Cineradiographic studies are reserved for patients whose symptoms and clinical examination suggest a diagnosis of internal rectal prolapse, which is treated in the same way as complete procidentia (Ihre and Seligson, 1975).

Neurological evaluation is indicated when a neurological lesion is suspected as the underlying causative factor. Radiographs of the lumbosacral spine, electromyography and computed tomography of the cauda equina may be necessary to assist the neurologist in achieving an accurate diagnosis. In our experience, anal manometric studies do not contribute additional diagnostic or therapeutic information to the routine evaluation of patients with rectal prolapse.

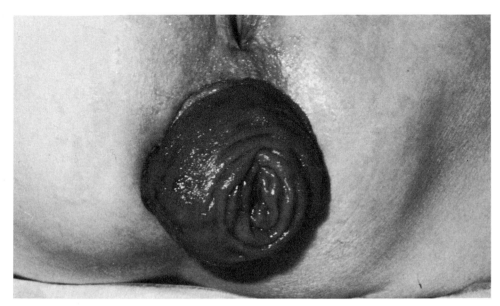

Figure 15.2. Typical rectal prolapse with concentric mucosal folds

Differential diagnosis

Only a few other conditions may be mistaken for true rectal prolapse. Large protruding haemorrhoids are the most frequent source of confusion. Prolapsing mucous membrane is usually related to the presence of third or fourth degree haemorrhoids, rectocele, perineal descent or weakness of the sphincter after fistula operation. Inspection and palpation should permit definition of a single layer of prolapsing material rather than the multiple layers of true rectal prolapse. In addition, the mucosal folds of a mucosal prolapse usually lie in a radial direction rather than in the concentric format seen in true rectal prolapse.

Both benign and malignant polypoid tumours may, although rarely, protrude through the anus and be mistaken for rectal prolapse. Inspection of the prolapsed mass should suffice for differentiation; the results of sigmoidoscopy and barium enema study, which are performed in all patients evaluated for rectal prolapse, will define the disease when the prolapsed neoplasm is not readily apparent.

Complications

Although serious complications of rectal prolapse are unusual, prompt recognition is essential to prevent serious morbidity and mortality. Irreducibility of rectal prolapse with progressive oedema and subsequent strangulation requires urgent surgical intervention. Strangulation may produce serious septic problems and death. Haemorrhage due to extensive ulceration of the exteriorized mucosa is sometimes seen. Rupture of the cul-de-sac with evisceration through the anus has also been reported on rare occasions (Wrobleski and Dailey, 1979).

B. Treatment

J. D. Watts, D. A. Rothenberger and S. M. Goldberg

Introduction

Rectal prolapse or rectal procidentia is an uncommon and disabling condition which evokes considerable controversy regarding its operative management. Despite the number of corrective procedures advocated in the literature, both patient and physician are too often dissatisfied because of persistent incontinence, bowel management problems or recurrence. Few studies adequately address the problem of incontinence, which remains the primary cause of persistent patient disability and dissatisfaction despite anatomical correction or procidentia.

Historical perspective

Moschcowitz (1912) described procidentia as a sliding hernia and for the first time attempted to establish sound anatomical principles regarding its management. Consistent with the principles of herniorrhaphy, attention was focused on correction of the pelvic floor defects and obliteration of the deep cul-de-sac. Subsequently, many authors focused on these and other anatomical defects characteristic of patients with rectal prolapse such as: (a) abnormally deep cul-de-sac, (b) diastasis of the levators, (c) loss of posterior fixation of the rectum with loss of horizontal position, (d) redundant rectosigmoid loop, and (e) patulous anal sphincter (Goldberg, Gordon and Nivatvongs, 1980) (*Figure 15.3*). Although some controversy may still exist, most would agree that the cineradiographic studies of Broden and Snellman (1968), as well as those of Theuerkauf, Beahrs and Hill (1970), confirm that prolapse is a rectorectal intussusception rather than a sliding hernia. The anatomical abnormalities are the result of the prolapse rather than its cause. Nevertheless, operations were developed to correct these anatomical abnormalities. The pelvic diaphragm was reconstructed to correct the sliding perineal hernia by obliteration of the deep cul-de-sac and repair of the levator hiatus. The abnormally mobile rectosigmoid was restored to its normal horizontal position and by various means firmly attached to the sacrum to prevent intussusception by means of suspension–fixation procedures. Redundancy in the left colon was eliminated in order to prevent intussusception, by performing a sigmoid or anterior resection. Most procedures still combine two or more of these principles. Further variation is introduced by altering the surgical approach which can be transabdominal, perineal or trans-sacral. In addition, with the suspension–fixation procedures a variety of autogenous and foreign materials have been utilized, such as fascia lata, omentum, Teflon, Dacron, Marlex, Mersilene, Ivalon sponge, silastic and nylon. Finally, there are the Thiersch or anal encirclement procedures which are aimed at narrowing the anal orifice, and a variety of foreign materials have been utilized with the various modifications of this procedure. Thus, Aminev and Malyshev (1964) reported that over 130 procedures have been described for the management of rectal prolapse. In reality, there are less than a dozen significantly different procedures currently utilized in the management of procidentia. In order to present a useful categorization of procedures for further discussion, we have adopted the classification in *Table 15.1*.

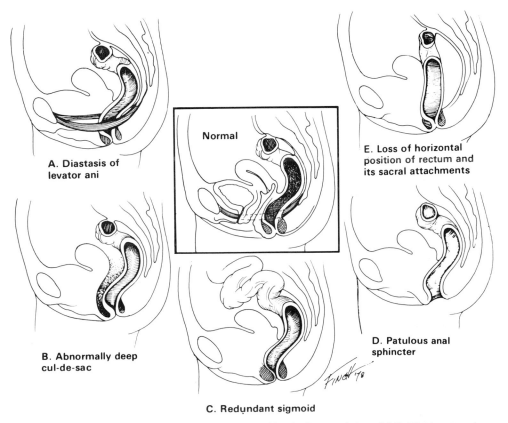

Figure 15.3. Pathological anatomy found in rectal procidentia (By permission of J. B. Lippincott and Harper and Row, publishers)

Transabdominal procedures: repair of the pelvic floor defects

Obliteration of the cul-de-sac (Moschcowitz)

The French surgeons Quenu and Duval first described an abdominal approach consisting of obliteration of the deep cul-de-sac frequently combined with colopexy for the management of prolapse (Goligher, 1980). However, it is Alexis Moschcowitz who is most frequently associated with this approach, as a result of his scholarly treatise on the subject of procidentia. He presented a paper before the New York Medical Society entitled 'The pathogenesis, anatomy, and cure of prolapse of the rectum', in which he attempted to establish sound anatomical principles for the management of rectal prolapse (Moschcowitz, 1912). He felt that prolapse was a sliding hernia and, therefore, consistent with the principles of herniorrhaphy, its management should include a repair of the pelvic floor and obliteration of the cul-de-sac. He felt that this was best accomplished by a transabdominal approach using concentric purse string sutures to obliterate the cul-de-sac and re-establish the pelvic floor (*Figure 15.4*). However, dismal recurrence rates such as those reported by Pemberton and Stalker (1939) of 63 per cent have subsequently cast doubt on his theory and relegated this procedure to one of historic interest only.

TABLE 15.1. Rectal procidentia

Classification of procedures	References	Literature results	
		No. of patients	Recurrence (per cent)
I. Transabdominal procedures			
A. Repair of pelvic floor defects			
1. Obliteration of cul-de-sac (Moschcowitz)	Theuerkauf et al. (1970)	115	48
2. Repair of levator diastasis (Graham–Goligher)	Theuerkauf et al. (1970)	213	8
3. Abdominoperineal levator repair (Hughes)	Hughes and Johnson (1980)	169	2
B. Suspension–fixation without foreign material			
1. Sigmoidopexy (Pemberton–Stalker)	Theuerkauf et al. (1970)	217	19
2. Presacral suture proctopexy (Kummel)	Aminev and Malyshev (1964)	591	12
3. Proctopexy and segmental resection (Frykman–Goldberg)*		138	2
4. Anterior resection (Muir)	Theuerkauf et al. (1970)	197	4
C. Suspension–fixation with foreign material			
1. Lateral strip rectopexy (Orr–Loygue)	Orr (1947); Christensen and Kirkegaard (1981b); Loygue et al. (1984)	226	4
2. Anterior sling rectopexy (Ripstein) (see *Table 15.2*)	Ripstein (1972); Jurgeleit et al. (1975); Biehl et al. (1978); Holmstrom et al. (1978); Failes et al. (1979); Morgan (1980); Launer et al. (1982)	840	3
3. Posterior sling rectopexy (Wells) (see *Table 15.5*)	Kupfer and Goligher (1970); Morgan et al. (1972); Penfold and Hawley (1972); Stewart (1972); Notaras (1973); Boutsis and Ellis (1974); Anderson et al. (1981); Keighley et al. (1983)	435	3
4. Puborectalis sling (Nigro)	Nigro (1978); Greene (1983)	65	0
D. Prevention of intussusception			
1. Rectal plication (Devadhar)	Devadhar (1967)	27	0
2. Ivalon stint (Wedell)	Wedell et al. (1980)	5	0

II. Perineal procedures		
A. Rectosigmoidectomy ± levator repair (see *Table 15.6*)	Hughes (1949); Porter (1962b); Theuerkauf et al. (1970); Altemeier et al. (1971); Friedman et al. (1983)	397	32
B. Rectal mucosectomy and plication (Rehne–Delorme) (see *Table 15.7*)	Aminev and Malyshev (1964); Nay and Blair (1972); Moskalenko (1973); Uhlig and Sullivan (1979); Christensen and Kirkegaard (1981a)	388	19
C. Perineal suspension–fixation (Wyatt)	Wyatt (1981)	22	5
D. Anal encirclement			
1. Thiersch	Theuerkauf et al. (1970)	114	68
2. Modified anal encirclement	Lomas and Cooperman (1972); Notaras (1973); Labow et al. (1980)	52	0
III. Trans-sacral procedures—suspension–fixation (Thomas)	Thomas (1975)	44	0

* Unpublished data, University of Minnesota affiliated hospitals.

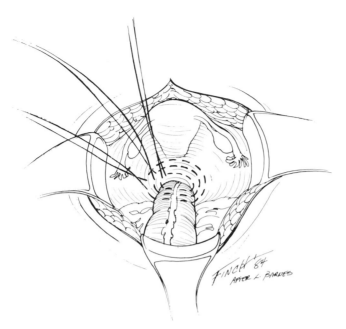

Figure 15.4. Moschcowitz procedure: obliteration of cul-de-sac (After Moschcowitz (1912), by permission of the publishers)

Repair of levator diastasis (Graham–Goligher)

Graham (1942) felt that, in order to cure procidentia, obliteration of the cul-de-sac alone was inadequate, and that an anterior repair of the levators was necessary to correct the pelvic floor defects adequately and thereby prevent recurrence. Following anterior mobilization of the rectum, the levator ani muscles were approximated with interrupted sutures, thereby forcing the rectum into the hollow of the sacrum (*Figure 15.5*). This repaired the anterior endopelvic defect as well as restoring the normal posterior angulation of the rectum. For additional support, the lateral rectal walls were sutured to the fascia overlying the levators and the pelvic floor was reperitonealized with obliteration of the cul-de-sac. Küpfer and Goligher (1970) then modified the Graham procedure to include complete posterior mobilization of the rectum and with this modification reported a recurrence rate of 8 per cent in 61 cases. On the other hand, utilizing the Graham–Goligher procedure, Kuijpers and Lubbers (1983) reported a recurrence rate of 27 per cent in 17 patients and recommended that the procedure be discontinued due to unacceptable recurrence rates.

Abdominoperineal levator repair (Hughes)

In 1957, Sir Edward Hughes described a combined abdominal–perineal approach to the Graham–Goligher procedure. McCann (1928) had described a perineal approach to suture the levator ani muscles, but a recurrence rate of 63 per cent was subsequently reported by Porter (1962b). Hughes based his operation on the premise that only by a combined approach could one adequately repair the levator hiatus. Hughes and Johnson (1980) reported 169 patients, managed in this fashion, and followed up for at

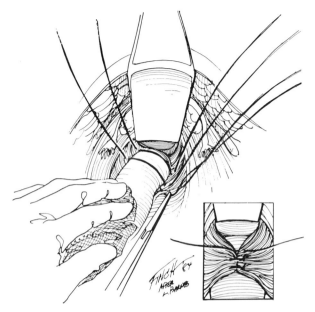

Figure 15.5. Graham procedure: repair of the endopelvic defect by anterior approximation of the levators

least 5 years. The recurrence rate was only 1.8 per cent. These are certainly impressive results. However, from a practical standpoint this procedure is technically too complex an approach ever to gain wide acceptance, when comparatively good results can be achieved by the transabdominal suspension–fixation procedures more familiar to most surgeons. Furthermore, it is probably not the levator repair that is the critical factor, but rather the suspension–fixation which is accomplished as a result of the complete posterior mobilization of the rectum, which if temporarily supported will become firmly adherent to the anterior sacrum, thereby preventing recurrence. Repair of the levators merely serves to support the rectum against the sacrum temporarily.

Transabdominal procedures: suspension–fixation without foreign material

Sigmoidopexy (Pemberton–Stalker)

Pemberton and Stalker (1939) pioneered suspension–fixation procedures in the management of complete rectal prolapse and emphasized the importance of complete posterior mobilization of the rectum. Colopexy was accomplished by suturing the sigmoid colon to the lateral abdominal wall and, in women, to the uterus (*Figure 15.6*). It was their view that the primary anatomical defect causing prolapse was an abnormally mobile rectosigmoid due to loss of its sacral attachment and of its horizontal position. Recurrences following simple sigmoidopexy were thought due to the difficulty encountered in permanently fixing the sigmoid to the parietal peritoneum. However, following complete posterior mobilization of the rectum with dissection in the presacral space, the rectum would become firmly and permanently scarred to the sacrum and its horizontal position re-established, thereby preventing recurrence. The

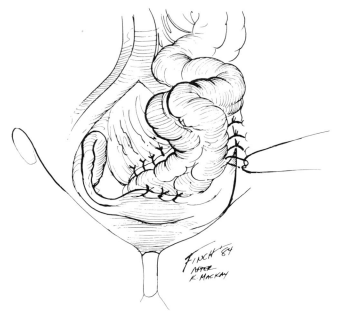

Figure 15.6. Pemberton–Stalker procedure: sigmoidopexy (After Pemberton and Stalker (1939), by permission of the publishers)

initial report of Pemberton and Stalker (1939) consisted of 6 cases without recurrence. However, later follow-up by Theuerkauf, Beahrs and Hill (1970) of the Mayo Clinic series, revealed a recurrence rate of 32 per cent in 68 cases. This procedure was most successful when the lateral peritoneal attachments of the rectum were sutured to the presacral fascia, as in the Frykman–Goldberg procedure, but even then the recurrence rate was 12.5 per cent.

Interesting similarities of procedures and results can be found in the Soviet literature. The Radizievsky operation, first described in 1934 by Aminev and Malyshev, was essentially a sigmoidopexy like the initial Pemberton–Stalker procedure, fixing the stretched sigmoid to the lateral abdominal wall. In a series of 220 cases, the recurrence rate was 23.6 per cent (Aminev and Malyshev, 1964).

Presacral suture proctopexy

Presacral proctopexy by simple suture was first advocated by Cutait, in 1959, but he did not report long-term results (Goligher, 1980). By 1964 the most popular and most successful treatment for prolapse in the USSR was the Kummel procedure which consists of fixation of the rectum to the presacral fascia. Recurrence rate was 12.3 per cent in 591 cases (Aminev and Malyshev, 1964). Goligher (1980) performed presacral suture proctopexy in 42 patients without recurrence, and Carter (1983) recently published a series of 32 patients managed in a similar fashion, with a recurrence rate of 3 per cent. This is a simple, effective procedure if the sigmoid redundancy is not over-prominent. Again, the key to success lies in a complete posterior mobilization of the rectum, with adequate fixation of its lateral peritoneal attachments to the presacral fascia.

Proctopexy plus resection (Frykman–Goldberg)

Frykman felt that 'of all the weaknesses or abnormalities required to produce rectal prolapse the only factor that can be controlled with certainty is the length of the colon' (Frykman and Goldberg, 1969). He therefore advocated combining a sigmoid resection with a suture proctopexy and anterior levator repair. In order to minimize morbidity and mortality, he advocated a sigmoid resection and anastomosis at a convenient level between fully peritonealized segments of bowel. Advocates of resection believe that elimination of redundancy in the left colon is an essential step in the treatment of procidentia. Resection prevents an early recurrence while the mobilized rectum is becoming firmly fixed to the sacrum by fibrous scar tissue. It is argued that shortening the left colon should permanently prevent recurrence irrespective of the multiplicity of aetiological factors that may be involved. Stress and strain may break down the rebuilt rectal support and again deepen the cul-de-sac, but the configuration of the shortened left colon will not change (Goldberg, Gordon and Nivatvongs, 1980). Furthermore, segmental resection is ideally suited for those patients with significant sigmoid diverticular disease. Retention of significant colon redundancy would certainly account for the persistence of bowel management problems common in these patients, while resection combined with proctopexy is beneficial in improving postoperative bowel habits. Patients with procidentia frequently exhibit chronic bowel management problems, with constipation and chronic straining being the most common problem. In our series of patients, 63 per cent complained of severe constipation prior to surgery, while following abdominal proctopexy and sigmoid resection, 56 per cent noted significant improvement. Although the addition of resection remains somewhat controversial, suspension–fixation procedures without resection are associated with recurrence rates of 0–18.9 per cent, while those with a resection have recurrence rates of 0–3.7 per cent (Broden and Snellman, 1968; Kupfer and Goligher, 1970; Theuerkauf, Beahrs and Hill, 1970; Morgan, Porter and Klugman, 1972; Penfold and Hawley, 1972; Stewart, 1972; Notaras, 1973; Boutsis and Ellis, 1974; Conyers and Cullen, 1974; Jurgeleit *et al.*, 1975; Holmstrom *et al.*, 1978; Failes, Stuart and Deluca, 1979; Anderson, Kennenmonth and Smith, 1981; Launer *et al.*, 1982; Friedman, Muggia-Sulam and Freund, 1983; Keighley, Fielding and Alexander-Williams, 1983). Theuerkauf, Beahrs and Hill (1970) reported 28 cases of proctopexy and resection from the Mayo clinic with a 3.7 per cent recurrence rate. Khubchandani and Bacon (1965) reported 29 cases, Conyers and Cullen (1974) 9 cases and Ferguson and Houston (1981) 10 cases, all without a recurrence.

At the University of Minnesota affiliated hospitals we have treated 138 patients with complete rectal prolapse by means of abdominal proctopexy and rectosigmoid resection. Thirty-six patients were lost to follow-up. Of the remaining 102 patients, 81 per cent were followed up for two or more years. Two patients developed a recurrence, an incidence of 1.9 per cent, one at 6 months and the other $2\frac{1}{2}$ yr postoperatively. There were no operative deaths and the average hospital stay was 10 d. Eighty per cent of patients considered their results to be excellent or good. We experienced a 4 per cent incidence of complications directly related to the anastomosis, half of which required further surgery for correction. Importantly, 38 per cent of the patients who were unacceptably incontinent preoperatively regained a satisfactory level of continence following surgery, and only 1 per cent of patients felt their level of continence diminished. Abdominal proctopexy and rectosigmoid resection is an ideal procedure for the good risk patient because it: (a) utilizes techniques familiar to all abdominal surgeons, (b) avoids the use of foreign material, (c) eliminates the risk of volvulus,

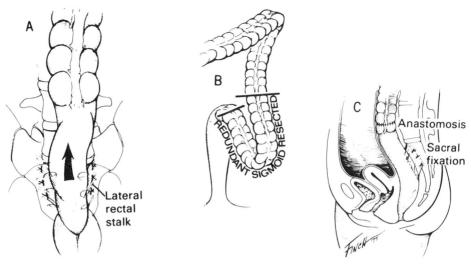

Figure 15.7. Abdominal proctopexy and rectosigmoid resection (Frykman–Goldberg procedure) (By permission of J. B. Lippincott and Harper and Row, publishers)

(d) promotes improved bowel habits, (e) has a low recurrence rate, (f) has a low morbidity and mortality, and (g) offers satisfactory maintenance or restoration of continence. We feel it is preferable to avoid the use of foreign material because of the risk of sepsis both in the postoperative period and over the long term—should the patient later develop a septic process such as diverticulitis. For all of these reasons, it remains our procedure of choice.

Technique

Abdominal proctopexy and rectosigmoid resection (*Figure 15.7*), as with any transabdominal repair of procidentia, requires complete posterior mobilization of the rectum with reduction and fixation to the presacral fascia. We perform this procedure through a transverse lower abdominal incision. The left colon is mobilized from mid-descending level to the level of the sacral promontory where the presacral space is entered. Posterior mobilization of the rectum is carried out to the level of the levator ani muscles. In the pelvis, the peritoneum is incised 1 cm lateral to either side of the rectum and dissection is carried distally with preservation of the lateral stalks. Anterior dissection is unnecessary, since repair of the levator diastasis has not proven of value. The rectum is elevated and its lateral peritoneal attachments are sutured to the presacral fascia beginning just below the sacral promontory. One or two sutures of 2–0 silk or Prolene on each side or on one side of the rectum is all that is necessary. If sutures are placed on both sides of the rectum, care must be taken not to place them too close to the bowel wall, since when tied an obstructing band may be formed across the anterior bowel wall (*Figure 15.8*). If this becomes a problem, it can be corrected by removing or replacing the suture. A segmental resection is performed, eliminating redundancy in the left colon. The anastomosis is performed at a convenient level without tension between two segments of peritonealized bowel, thus hopefully avoiding complications associated with low anterior resection. No attempt is made to obliterate the deep cul-de-sac or repair the levator hiatus.

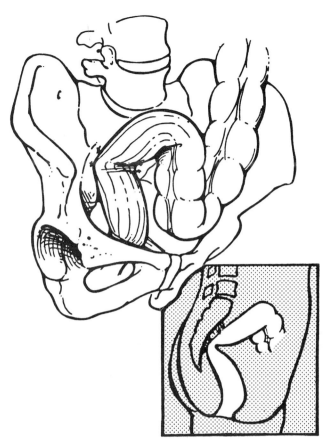

Figure 15.8. An obstructing band may result when sutures are placed on both sides of the rectum

Anterior resection (Muir)

Stabins (1951) reported the first successful use of anterior resection in the management of procidentia. Muir (1962) observed that the rectum was firmly fixed to the sacrum when he re-explored a patient who had previously undergone an anterior resection. He reasoned that anterior resection would be useful in the management of prolapse and in 1962 reported 48 cases with a 2.1 per cent mortality and 4.3 per cent recurrence rate. The demonstration that procidentia is due to a rectorectal intussusception makes this approach even more appealing since the intussusception itself is resected. However, most series of anterior resection appearing in the literature are associated with a significant incidence of complications. Furthermore, anterior resection may diminish reservoir capacity, thereby adversely affecting continence.

Transabdominal procedures: suspension–fixation with foreign material

Lateral strip rectopexy (Orr–Loygue)

Thomas Orr (1947) expanded the scope of the Pemberton–Stalker suspension–fixation procedure and led the way to subsequent modifications such as the Ripstein and Wells

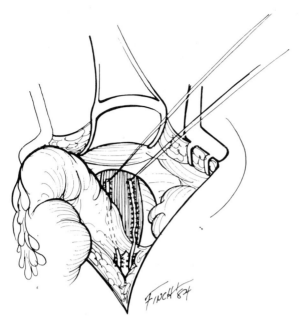

Figure 15.9. Orr procedure (After Orr (1947), by permission of the publishers)

procedures. He reported the successful management of four cases of complete rectal prolapse employing the principles of suspension–fixation. Without prior mobilization, the rectum was elevated and suspended by two strips of fascia lata which were sutured superiorly to the presacral fascia and inferiorly along the lateral aspects of the rectum (*Figure 15.9*). The cul-de-sac was obliterated and the pelvic peritoneum was sutured along each side of the rectum covering the fascial strips. Loygue *et al.* (1984), in Paris, employed a modification of this technique in which complete posterior mobilization of the rectum was carried out, using suspension with nylon strips rather than fascia lata. They recently published a series of 257 patients operated on from 1953 to 1982, with a recurrence rate of 5.6 per cent. In the earlier patients where fascia lata had been used, the recurrence rate was 10.2 per cent, while in those using nylon it was only 4.3 per cent, with nylon being used exclusively since 1962 (Loygue *et al.*, 1984). Three patients developed an intervertebral disc infection, which Loygue points out should be avoided by placing sutures into the presacral fascia and not the intervertebral disc. Christensen and Kirkegaard (1981b) published a series of 24 patients treated by the Orr procedure, using fascia lata for suspension, with a recurrence rate of 8 per cent. Loygue's use of nylon rather than fascia lata seems appropriate from both a practical as well as a technical standpoint. Furthermore, the sling problems common to the Ripstein procedure do not appear to represent a significant problem following the Orr–Loygue suspension with lateral fixation.

Anterior sling rectopexy (Ripstein)

The Ripstein procedure is currently the most commonly used procedure in the USA for the management of procidentia. In 1952, Charles Ripstein reported the successful management of four cases of rectal prolapse (Ripstein, 1952). He felt that prolapse began as a sliding hernia passing through the anterior pelvic floor defect created by the levator diastasis and then continued through the anus as an intussusception of the abnormally mobile rectosigmoid. He pointed out that in patients with procidentia the rectum had lost its posterior fixation and on straining assumed a straight course through the pelvis, such that any increased intra-abdominal pressure would encourage intussusception. Furthermore, he felt that the levators were generally atrophic and that simple suture repair, as accomplished in the Graham procedure, would not result in adequate anterior support. Therefore, his initial procedure consisted of suture repair for the levators anterior to the rectum and reinforcement of the resultant pelvic floor with a V-shaped graft of fascia lata (Ripstein, 1952). The graft was sutured anteriorly to the fascia at the base of the bladder and posteriorly to the presacral fascia about the rectum, thereby fixing the rectum to the sacrum. His early cases were managed in this fashion, but later he used Teflon mesh instead of fascia lata.

In a later paper, Ripstein (1972) made no mention of repairing the pelvic floor, but rather described his procedure as an anterior sling rectopexy. At this time he emphasized that prolapse was primarily an intussusception and that the pelvic floor defects were secondary to the intussusception. He suggested that a successful repair required adequate posterior fixation of the rectum and re-establishment of its normal horizontal position. The technique involves complete posterior mobilization of the rectum. A 5 cm band of Teflon or Marlex mesh is placed anteriorly around the rectum and the free ends are sutured to the presacral fascia 5 cm below the sacral promontory (*Figure 15.10*). Non-absorbable sutures are placed about 1 cm from the midline in order to avoid the presacral vessels. As the rectum is pulled upward, the upper and lower borders of the sling are sutured to its anterior wall to prevent displacement of the sling. The sling must be loose enough to allow two to three fingers to pass between the rectum and the sacrum. If it is too snug, it may cause stricture, stenosis or faecal impaction. If angulation of the rectum by the sling is apparent, a 'hitch' suture can be placed between the anterior surface of the presacral fascia and the mesorectum (Goldberg, Gordon and Nivatvongs, 1980). The pelvic floor is reperitonealized above in order to prevent adhesions to the sling. As of 1972, Ripstein had operated on 289 patients with apparently 1 death and 1 recurrence, but no mention is made of follow-up results or other problems (Ripstein, 1972). Morgan (1980) reported that Ripstein had performed 500 procedures with only 2 recurrences.

Review of the literature reveals that recurrence following the Ripstein procedure ranges from 5 to 13 percent, with a current composite of 6 per cent (Jurgeleit *et al.*, 1975; Biehl, Ray and Gathright, 1978; Holmstrom *et al.*, 1978; Failes, Stuart and Deluca, 1979; Morgan, 1980; Launer *et al.*, 1982) (*Table 15.2*). It is also apparent that there is a significant learning curve associated with this procedure that is reflected in recurrence rates and complications. During their first 10 years' experience of the Ripstein procedure, the Lahey Clinic group (Jurgeleit *et al.*, 1975) experienced a recurrence rate of 7.5 per cent and the Cleveland Clinic group (Launer *et al.*, 1982) a recurrence rate of 24 per cent. Both groups noted that in more recent experience their recurrence rate had dropped to 3 per cent. Most would agree that the Ripstein procedure can be performed with minimum mortality in the elderly patient population who most commonly exhibit prolapse and that, after some experience, the procedure can be performed with acceptably low recurrence rates. However, the major drawback to this procedure lies in its significant postoperative morbidity, consisting of sepsis, stenosis, sling obstruction, faecal impaction and bowel management problems. Gordon and Hoexter (1978) collected a series of 1111 cases of rectal prolapse managed by the Ripstein procedure by polling the members of the American Society of Colon and Rectal Surgeons. This

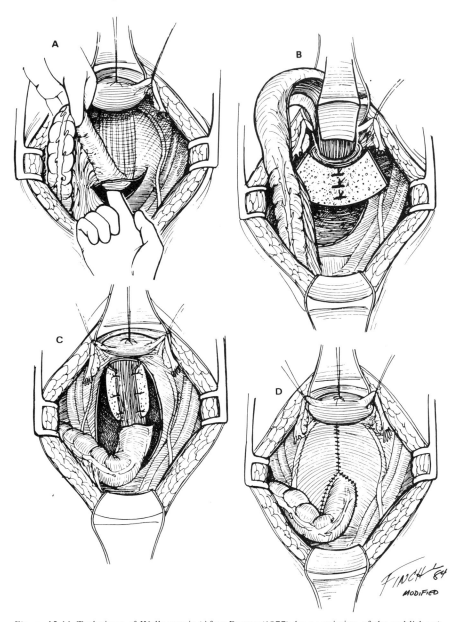

Figure 15.11. Technique of Wells repair (After Porter (1977), by permission of the publishers)

posteriorly about the rectum (*Figure 15.11*). This modification leaves the anterior one-third to one-quarter of the bowel free and thereby has eliminated the problems of stenosis, faecal impaction and sling obstruction not infrequently encountered with the Ripstein procedure. This procedure is associated with a low mortality rate comparable with that of the Ripstein procedure, while morbidity seems significantly less. Concern was initially focused on the fact that Ivalon sponge was known to be associated with the development of sarcoma in mice, but this has never been reported to occur in man.

Ivalon sponge was selected because of its propensity to induce reactive fibrosis which would assure permanent fixation of the rectum to the hollow of the sacrum. However, in the few cases which have been reoperated following the Ivalon sponge procedure, it has been found that minimal scarring has occurred and dissection of the rectum from the sacrum can be carried out without difficulty. Furthermore, we know that Ivalon sponge tends to fragment and that infection in the presence of Ivalon is a serious problem requiring its removal. For these reasons, some surgeons have utilized Marlex or Mersilene mesh instead of Ivalon sponge. Review of the literature reveals recurrence rates of 0–11.5 per cent, with a current composite recurrence rate of 3 per cent (*Table 15.5*). A recent series published by Keighley, Fielding and Alexander-Williams (1983) reported 100 consecutive patients who had undergone a Wells suspension–fixation

TABLE 15.5. Recurrence after Wells procedure

Reference	Material	No. patients Recurrence/ operated	Recurrence (per cent)
Anderson *et al.* (1981)	Ivalon	1/40	3
Boutsis and Ellis (1974)	Ivalon	3/26	12
Keighley *et al.* (1983)	Marlex	0/100	0
Kupfer and Goligher (1970)	Ivalon	0/21	0
Morgan *et al.* (1972)	Ivalon	3/93	3
Notaras (1973)	Mersilene	0/19	0
Penfold and Hawley (1972)	Ivalon	3/95	3
Stewart (1972)	Ivalon	3/41	7
		Total = 13/435 Average = 3	

procedure utilizing Marlex mesh. Eighty-six per cent of the patients have been followed for greater than 2 years with no known recurrence. Of the suspension–fixation procedures utilizing foreign material, this appears to be superior to the others, and by leaving one-third to one-quarter of the anterior wall of the rectum free, the incidence of bowel management and sling problems encountered with the Ripstein procedures diminished. Furthermore, the use of Marlex or Mersilene mesh instead of Ivalon sponge makes sense from the standpoint of permanency and better tolerance toward infection.

Technique

The Wells procedure involves complete posterior mobilization of the rectum. A rectangular sheet of Ivalon sponge (polyvinyl alcohol) is sutured to the periosteum of the sacrum by means of non-absorbable sutures. The rectum is then drawn upward and fixed in place by suturing the lateral extremities of the Ivalon sheet to the anterior rectal wall so as to form a trough leaving one-third to one-quarter of the circumference of the rectum free. The pelvic floor is reperitonealized above to prevent adhesions to the sling. Haemostasis must be meticulous, as subsequent haematoma formation might predispose toward infection in the presence of Ivalon sponge.

Puborectalis sling procedure (Nigro)

This procedure, originally described by Nigro (1958), was designed as a suspension–fixation procedure that would support and stabilize the rectum by simulating the normal puborectalis sling. The procedure accomplishes two important things as far as the management of prolapse is concerned. First, the sling elevates and fixes the rectum to the sacrum. Secondly, it re-creates the anorectal angle and in doing so theoretically improves the patient's continence. Parks, Porter and Hardcastle (1966) and Parks (1967) emphasized the importance of the anorectal angle in the mechanism of continence. This angle and the horizontal position of the rectum are lost in prolapse patients who demonstrate varying degrees of incontinence.

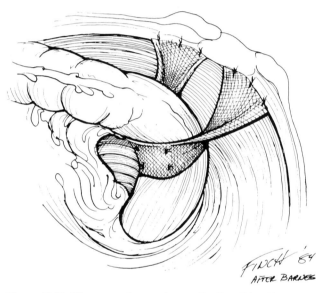

Figure 15.12. Nigro procedure: puborectalis sling (After Corman (1984), by permission of the publishers)

The procedure utilizes a Teflon sling which is fixed posteriorly around the lower rectum and anteriorly to the pubic tubercles (*Figure 15.12*). Nigro initially used a perineal transcoccygeal approach, but later found the transabdominal approach to be more appropriate. Once the rectum has been mobilized posteriorly, the prevesicle space is opened anteriorly to expose the pubic tubercles. A 3 × 20 cm strip of Marlex or Teflon is used for the sling. The mid-portion of the sling is sutured to the posterior and lateral aspects of the rectum. Using a large curved clamp, a tunnel is made from each pubic tubercle down to the level of the obturator foramen and then posteriorly to the retrorectal space. The ends of the sling are grasped with the clamp, drawn through the retroperitoneal tunnels and sutured to their respective pubic tubercles, so as to elevate the rectum out of the pelvis and recreate the acute anorectal angle (Greene, 1983). Nigro (1978) reports excellent results in over 60 patients in whom there have been no recurrences. Greene (1983) published a report of 15 patients managed by means of transabdominal placement of a puborectalis sling using Marlex mesh. The follow-up period ranged from 6 months to 4 yr with no recurrence. In addition, he noted that preoperatively 53 per cent of patients were incontinent while postoperatively all regained continence. An intriguing aspect of this procedure is its corrective effect on incontinence due to restoration of the anorectal angle, similar to the effect produced by a Parks postanal repair. Furthermore, as noted by Nigro, urinary incontinence is also improved.

Transabdominal procedures: prevention of intussusception

Devadhar (1965) and Wedell, ZuEissen and Fiedler (1980) emphasized that prolapse is an intussusception and not a sliding hernia. Therefore, they reasoned the repair of procidentia should be aimed at the prevention of intussusception, not the repair of pelvic floor defects which are secondary to the prolapse. These authors approach the technical aspects of treatment differently, but with a similarity of concept.

Rectal plication (Devadhar)

Devadhar (1965, 1967) feels that the primary pathology in patients with prolapse resides in the rectum which is hyposensitive. This leads to increased proximal peristalsis converging on a 'crucial point' of the rectum about 2 in (50 mm) below the sacral promontory. He feels this is the site of the rectorectal intussusception and can be identified at surgery by palpation of the transition between the thickened distal rectum and the normal proximal rectum. Frequently, this point is identifiable by a white fibrous band on the anterior wall of the bowel. His method of treatment consists of creating a reverse intussusception at this 'crucial point' by plicating proximal rectum over distal rectum with anteriorly placed Lembert sutures and laterally placed reefing sutures (*Figure 15.13*). This reversed intussusception is effected only in the anterior two-thirds of the rectum. The purpose of the lateral plicating sutures is to shorten the rectum longitudinally and 'splint' the rectal wall to further discourage intussusception. No posterior mobilization is necessary. Devadhar (1967) reported 27 cases followed over an average of 5 yr with no recurrence. He further points out that in accordance with his theory, the Ripstein and the Wells procedures obtain their excellent results because of the stinting effect of the sling on the rectum, rather than any fixation to the presacral fascia. Penfold and Hawley (1972) observed that on reoperation of patients with implanted Ivalon sponge there was minimal fibrous tissue formed between the sacrum and the rectum and, therefore, the success of the operation in controlling prolapse was probably due to stinting of the rectal walls, which prevented intussusception.

Ivalon stint (Wedell)

That stinting of the rectal wall can prevent prolapse would appear to be further substantiated by Wedell, ZuEissen and Fiedler (1980), who reported 5 cases of procidentia successfully managed by wrapping Ivalon sponge partially around the mobilized rectum as in the Wells procedure, but without sacral fixation (*Figure 15.14*). In addition, a prolapsing colostomy was successfully corrected in a similar fashion by wrapping the distal colon in a sleeve of Ivalon just proximal to its exit through the abdominal wall. Wedell reports no recurrence, but his follow-up is short.

This concept is certainly provocative and the management innovative. However, the reported series is small and at present unconfirmed by others.

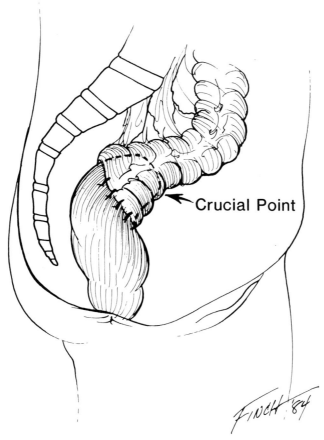

Figure 15.13. Devadhar procedure: a reverse intussusception (After Devadhar (1967), by permission of the publishers)

Perineal procedures: rectosigmoidectomy

Amputative rectosigmoidectomy was described by Mikulicz in 1889, and in 1933 was championed by Miles for the management of rectal cancer (Goligher, 1980). The application of this procedure to the management of procidentia is attractive from the standpoint that it is tolerated very well by the elderly and debilitated patients. The names of Altemeier, Auffret, Mikulicz and Miles are frequently associated with a particular modification of this general approach. Altemeier felt strongly that for the management of procidentia this procedure should include: (a) resection of redundant rectosigmoid, (b) anterior suture repair of the levator ani and puborectalis, and (c) obliteration of the deep cul-de-sac. This is consistent with his belief that in the majority of cases procidentia is a sliding hernia. Altemeier *et al.* (1971) reported a series of 106 patients managed in this fashion with a recurrence rate of 2.8 per cent. Unfortunately, no one has been able to duplicate these results in a similarly large series of patients (*Table 15.6*). Hughes (1949) published a series of 150 patients at St Mark's Hospital, London, who underwent perineal rectosigmoidectomy for the management of procidentia. He reported a recurrence rate of over 60 per cent and more than half of the

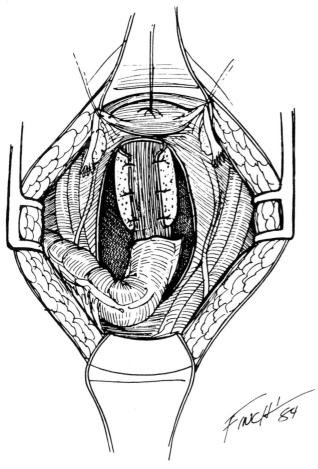

Figure 15.14. Wedell procedure: rectal stint to prevent intussusception (After Wedell, Zu Eissen and Fiedler (1980), by permission of the publishers)

TABLE 15.6. Recurrence after perineal rectosigmoidectomy*

Reference	No. patients Recurrence/operated	Recurrence (per cent)
Altemeier *et al.* (1971)	3/106	3
Friedman (1983)	13/27	50
Hughes (1949)	55/108	60
Porter (1962b)	52/110	58
Theuerhauf *et al.* (1970)	3/13	39
Authors' series	0/33	0
	Total = 126/397	Average = 32

* See text for discussion regarding discrepant recurrence rates reported after this operation.

patients were incontinent. Porter (1962) reported an additional 110 patients in the St Mark's series who in addition to rectosigmoidectomy had repair of the levator hiatus and suture of the puborectalis muscles. The results did not seem to be improved by repair of the levators since recurrence developed in 58 per cent.

At the University of Minnesota affiliated hospitals we have performed a perineal rectosigmoidectomy in 33 patients with an average age of 78 yr. These patients were followed from 1 to 6 yr with no recurrence, no mortality and excellent or good results in 73 per cent. Fair or poor results were present in 28 per cent because of incontinence. We do not routinely repair the levators nor suture the puborectalis muscle. This is our procedure of choice for the elderly, debilitated patient who, in fact, tolerates this operation so well that we have not found it necessary to perform anal encirclement procedures. However, we have limited perineal rectosigmoidectomy to this category of patient because of our concern over the high recurrence rates reported by others, and the chance that resection of distal anorectum may interfere with continence (Hughes, 1949; Porter, 1962b; Theuerkauf, Beahrs and Hill, 1970; Altemeier *et al.*, 1971; Friedman, Muggia-Sulam and Freund, 1983). O'Carroll (1949) observed that, following perineal rectosigmoidectomy, patients had an afferent sensory alteration in their mechanism of continence. Theoretically, reduction of the ampullary reservoir secondary to resection in addition to this sensory change could result in diminished continence. In our series of 33 patients, now 1–6 yr after perineal rectosigmoidectomy, only 6 per cent felt their level of continence had improved, while 22 per cent felt it had diminished.

Technique

Perineal rectosigmoidectomy (*Figure 15.15a*) can be performed in either the prone jack-knife or dorsal lithotomy position. It requires that the rectum can be prolapsed a minimum of 5 cm through the anal verge. Two to three centimetres proximal to the dentate line, the mucosa and submucosa are infiltrated with a solution containing 1:200 000 units of adrenaline. A circumferential full thickness incision is made completely incising the outer cylinder of bowel. The rectosigmoid is mobilized by opening the peritoneum and taking down its posterior and lateral mesenteric attachments. This procedure is continued until the redundant bowel cannot be pulled down any further. Approximately 2 cm distal to the anus the everted inner cylinder of bowel is transsected. A redundant segment of 6–25 cm is resected and the anastomosis is performed 1–2 cm proximal to the dentate line, either with interrupted sutures or with an intraluminal stapling device. When stapling devices are used, the bowel should be transsected 1 cm longer to allow for the cuff resected with these instruments (Uhlig and Sullivan, 1979) (*Figure 15.15b*).

Perineal procedures: Delorme procedure

The Delorme procedure is based on the principle of stripping the mucosa from the redundant prolapsed rectum over a distance of several centimeters, and then plicating the denuded bowel wall to form a supralevator muscular pessary which prevents further prolapse. In addition, Uhlig and Sullivan (1979) recommend plication of the external sphincter, repair of the levator diastasis and any other pelvic floor defects which may be present, such as a rectocele. They perform the mucosal stripping and plication through the anal orifice with the prolapse reduced rather than everted.

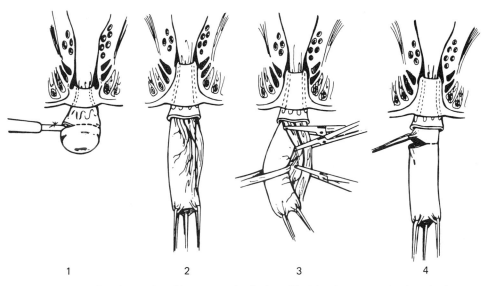

Figure 15.15(a). Perineal rectosigmoidectomy: 1, beginning of incision 2–3 cm proximal to the dentate line; 2, unfolding of prolapsing segment; 3, division of mesentery; 4, division of inner cylinder of intestine

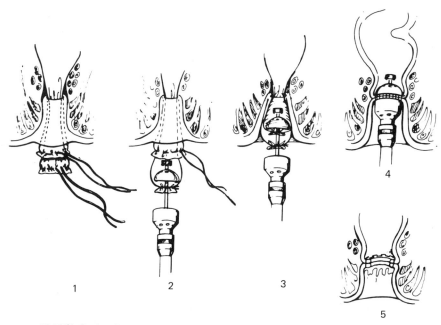

Figure 15.15(b). Perineal rectosigmoidectomy — anastomosis utilizing an intraluminal stapling device: 1, placement of purse-string sutures; 2, proximal purse-string suture secured around anvil; 3, distal purse-string suture secured; 4, closure of instrument, ready for firing; 5, completed anastomosis (After Vermuelen *et al.* (1983), by permission of the publishers)

TABLE 15.7. Recurrence after Delorme procedure

Reference	No. patients Recurrence/operated	Recurrence (per cent)
Aminev and Malyshev (1964)	67/281	24
Christensen and Kirkegaard (1981a)	1/12	17
Moskalenko (1973)	0/21	0
Nay and Blair (1972)	3/30	10
Uhlig and Sullivan (1979)	3/44	7
	Total = 74/388	Average = 11

Review of the literature reveals that recurrence rates range from 0 to 24 per cent following the Delorme procedure (Aminev and Malyshev, 1964; Nay and Blair, 1972; Uhlig and Sullivan, 1979; Labow *et al.*, 1980; Christensen and Kirkegaard, 1981b) (*Table 15.7*). Like the perineal rectosigmoidectomy, the Delorme procedure is usually performed under general or regional anaesthesia, but can be performed under local anaesthesia. Unlike the perineal rectosigmoidectomy, it is applicable to the hidden or occult procidentia which has not yet reached the stage of development where it can be prolapsed through the anus. The Delorme procedure may be an attractive alternative to perineal rectosigmoidectomy, and Uhlig and Sullivan (1979) have been pleased with results in the elderly, poor risk patient. They have reported good functional results and a recurrence rate of 6.8 per cent in 44 patients followed up 2–10 yr.

Technique

The Delorme procedure is performed either in the prone jack-knife or lithotomy position. A circumferential incision is made 1 cm proximal to the dentate line and a plane is developed between the mucosa and the circular muscle layer of the bowel wall. This dissection is facilitated and haemostasis promoted by a submucosal injection of a solution containing 1:200 000 units of adrenaline. Upward dissection continues until traction on the mucosal sleeve gives resistance. At this stage, Uhlig and Sullivan (1979) recommend a multiphasic repair consisting of repair of the perineal body and rectocele defect, repair of anal sphincter defects, longitudinal plication of the circular muscle of the rectum, excision of the mobilized mucosa, and finally anastomosis of the mucosa at the dentate line.

Perineal procedures: suspension–fixation (Wyatt procedure)

Posterior rectopexy from a perineal approach was one of the earliest forms of treatment for procidentia. Methods to accomplish this by suture of the rectal wall to the sacrum were described by Lang in 1887, Tuttle in 1903 and Grant in 1923, but because of dismal recurrence rates, fell into disrepute (Goligher, 1980). Wyatt (1981) described a modification of the Wells procedure using a perineal approach to suspension–fixation of the rectum. The anococcygeal ligament is incised, the levators separated to gain access to the retrorectal space and the rectum mobilized up to Waldeyer's fascia. In some patients the coccyx is removed in order to gain added exposure. A sheet of Mersilene mesh is fixed to the presacral fascia and then wrapped partially about the rectum in a fashion similar to the Wells procedure. Difficulty is occasionally encountered with the deep placement of the anchoring sutures to fix the Mersilene mesh to the presacral fascia, so a special stapling device was developed for this purpose. Wyatt performed this procedure in 22 patients with 1 recurrence, which was due to the mesh becoming detached from the sacrum. Again, the anatomical approach is unfamiliar to most and is unlikely ever to gain popularity. Furthermore, the use of foreign material through a perineal incision is unattractive from the standpoint of its potential for infection.

Perineal procedures: anal encirclement procedures (Thiersch and modifications)

The classic Thiersch procedure, originally described in 1891 by Thiersch and popularized by Gabriel in 1951, utilized a subcutaneous stainless steel wire which encircled and partially obstructed the anal outlet (Goligher, 1980) (*Figure 15.16*). Theoretically, the wire would evoke a tissue reaction resulting in a fibrous ring which would ensure long-term success even after removal of the wire. However, practically speaking, the procedure did nothing for the underlying pathology of procidentia, but merely kept the prolapse hidden above the perineum. Furthermore, the wire failed to cause fibrosis and frequent problems of breakage, erosion or protrusion led to removal of the wire with recurrence of the prolapse. Bowel management and nursing care problems were frequently aggravated rather than improved, with faecal impaction becoming a frequent and formidable problem. The primary advantage of this procedure was that it could be performed easily and quickly under local anaesthesia in the poor risk patient.

Many modifications have been proposed using various materials. The materials are inert in order to resist infection, pliable to eliminate the problem of fracture, soft to

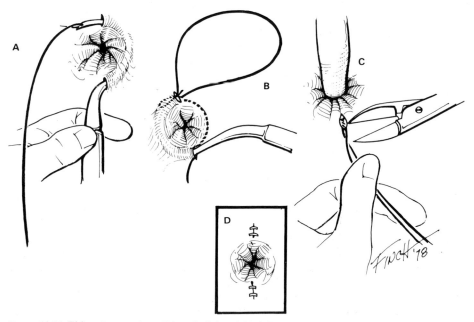

Figure 15.16. Thiersch procedure (After Goligher (1980), by permission of the publishers)

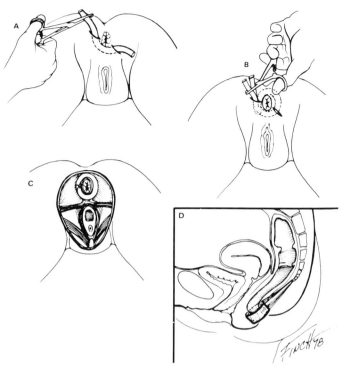

Figure 15.17. Lomas and Cooperman modification of the Thiersch procedure (After Lomas and Cooperman (1972), by permission of the publishers)

avoid erosion and, in some cases, semi-elastic to allow expansion of the anal canal with bowel movements. These modifications place a synthetic cuff about the anal canal anywhere from a supralevator location proposed by Notaras (1973) to a mid-anal canal level proposed by others (Lomas and Cooperman, 1972; Labow *et al.*, 1980) (*Figure 15.17*). This 0.5–1.5 cm wide synthetic cuff functionally narrows and lengthens the anal canal, supports the patulous external sphincter and not only prevents prolapse, but also supposedly assists in maintaining continence. In fact, Corman (1984) has recently proposed using a silastic impregnated Dacron cuff in the management of selected cases of idiopathic incontinence. By expanding the scope of this procedure, these modifications have also expanded the magnitude of the procedure. Patients undergo mechanical and antibiotic bowel preparation preoperatively and receive parenteral antibiotics postoperatively. These procedures are frequently performed under general, caudal or low spinal anaesthesia, but can occasionally be done with local anaesthesia supplemented by sedation. The results have been satisfactory in a series of 25 patients reported by Lomas and Cooperman (1972) utilizing a strip of Marlex mesh. In 2 cases, healing progressed in the face of a wound infection without removal of the Marlex. Labow *et al.* (1980) reported excellent results in 9 patients using a 1–1.5 cm wide strip of Dacron-impregnated silastic which has elastic characteristics and would seem ideally suited to this purpose. In no patients was infection, erosion or impaction a problem. The newer modifications may represent an improvement over the original Thiersch procedure, but require a more formidable surgical/anaesthetic intervention. Furthermore, the placement of a foreign material in a perineal wound is unattractive from the standpoint of its potential for infection. It has been our experience that the poor risk patient tolerates perineal rectosigmoidectomy or the Delorme procedure so well that there has been no need to use the anal encirclement procedures.

Trans-sacral approach: suspension–fixation (Thomas procedure)

The trans-sacral approach has been recommended by Thomas (1975) and Davidian and Thomas (1972) as well as by Hagihara and Griffen (1975), in the management of procidentia. It is their feeling that this approach is advantageous because it is well tolerated by the elderly, debilitated patient and lends itself well to correction of associated abnormalities such as levator diastasis, deep cul-de-sac and redundant rectosigmoid. The patient is placed in a prone jack-knife position and the incision is made lateral to the sacrum extending from the coccyx to the third sacral vertebra. The coccyx and fifth sacral segment are removed and the redundant rectum is delivered through the wound. The repair consists of anterior approximation of the levators, obliteration of the cul-de-sac and suture fixation of the rectum to the presacral fascia. Resection is performed only if there is marked redundancy and concern over volvulus. Thomas (1975) reported 44 cases managed in this fashion without a recurrence. However, postoperative morbidity of 38 per cent occurred, with the most common problem being wound infection in 20 per cent of the patients. In addition, 25 per cent of those (Browning and Parks, 1983) who underwent a segmental resection developed a leak of the anastomosis. This procedure has not gained popularity because the anatomical approach is unfamiliar to most surgeons and has historically been associated with a significant incidence of local wound problems. Low resection performed through this approach continues to be associated with a significant incidence of leak with formation of a faecal fistula and should be performed with caution. In our view, the trans-sacral approach popularized by Kraske is associated with significant morbidity and has been appropriately discarded by most surgeons.

Occult prolapse

Occult or hidden prolapse refers to that condition in which the prolapse occupies the rectal ampulla and has not yet protruded through the anus. This probably represents an early stage in the development of complete procidentia. This condition gives rise to the symptoms of constipation, obstruction, tenesmus, pain, mucous discharge and, occasionally, incontinence. Examination is frequently unremarkable except for evidence of irritation of the anterior rectum consisting of oedema, petechiae and, occasionally, frank ulceration compatible with 'solitary rectal ulcer syndrome'. However, if the patient is asked to bear down, the intussuscepting mass and the descending perineum will be appreciated (Goldberg, Gordon and Nivatvongs, 1980). Ihre and Seligson (1975) reviewed 90 cases of occult prolapse and treated 40 by means of a Ripstein procedure. They found that 64 per cent were subjectively improved, 26 per cent were unchanged and 10 per cent were worse. Of the 14 patients whose main complaint had been pain, tenesmus or obstruction, only 36 per cent were improved. However, of those patients who were incontinent preoperatively, 75 per cent regained continence. Therefore, Ihre and Seligson recommend that with occult prolapse, unless the patient develops incontinence, a trial of conservative management should be attempted consisting of bulk agents, high fibre diet, stool softeners, and avoidance of frequent and excessive straining at stool. Of interest is the fact that some of Ihre and Seligson's untreated patients went on to develop complete rectal prolapse, confirming the concept that this is a part of the spectrum of procidentia. Ripstein (1975) treated 12 patients with occult procidentia, and 11 became asymptomatic. Certainly, in the absence of incontinence a trial of conservative management is warranted, but if this fails to significantly alleviate symptoms, operation is advised.

Incontinence

Published series indicate that the incidence of incontinence associated with procidentia varies from 11 to 81 per cent (*Table 15.8*). Approximately half of those patients who are incontinent will improve following a transabdominal repair of the prolapse, but this may require 6–12 months. Persistence of incontinence despite anatomical correction of the prolapse represents the major cause of postoperative patient disability and dissatisfaction. Few studies have addressed the problem of incontinence to any depth. For some time it was felt that the mechanical stretching of the sphincter with prolapse caused the incontinence. However, Parks, Porter and Hardcastle (1966) pointed out that patients with incontinence, either idiopathic or associated with prolapse, all demonstrated abnormal perineal descent on straining. EMG and biopsy studies confirmed Parks's theory that incontinence was the result of this abnormal perineal descent which led to a traction injury of the pudendal and perineal nerves, resulting in denervation of the pelvic floor musculature and sphincters (Parks, Swash and Urich, 1977). This may explain the persistence of incontinence in some patients, despite anatomical correction of procidentia. Following transabdominal procedures for the correction of procidentia, incontinence improves in 40–64 per cent of patients (*Table 15.8*). Following perineal rectosigmoidectomy, incontinence improves in only 6–20 per cent of the patients and, in this respect, the functional results of transabdominal procedures are superior to the perineal rectosigmoidectomy (*Table 15.8*). When selecting the appropriate procedure for correction of prolapse, it is important to consider the potential effect on continence. Ideally, the corrective procedure should maintain or restore continence. In our experience 38 per cent of the patients with unacceptable incontinence preoperatively regained an acceptable level of continence following proctopexy and rectosigmoid resection. Overall, 69 per cent of patients remain unchanged, 29 per cent improved and only 2 per cent felt their level of continence had diminished. However, following perineal rectosigmoidectomy, 72 per cent remained unchanged, only 6 per cent improved and 22 per cent complained of diminished continence (*Table 15.8*). From the work of Keighley, Matheson and Duncan (1981) and Keighley and Fielding (1983) it appears that preoperative anal manometry is of no predictive value in determining which patients will regain acceptable levels of continence following correction of prolapse. It is further apparent that rectopexy has no effect on basal resting or maximal squeeze pressures. Parks, Porter and Hardcastle (1966) and Parks (1967) emphasized the importance of the puborectalis muscle in the maintenance of continence. This muscle normally displaces the rectum anteriorly and upward, creating the acute anorectal angle and flap valve configuration so important in the maintenance of normal continence. Frequently, this angle and the horizontal position of the rectum are lost in prolapse patients with abnormal perineal descent and varying degrees of incontinence. The Parks postanal repair restored satisfactory continence in more than 80 per cent of patients in whom incontinence persisted following anatomical correction of prolapse (Keighley, Matheson and Duncan, 1981;

TABLE 15.8. Restoration of continence vs. type of repair

Reference	Procedure	No. patients	Incontinence		Improvement (per cent)
			Preoperative	Postoperative	
	Transabdominal:				
Holmstrom et al. (1978)	Ripstein	59	54	22	59
Keighley et al. (1983)	Wells	100	67	24	64
Morgan et al. (1972)	Wells	103	81	39	52
Christensen and Kirkegaard (1981b)	Orr–Loygue	24	46	25	46
Authors' series*	Frykman–Goldberg	61	24	15	38
	Perineal:				
Friedman et al. (1983)	Rectosigmoidectomy	27	41	33	20
Theuerkauf et al. (1970)	Rectosigmoidectomy	10	50	40	20
Christensen and Kirkegaard (1981a)	Delorme	12	50	33	33
Authors' series*	Rectosigmoidectomy	18	12	28	−16

* Unpublished data. University of Minnesota affiliated hospitals (major or total incontinence only).

Keighley and Fielding, 1983). This repair consists of a postanal intersphincteric approach to the levators with posterior plication of the levators, puborectalis and deep external sphincter, so as to recreate the acute anorectal angle. Browning and Parks (1983) point out that, following postanal repair, those patients regaining continence demonstrate functional lengthening of the anal canal as well as increased basal and maximal squeeze pressures.

Postoperative regulation of bowel habits by use of a high fibre diet, bulk agents, avoidance of diarrhoea and correction of mucosal prolapse, if present, will correct minor degrees of incontinence. Mucosal prolapse occurs in 5–13 per cent of patients following any of the various procedures for correction of full thickness rectal prolapse (Kupfer and Goligher, 1970; Morgan, Porter and Klugman, 1972; Goldberg and Gordon, 1975). This can frequently be managed with simple rubber band ligation and rarely requires an excisional type of proctoplasty. It is important to correct this problem because this in itself can improve the patient's results by eliminating irritating mucus soilage and minor degrees of incontinence.

Conclusions

Controversy regarding the ideal operation for procidentia of the rectum persists. Mature judgement is required to properly match the patient to the appropriate procedure. One must consider the operative and anaesthetic risk factors of the patient, the extent of the prolapse and the preoperative state of anal continence.

These factors are then balanced against the characteristics of a given procedure, i.e. its recurrence rate, morbidity, mortality and odds of improving or maintaining continence.

In spite of all the controversies associated with its management, the following conclusions have guided our approach to procidentia:

1. The good risk patient should be managed by a transabdominal suspension–fixation procedure with or without resection.
2. Complete posterior mobilization of the rectum is essential to any transabdominal repair of procidentia.
3. Anterior mobilization, repair of the levators and obliteration of the cul-de-sac are unnecessary.
4. The need for resection should be individualized and is relatively contraindicated when using foreign material.
5. The posteriorly placed, partially-surrounding, Wells-type fixation is preferred to the anterior Ripstein-type sling which is associated with a significant incidence of problems such as stenosis, faecal impaction and sling obstruction.
6. Of all the foreign material used, Ivalon sponge appears to be the least appropriate due to poor tolerance for infection and lack of permanency, while Marlex and Mersilene mesh would appear to be better choices.
7. The poor risk patient is best managed by either a perineal rectosigmoidectomy or Delorme procedure.
8. The anal encirclement procedures have a very limited place in the modern management of rectal prolapse.
9. Incontinence, not infrequently associated with procidentia, represents a major aspect in the overall management of patients with prolapse, and is more likely to improve following transabdominal repairs than after perineal repairs.

10. Those patients who are unacceptably incontinent 6–12 months following correction of procidentia should be treated by a Parks postanal repair.

References

ALTEMEIER, W. A., CUTHBERTSON, W. R., SCHOWENGERDT, C. and HUNT, J. (1971). Nineteen years experience with the one-stage perineal repair of rectal prolapse. *Annals of Surgery*, **173**, 993–1006

AMINEV, A. M. and MALYSHEV, J. U. I. (1964). Rectal prolapse: a comparative evaluation of some operative methods of treatment concerning late observations made by the surgeons of the Soviet Union. *American Journal of Proctology*, **15**, 355–360

ANDERSON, J. R., KENNENMONTH, A. W. G. and SMITH, A. N. (1981). Polyvinyl alcohol sponge rectopexy for complete rectal prolapse. *Journal of the Royal College of Surgeons of Edinburgh*, **26**, 292–294

BIEHL, A. G., RAY, J. E. and GATHRIGHT, J. B. (1978). Repair of rectal prolapse: experience with the Ripstein sling. *Southern Medical Journal*, **71**, 923–925

BOMAR, R. L. and SAWYERS, J. L. (1977). Transabdominal proctopexy (Ripstein procedure) for massive rectal prolapse. *American Surgeon*, **43**, 97–100

BOUTSIS, C. and ELLIS, H. (1974). The Ivalon-sponge-wrap operation for rectal prolapse: an experience with 26 patients. *Diseases of the Colon and Rectum*, **17**, 21–37

BRITTEN-JONES, R. (1977). In *Operative Surgery*, p. 228 (I. P. Todd, Ed.). London; Butterworths

BRODEN, B. and SNELLMAN, B. (1968). Procidentia of the rectum studied with cineradiography: a contribution to the discussion of causative mechanism. *Diseases of the Colon and Rectum*, **11**, 330–347

BROWNING, G. G. P. and PARKS, A. G. (1983). Postanal repair for neuropathic faecal incontinence: correlation of clinical result and anal canal pressures. *British Journal of Surgery*, **70**, 101–104

CARTER, A. E. (1983). Rectosacral suture fixation for complete rectal prolapse in the elderly, the frail, and the demented. *British Journal of Surgery*, **70**, 522–523

CHRISTENSEN, J. and KIRKEGAARD, P. (1981a). Delorme's operation for complete rectal prolapse. *British Journal of Surgery*, **68**, 537–538

CHRISTENSEN, J. and KIRKEGAARD, P. (1981b). Complete prolapse of the rectum treated by modified Orr operation. *Diseases of the Colon and Rectum*, **24**, 90–92

CONYERS, C. L. and CULLEN, P. K. (1974). Correction of rectal prolapse by anterior resection. *Western Journal of Medicine*, **121**, 270–273

CORMAN, M. L. (1984). *Colon and Rectal Surgery*, 1st edn, pp. 134–137. Philadelphia; Lippincott

DAVIDIAN, V. A. and THOMAS, C. G. (1972). Transsacral repair of rectal prolapse. *American Journal of Surgery*, **123**, 231–235

DEVADHAR, D. S. C. (1965). A new concept of mechanism and treatment of rectal procidentia. *Diseases of the Colon and Rectum*, **8**, 75–77

DEVADHAR, D. S. C. (1967). Surgical correction of rectal procidentia. *Surgery*, **62**, 847–852

EFRON, G. (1977). A simple method of posterior rectopexy for rectal procidentia. *Surgery, Gynecology and Obstetrics*, **145**, 75–76

FAILES, D., STUART, M. and DELUCA, C. (1979). Rectal prolapse. *Australian and New Zealand Journal of Medicine*, **49**, 72–75

FERGUSON, E. F. and HOUSTON, C. H. (1981). Omental pedicle graft rectopexy for rectal procidentia. *Diseases of the Colon and Rectum*, **24**, 417–421

FRIEDMAN, R., MUGGIA-SULAM, J. and FREUND, H. R. (1983). Experience with the one-stage perineal repair of rectal prolapse. *Diseases of the Colon and Rectum*, **26**, 789–791

FRYKMAN, H. M. and GOLDBERG, S. M. (1969). The surgical treatment of rectal procidentia. *Surgery, Gynecology and Obstetrics*, **129**, 1225–1230

GOLDBERG, S. M. and GORDON, P. H. (1975). Treatment of rectal prolapse. *Clinics of Gastroenterology*, **4**, 489–504

GOLDBERG, S. M., GORDON, P. H. and NIVATVONGS, S. (1980). *Essentials of Anorectal Surgery*, pp. 248–268. Philadelphia; Lippincott

GOLIGHER, J. C. (1980). *Surgery of the Anus, Rectum and Colon*, 4th edn, pp. 224–258. New York; Macmillan

GOLIGHER, J. (1984). *Surgery of the Anus, Rectum and Colon*, 5th edn, pp. 246–284. London; Baillière, Tindall

GORDON, P. H. and HOEXTER, B. (1978). Complications of the Ripstein procedure. *Diseases of the Colon and Rectum*, **21**, 277–280

GRAHAM, R. R. (1942). The operative repair of massive rectal prolapse. *Annals of Surgery*, **115**, 1007–1014

GREENE, F. L. (1983). Repair of rectal prolapse using a puborectalis sling procedure. *Archives of Surgery*, **118**, 398–400

HAGIHARA, P. F. and GRIFFEN, W. O. (1975). Transsacral repair of rectal prolapse. *Archives of Surgery*, **110**, 343–344

HOLMSTROM, B., AHLBERG, J., BERGSTRAND, O., GORAN, B. and EWERTH, S. (1978). Results of the treatment of rectal prolapse operated according to Ripstein. *Acta Chirurgica Scandinavica*, Supplement, **482**, 51–52

HUGHES, E. S. R. (1949). In discussion on rectal prolapse. *Proceedings of the Royal Society of Medicine*, **42**, 1007–1011

HUGHES, E. S. R. and JOHNSON, W. R. (1980). Abdominoperineal levator ani repair for rectal prolapse: technique. *Australian and New Zealand Journal of Medicine*, **50**, 117–120

IHRE, T. and SELIGSON, U. (1975). Intussusception of the rectum—internal procidentia: treatment and results in 90 patients. *Diseases of the Colon and Rectum*, **18**, 391–396

JURGELEIT, H. C., CORMAN, M. L., COLLER, J. A. and VEIDENHEIMER, M. C. (1975). Procidentia of the rectum: Teflon sling repair of rectal prolapse, Lahey Clinic experience. *Diseases of the Colon and Rectum*, **18**, 464–467

KEIGHLEY, M. R. B. and FIELDING, J. W. L. (1983). Management of faecal incontinence and results of surgical treatment. *British Journal of Surgery*, **70**, 463–468

KEIGHLEY, M. R. B., FIELDING, J. W. L. and ALEXANDER-WILLIAMS, J. (1983). Rectopexy for rectal prolapse in 100 consecutive patients. *British Journal of Surgery*, **70**, 229–232

KEIGHLEY, M. R. B., MATHESON, D. M. and DUNCAN, M. M. (1981). Results of treatment for rectal prolapse and fecal incontinence. *Diseases of the Colon and Rectum*, **24**, 449–453

KENNEDY, D. K., HUGHES, E. S. R. and MASTERTON, J. P. (1977). The natural history of benign ulcer of the rectum. *Surgery, Gynecology and Obstetrics*, **144**, 718–720

KHUBCHANDANI, I. T. and BACON, H. E. (1965). Complete prolapse of the rectum and its treatment. *Archives of Surgery*, **90**, 337–340

KUIJPERS, J. H. C. and LUBBERS, E. J. C. (1983). The Roseoc Graham–Goligher procedure in the treatment of complete rectal prolapse. *Netherlands Journal of Surgery*, **35**, 24–26

KUPFER, C. A. and GOLIGHER, J. C. (1970). One hundred consecutive cases of complete prolapse of the rectum treated by operation. *British Journal of Surgery*, **57**, 481–487

LABOW, S., RUBIN, R., HOEXTER, B. and SALVATI, E. (1980). Perineal repair of procidentia with an elastic fabric sling. *Diseases of the Colon and Rectum*, **23**, 467–469

LAUNER, D. P., FAZIO, V. W., WEAKLEY, F. L., TURNBULL, R. B., JAGELMAN, D. G. and LAVERY, I. C. (1982). The Ripstein procedure: a 16 year experience. *Diseases of the Colon and Rectum*, **25**, 41–45

LESCHER, T. J., CORMAN, M. L., COLLER, J. A. and VEIDENHEIMER, M. C. (1979). Management of late complications of Teflon sling repair for rectal prolapse. *Diseases of the Colon and Rectum*, **22**, 445–447

LOMAS, M. I. and COOPERMAN, H. (1972). Correction of rectal procidentia by use of a polypropylene mesh (Marlex). *Diseases of the Colon and Rectum*, **15**, 416–419

LOYGUE, J., NORDLINGER, B., CUNEI, O., MALAFOSSE, M., HUGUET, C. and PARC, R. (1984). Rectopexy to the promontory for the treatment of rectal prolapse. *Diseases of the Colon and Rectum*, **27**, 356–359

McCANN, F. J. (1928). Note on an operation for the cure of prolapse of the rectum. *Lancet*, **214**, 1072–1073

MOORE, H. D. (1977). The results of treatment for complete prolapse of the rectum in the adult patient. *Diseases of the Colon and Rectum*, **20**, 566–569

MORGAN, B. (1980). The Teflon sling operation for repair of complete rectal prolapse. *Australian and New Zealand Journal of Medicine*, **50**, 121–123

MORGAN, C. N., PORTER, N. H. and KLUGMAN, D. J. (1972). Ivalon (polyvinyl alcohol) sponge in the repair of complete rectal prolapse. *British Journal of Surgery*, **59**, 841–846

MOSCHCOWITZ, A. V. (1912). The pathogenesis, anatomy, and cure of prolapse of the rectum. *Surgery, Gynecology and Obstetrics*, **15**, 7–21

MOSKALENKO, V. W. (1973). Modification of Delorme's resection of rectal mucosa for prolapse of the rectum. *International Surgery*, **58**, 192–194

MUIR, E. G. (1962). Treatment of complete rectal prolapse in the adult. *Proceedings of the Royal Society of Medicine*, **55**, 1086

NAY, H. R. and BLAIR, C. R. (1972). Perineal surgical repair of rectal prolapse. *American Journal of Surgery*, **123**, 577–579

NEILL, M. E., PARKS, A. G. and SWASH, M. (1981). Physiological studies of the anal sphincter musculature in faecal incontinence and rectal prolapse. *British Journal of Surgery*, **68**, 531–536

NIGRO, N. D. (1958). Restoration of the levator sling in the treatment of rectal procidentia. *Diseases of the Colon and Rectum*, **1**, 123–127

NIGRO, N. D. (1966). An evaluation of the cause and mechanism of complete rectal prolapse. *Diseases of the Colon and Rectum*, **9**, 391–398

NIGRO, N. D. (1978). Symposium on colon and rectal surgery: procidentia of the rectum. *Surgical Clinics of America*, **58**, 539–554

NOTARAS, M. J. (1973). The use of Mersilene mesh in rectal prolapse repair. *Proceedings of the Royal Society of Medicine*, **66**, 684–686

O'CARROLL, C. B. (1949). *Proceedings of the Royal Society of Medicine*, **42**, 1014–1015

ORR, T. G. (1947). A suspension operation for prolapse of the rectum. *Annals of Surgery*, **126**, 833–840

PARKS, A. G. (1967). Post-anal perineorrhaphy for rectal prolapse. *Proceedings of the Royal Society of Medicine*, **60**, 920–921

PARKS, A. G., PORTER, N. H. and HARDCASTLE, J. (1966). The syndrome of the descending perineum. *Proceedings of the Royal Society of Medicine*, **59**, 477–482

PARKS, A. G., SWASH, M. and URICH, H. (1977). Sphincter denervation in anorectal incontinence and rectal prolapse. *Gut*, **18**, 656–665

PEMBERTON, J. de J. and STALKER, L. K. (1939). Surgical treatment of complete rectal prolapse. *Annals of Surgery*, **109**, 799–808

PENFOLD, J. C. B. and HAWLEY, P. R. (1972). Experience of Ivalon sponge implant for complete rectal prolapse at St Mark's Hospital, 1960–70. *British Journal of Surgery*, **59**, 846–848

PORTER, N. H. (1962a). A physiological study of the pelvic floor in rectal prolapse. *Annals of the Royal College of Surgeons of England*, **31**, 379–404

PORTER, N. H. (1962b). Collective results of operations for rectal prolapse. *Proceedings of the Royal Society of Medicine*, **55**, 1090

PORTER, N. H. (1977). In *Operative Surgery*, pp. 222–224 (I. P. Todd, Ed.). London; Butterworths

RIPSTEIN, C. B. (1952). Treatment of massive rectal prolapse. *American Journal of Surgery*, **83**, 68–71

RIPSTEIN, C. B. (1972). Procidentia: definitive corrective surgery. *Diseases of the Colon and Rectum*, **15**, 334–336

RIPSTEIN, C. B. (1975). Procidentia of the rectum: internal intussusception of the rectum. *Diseases of the Colon and Rectum*, **18**, 458–460

RIPSTEIN, C. B. and LAUTER, B. (1963). Etiology and surgical therapy of massive prolapse of the rectum. *Annals of Surgery*, **157**, 259–264

ROSEMAN, D. L., de PEYSTER, F. A. and GILCHRIST, R. K. (1975). Benign diseases of the anorectum, in *General Surgery 2* (J. J. Byrne, Ed.). In the series *Practice of Surgery*, pp. 55–57 (H. S. Goldsmith, Ed.). Philadelphia; Harper and Row

RUTTER, K. R. P. (for Parks, A. G.) (1974). Electromyographic changes in certain pelvic floor abnormalities. *Proceedings of the Royal Society of Medicine*, **67**, 53–56

SCHWEIGER, M. and ALEXANDER-WILLIAMS, J. (1977). Solitary-ulcer syndrome of the rectum: its association with occult rectal prolapse. *Lancet*, **1**, 170

STABINS, S. J. (1951). A new surgical procedure for complete rectal prolapse in the mentally ill patient (case report). *Surgery*, **29**, 105–108

STEWART, R. (1972). Long term results of Ivalon wrap operation for complete rectal prolapse. *Proceedings of the Royal Society of Medicine*, **65**, 777

THEUERKAUF, F. J., BEAHRS, O. H. and HILL, J. R. (1970). Rectal prolapse: causation and surgical treatment. *Annals of Surgery*, **171**, 819–835

THOMAS, C. G. (1975). Procidentia of the rectum: transsacral repair. *Diseases of the Colon and Rectum*, **18**, 473–477

UHLIG, B. E. and SULLIVAN, E. S. (1979). The modified Delorme operation: its place in surgical treatment for massive rectal prolapse. *Diseases of the Colon and Rectum*, **22**, 513–521

VERMEULEN, F. D., NIVATVONGS, S., FANG, D. T., BALCOS, E. G. and GOLDBERG, S. M. (1983). A technique for perineal rectosigmoidoscopy using autosuture devices. *Surgery, Gynecology and Obstetrics*, **156**, 85–86

WEDELL, J., ZuEISSEN, P. M. and FIEDLER, R. (1980). A new concept for the management of rectal prolapse. *American Journal of Surgery*, **139**, 723–725

WELLS, C. (1959). New operation for rectal prolapse. *Proceedings of the Royal Society of Medicine*, **52**, 602–603

WROBLESKI, D. E. and DAILEY, T. H. (1979). Spontaneous rupture of the distal colon with evisceration of small intestine through the anus: report of two cases and review of the literature. *Diseases of the Colon and Rectum*, **22**, 569–572

WYATT, A. P. (1981). Perineal rectopexy for rectal prolapse. *British Journal of Surgery*, **68**, 717–719

Chapter 16

Pathogenesis and treatment of anal fissure

R. W. Motson and M. A. Clifton

Introduction

A true primary anal fissure appears as a painful split in the lining of the anal canal. Although this may resolve spontaneously or in response to appropriate treatment, it may progress to a chronic form characterized by fibrous induration of the lateral edges of the fissure, the presence of a tag-like swelling at the anal verge—the 'sentinel pile'— and a hypertrophied anal papilla or polyp at the pectinate line. It is with this latter type of fissure that this chapter is concerned.

Fissures may also appear in the anal canal as a result of local lesions such as carcinoma, chancre, tuberculosis or ulcerated piles, or as a local manifestation of a more generalized process such as ulcerative colitis, proctocolitis or Crohn's disease. The natural history and treatment of such lesions is quite unlike that of primary anal fissures and depends upon the underlying condition.

Pathogenesis

Many theories have been advanced to explain the origin of anal fissures, some more elaborate than others, but in all, trauma from a faecal mass is thought to be an important factor.

One suggestion, still sometimes quoted, is that made by Sir Charles Ball, who was convinced that an anal valve was torn down by the stool. The repeated trauma of defaecation served to reopen the fissure, causing pain and preventing healing. He thought that the torn-down valve became oedematous and, situated as it was at the anal margin, was identified as the sentinel pile. This condition, which he likened to the torn skin sometimes seen at the edge of a fingernail, could be treated in like manner by simple excision of the tag, more elaborate treatments being unnecessary. Spontaneous cure could be effected by the repeated dilatation afforded by defaecation, which caused the rent to tear down further so that the tag was no longer subjected to trauma, a situation that could also be achieved surgically by forcible stretching of the sphincters (Ball, 1908). This ingenious theory overlooked the fact that the fissure, if it were caused in this way, would always extend to the pectinate line, which is seldom the case, and failed to explain the tendency for fissures to develop in the anterior and posterior midlines. Furthermore, the anal valve may be seen to be intact and the anal papilla may be hypertrophied at the pectinate line.

Another popular theory has been that the pecten band, a condensation of fibrous tissue in the submucosal layer of the anal canal thought to develop because of varicose veins in this region (Miles, 1919), might be more susceptible to trauma. In fact, it was thought that fissures seldom developed in patients in whom this band was not present (Abel, 1932). The treatment recommended was division of the white fibres of the pecten band, preserving the external sphincter. It has since been suggested that this band may have been the lower fibres of the internal sphincter, division of which would have amounted to an internal sphincterotomy (Eisenhammer, 1953).

The pathological substrate of anal fissure has also been thought to be a varicose ulcer, the condition arising as a result of trauma, but secondary to previously existing infections of the tissues about the anal margin (Rankin, Bargen and Buie, 1932). According to this theory the fissure develops because of infection in the anal crypts and becomes intractable because of phlebitis developing in the underlying varicosities. The overlying skin then becomes diseased and less resistant to trauma. The posterior situation of most fissures was thought to be due to the susceptibility of the anorectal angle to trauma at defaecation, although this would seem to conflict with the assertion that fissures rarely extend internally even as far as the pectinate line. It was suggested that the lesion did not differ from an ulcer in any other part of the body and that cure could be accomplished by excision of the tag and fissure, removing the skin only as far as the pectinate line and suturing the mucosa to the underlying muscle.

Blaisdell (1937) drew attention to the fact that fissures frequently occurred posteriorly, occasionally anteriorly and seldom elsewhere, whereas other pathological lesions, crypts, haemorrhoids, hypertrophied papillae and varicosities, which theoretically might cause fissures, were noticeably inconspicuous either anteriorly or posteriorly. If the lesion were due to a torn crypt then it should occur at other sites around the circumference and if due to haemorrhoids or varicosities then why were these rarely found where fissures are constantly found?

Blaisdell incriminated the anatomical arrangement of the sphincter muscles, pointing out that the main bulk of the external sphincter does not completely encircle the anal canal but decussates to form a 'Y' configuration posteriorly. The subcutaneous part of the external sphincter, however, does completely encircle the anus. Thus, between these two muscles at the level of the anal intermuscular septum there is a triangular area where the anal mucosa may be less well supported, and more liable to trauma.

In view of this possible mechanism, it was suggested that excision of the ulcer with division of the subcutaneous part of the external sphincter would ensure recovery. Blaisdell scorned the idea of sphincter rest being provided by anything less than its complete division, pointing out that such rest is not necessary anyway, for if it were, then surely the wounds of haemorrhoidectomy would never heal.

Others have supported the concept of the subcutaneous external sphincter as the structural cause of fissure. Milligan (1942) suggested that the accidental passage of a hard stool pushed the undilated muscle in front of it, stretching the delicate skin of the anal canal and causing a breach. Lesions in this delicate skin caused pain and spasm. Division of this part of the external sphincter would cure the fissure which would then not recur.

Gabriel (1945), too, accepted the idea of 'Blaisdell's bar' and advocated division of the subcutaneous external sphincter in its treatment. He described the natural history of the lesion, with its initial linear shape which later becomes indurated, with a tag forming due to oedema.

A further change in ideas about the aetiology of fissure-in-ano was brought about by the work of Eisenhammer (1953) who described persistent spasm of the internal sphincter leading to a contracture. The overlying mucosa then changed and became rigid, allowing a tear to develop at the unsupported posterior position. This led to the suggestion of internal sphincterotomy to treat the condition, but now preserving the subcutaneous external sphincter to guard against a patulous anal verge. The base of a chronic fissure was thought to be formed by the lower inner surface of the internal sphincter and not, as often stated, by the subcutaneous external sphincter.

More recently, attention has been drawn to the mechanism of defaecation in which there is seen to be initial prolapse of the pecten and a fringe of mucosa, which lies below the sphincter when the stool passes. Straining produces a perineal bulge between the coccyx and the anus, stool passes through the pecten ring obliquely, and the ring of skin which lies horizontally is tilted so that the front is supported by the tissues of the perineum whereas the posterior part, which is lower, is devoid of tissue support and easily torn. If this is true, then treatment should be directed to widening the ring of skin in the pectinate portion of the anal canal, which might be compared in its effect with an episiotomy (Graham-Stewart, Greenwood and Lloyd-Davies, 1961).

Pathophysiology

Physiological studies have yielded conflicting results about sphincter pressures in this condition. A study of 8 patients with active fissures failed to support the idea that anal sphincter spasm was a constant accompaniment of a fissure-in-ano undisturbed by distension of the anal canal; sphincter spasm was present, however, on digital examination and was presumed to occur during the painful stimulus of defaecation. Pressures dropped a little after anal dilatation but returned to normal after 1 week (Duthie and Bennett, 1964). These investigators felt that the increased resistance during the passage of the stool probably increased the tearing force of the stool on the overlying fissured anal skin, thus delaying healing and producing more pain, any undesirable effects attributable to muscle spasm probably being restricted to the time of defaecation. The success of treatment was due not so much from the reduction of resting sphincter pressure, as from preventing spasm in response to the stimulus of defaecation.

In a subsequent study, Nothmann and Schuster (1974) reported an abnormal internal anal sphincter reflex in response to rectal distension, producing an overshoot contraction immediately after the initial relaxation. This situation returned to normal after successful treatment. They also demonstrated a higher resting pressure in the internal sphincter in those patients with fissure-in-ano, but this may have been because of a higher distension pressure than that used by Duthie and Bennett (1964) in their experiments. They concluded that the resting pressure in the unstimulated sphincter is normal, but that sphincter spasm may result from rectal stimulation such as may occur when stool enters the rectum or during defaecation.

Anal sphincter pressure may vary with different measurement techniques. The rate of perfusion may affect the recorded levels when open perfused tube techniques are used; on the other hand, a balloon probe causes some dilatation, thus failing to measure the pressure in the truly unstimulated sphincter. The diameter of the balloon probe is less critical if it is left *in situ* for 15 min before measurements are taken (Hancock, 1976).

Anal pressure measurements on 14 patients with fissures, using a balloon probe rather than the open-ended capillary tube used by Duthie, has demonstrated a mean maximal resting anal pressure which was significantly higher in 14 patients with fissures than in normal controls (Hancock, 1977). The presence of ultra-slow waves has also been demonstrated more often than in controls. The pressure was highest in those patients who suffered most pain and both pressure and slow waves were reduced by sphincterotomy or dilatation of the anus. It was not possible to determine in these experiments whether this overactivity was the cause or the effect of the condition (Hancock, 1977). In a much larger series of 78 patients with anal fissures, resting anal pressures were measured with a balloon probe after preliminary proctoscopy and found to be significantly higher than in control subjects (Arabi, Alexander-Williams and Keighley, 1977). These findings are different from the earlier findings of the same group, who found no difference in pressure compared with controls in 7 patients with chronic fissures, but an increased pressure in 2 patients with acute fissures (Keighley, Arabi and Alexander-Williams, 1976).

It is reasonable to conclude that the initial lesion in anal fissure is a tear in the anoderm caused by overstretching of the anal canal, presumably by a faecal bolus. This tear occurs most commonly in the posterior midline because this is where the skin of the anal canal is most stretched during defaecation, the anterior margin being stretched to a lesser extent. Spasm of the sphincters may well be secondary to the pain of this stretching and the spasm may make the pain worse. Procedures designed to reduce this spasm reduce the pain of the condition but do not allow the sphincter to 'rest', even if this were a prerequisite of successful healing (which it is not). Cure may be effected by any of the current treatments which allow the anal canal to dilate more easily during defaecation, thus preventing further tearing of the fissure.

Diagnosis

The diagnosis of anal fissure is usually clear from the history and patients with an acute fissure, not surprisingly, are apprehensive of rectal examination. The examination does not necessarily have to be complete; once the diagnosis is confirmed by seeing the lower border of the fissure or a sentinel tag on retraction of the buttocks, then further examination can be deferred to the time of treatment. If no external evidence is visible, then rectal examination should be performed gently. Tenderness is localized to the site of the fissure and since the majority lie posteriorly it is helpful to introduce the examining finger pressed forwards against the anterior wall of the anal canal. Proctoscopy and sigmoidoscopy can usually be deferred if digital examination is painful. However, if the diagnosis remains doubtful, proctoscopy may demonstrate the fissure or other causes for the symptoms such as haemorrhoids, solitary ulcer or proctitis.

Treatment

There are several methods of treatment for anal fissure which have been employed successfully for many years. Recent evidence from controlled trials has clarified the more anecdotal results of earlier reports describing the different techniques.

Non-operative treatment

Avoidance of constipation

The passage of a hard faecal bolus is the probable initiating factor in most cases. It is logical to advise the avoidance of constipation by the use of a high roughage diet or stool bulking agents. In the very early case, avoidance of constipation alone may be all that is needed for healing to take place.

Local anaesthetic

Local anaesthetic cream or ointment inserted into the anal canal may also help to lessen the symptoms but will not, of course, have any direct effect on healing. Excessive use can lead to dermatitis and perianal fissuring.

Anal dilatation

Apart from being a convenient instrument for introducing local anaesthetic for symptomatic relief, the dilator is probably of little value. Stretching of the anal canal by the dilator is unlikely to have as great an effect as an anal stretch under anaesthetic. In a selected series of patients at St Mark's Hospital, in whom conservative treatment was used, only 50 per cent healed with the use of the dilator and anaesthetic gel, but only half of these patients remained healed 4 years later (Lock and Thomson, 1977).

A subsequent study, also from St Mark's Hospital, specifically examined the role of the dilator. There was no significant difference in the rate of healing or the number of patients referred for surgery whether a dilator was used or not (McDonald, Driscoll and Nicholls, 1983). It seems very likely that patients whose fissures heal with this method of treatment would have healed merely by avoidance of constipation alone, and indeed greater dilatation will occur with the passage of stool than with a dilator.

Operative treatment

Excision of the fissure (Gabriel, 1945) is now very rarely performed. Although such excision is effective, the large wound is slow to heal. The technique was modified by skin grafting to reduce the time for healing (Hughes, 1953), but inpatient stay is still considerably longer than with the methods described below.

Anal dilatation

The patient is placed in lithotomy under general anaesthesia and after examination with the index finger, two, three and finally four fingers are gently introduced into the anal canal. The dilatation is maintained for 3–4 min. The procedure is quick and easy to perform, hospital inpatient time is short and the procedure can be easily performed on a day case basis. Serious injury to the sphincter is rare.

Randomized controlled trials have shown there to be a higher incidence of recurrent fissure after simple anal stretch than after sphincterotomy (Hawley, 1969; Jensen *et al.*, 1984). In a more recent study, maximal dilatation of the anus under general anaesthetic (six-finger stretch) has been compared with lateral subcutaneous sphincterotomy under local anaesthetic (Marby *et al.*, 1979). Although in this study the results were slightly better after maximal dilatation, the same group has subsequently shown that lateral subcutaneous sphincterotomy has a much higher recurrence rate when performed under local rather than general anaesthetic (Keighley *et al.*, 1981).

Posterior (open) sphincterotomy

Posterior open sphincterotomy was popularized by Eisenhammer (1953, 1959). The procedure is performed with the patient in the lithotomy position and the posterior wall of the anal canal is exposed using an anal retractor. The internal sphincter is usually visible as the incision with the scalpel is made. All the internal sphincter distal to the dentate line is divided, and care must be taken to extend the incision into the perianal skin so that there is no overhanging edge under which the stool can be driven.

As with simple anal stretch, the relief of pain is almost immediate, but complete healing of the wound is sometimes slow and may take several weeks. The healed wound sometimes leaves a gutter which may be responsible for poor control of flatus, mucus leakage or soiling in some patients (Hardy, 1967). Recurrence of the fissure is relatively infrequent and less than after simple anal dilatation.

Lateral subcutaneous sphincterotomy

The imperfections of posterior sphincterotomy led surgeons to look for an alternative technique (Eisenhammer, 1959; Bennett and Duthie, 1964). Lateral sphincterotomy through a circumanal incision (Parks, 1967) has the advantage that there is no wound in the anal canal and a sphincterotomy can be performed under direct vision. Lateral sphincterotomy can also be performed by a closed technique using a tenotomy knife (Notaras, 1969). These two techniques are now the most widely used and both will therefore be described.

Open lateral subcutaneous sphincterotomy (Figure 16.1).   The patient is placed in the lithotomy position under general anaesthetic. Although the procedure can be performed under local anaesthetic, there is evidence that the incidence of recurrent fissure is higher (Keighley *et al.*, 1981).

The lower border of the sphincter is palpated and the subcutaneous tissues on the lateral side of the anal canal are infiltrated with adrenaline in saline (1:200 000). A circumferential incision 2–3 cm in length is made over the previously palpated sphincter which is then exposed. The intersphincteric plate is opened up with scissors and the internal sphincter is then divided up to the level of the dentate line, exposing the longitudinal fibres overlying the external sphincter. There is usually little or no bleeding, but any that occurs should be controlled with diathermy before wound closure with interrupted catgut or subcutaneous Dexon sutures. Packs within the anal canal are unnecessary and uncomfortable.

Closed lateral subcutaneous sphincterotomy (Figure 16.2).   The procedure may be performed either in lithotomy or in the left lateral position under local or general anaesthetic. Local anaesthesia is achieved by bilateral haemorrhoidal nerve block. The anal canal is gently dilated with an anal retractor which makes it easier to palpate the internal sphincter. Once the internal sphincter is identified a narrow-blade scalpel (Swann Morton no. 11 or Beaver no. 52L) is introduced through the perianal skin with the flat of the blade between the anal skin and the sphincter. The blade is then turned through 90° and sphincterotomy performed by incising outwards and laterally. As the sphincterotomy is performed the resistance to the scalpel can be felt to diminish. The

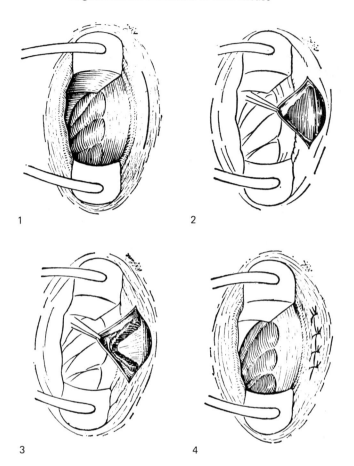

1

2

3

4

Figure 16.1. Open lateral subcutaneous sphincterotomy. A circumanal incision is made over the lower border of the sphincter (1) and the internal sphincter exposed (2). The internal sphincter is divided up to the level of the dentate line (3), and after haemostasis the wound is closed with chromic catgut or subcuticular polyglycolic acid sutures (4) (From Parks (1967), by permission of the publishers)

scalpel is withdrawn and the puncture wound left open to drain. A modification of the technique has been described by Hoffmann and Goligher (1970), in which the knife is introduced between the internal and external sphincters and the sphincterotomy performed by cutting towards, rather than away from, the anal canal. There is no difference in the extent of the division and the direction of incision is one of personal preference.

After sphincterotomy by either technique, simple analgesics for a few days and stool softener to assist with regular defaecation are usually necessary.

Results

In most cases, the results of treatment for fissure are very satisfactory, regardless of the technique chosen. As previously stated, the incidence of recurrence after simple anal stretch is a little higher than with techniques in which the sphincter is formally divided.

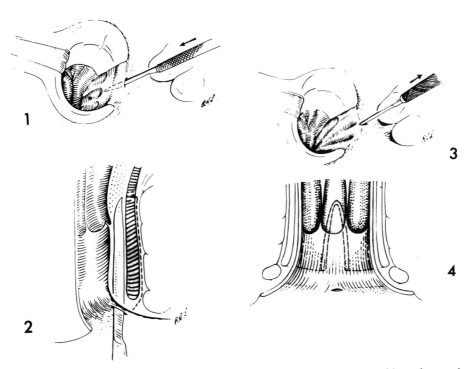

Figure 16.2. Closed lateral subcutaneous sphincterotomy. A small puncture wound is made over the lower border of the internal sphincter and the narrow-blade scalpel introduced, with blade lying flat between the mucosa of the anal canal and the internal sphincter (1). The blade is then turned outwards through 90° (2) and the lower half of the internal sphincter is divided as the knife is withdrawn (3), leaving a palpable defect in the lateral wall (4) (From Notaras (1983), by permission of the publishers)

TABLE 16.1. Results of lateral subcutaneous sphincterotomy

Reference	No. cases	Success		Recurrence		Complications	
		No.	(per cent)	No.	(per cent)	No.	(per cent)
Hawley (1969)	24	24	100.0	0	0.0	0	0.0
Hoffmann and Goligher (1970)	99	96	96.9	3	3.1	12	12.1
Notaras (1971)	73	73	100.0	0	0.0	7	9.6
Millar (1971)	99	99	100.0	0	0.0	3	3.0
Ray *et al.* (1974)	21	21	100.0	0	0.0		
Rudd (1975)	200	199	99.5	1	0.5	1	0.5
Bailey *et al.* (1978)	418	399	93.3	19	4.5		
Abcarian (1980)	150	149	99.7	2	0.6	0	0.0
Marya *et al.* (1980)	100	98	98.0	2	2.0	5	5.0
Oh (1982)	550	548	99.6	2	0.4	38	6.9
Ravikumar *et al.* (1982)	60	58	96.7	2	3.3	3	5.0
Boulos and Aranjo (1984)	14	14	100.0	0	0.0	3	21.4
Total	1808	1778	97.7	31	1.8	72	4.0

Mucus leakage and occasional soiling are both more common after open sphincterotomy. Lateral subcutaneous sphincterotomy has the highest degree of success and is rarely complicated by any of the minor incontinence associated with the open technique (*Table 16.1*). The raised maximal anal pressure in patients with anal fissure (Nothmann and Schuster, 1974; Arabi, Alexander-Williams and Keighley, 1977; Hancock, 1977) is reduced by 50 per cent after sphincterotomy. The reduction is of a similar degree with both open and subcutaneous sphincterotomy (Boulos and Araujo, 1984). Although there is no doubt that open sphincterotomy produces satisfactory results, lateral subcutaneous sphincterotomy is equally effective in providing rapid relief of pain with a very low incidence of recurrent fissure (*Table 16.1*). Furthermore, lateral subcutaneous sphincterotomy does not lead to the delayed wound healing and minor degrees of mucus or faecal incontinence that occasionally occur after the open technique. It must now be regarded as the preferred method in all patients except those in whom the fissure is associated with an intersphincteric abscess. In these cases, drainage of the abscess can only be effectively performed by the open sphincterotomy technique.

References

ABCARIAN. H. (1980). Surgical correction of chronic anal fissure: results of lateral internal sphincterotomy vs. fissurectomy–midline sphincterotomy. *Diseases of the Colon and Rectum*, **23**, 31–36

ABEL, A. L. (1932). The pecten: the pecten band: pectenosis and pectenotomy. *Lancet*, **1**, 714–718

ARABI. Y.. ALEXANDER-WILLIAMS. J. and KEIGHLEY. M. R. B. (1977). Anal pressures in hemorrhoids and anal fissure. *American Journal of Surgery*, **134**, 608–610

BAILEY. R. V.. RUBIN. R. J. and SALVATI. E. P. (1978). Lateral internal sphincterotomy. *Diseases of the Colon and Rectum*, **21**, 584–586

BALL. C. (1908). *The Rectum, Its Diseases and Developmental Defects*, pp. 146–152. London; Hodder and Stoughton

BENNETT. R. C. and DUTHIE. H. L. (1964). The functional importance of the internal anal sphincter. *British Journal of Surgery*, **51**, 355–357

BLAISDELL. P. C. (1937). Pathogenesis of anal fissure and implications as to treatment. *Surgery, Gynecology and Obstetrics*, **65**, 672–677

BOULOS. P. B. and ARAUJO. J. G. C. (1984). Adequate internal sphincterotomy for chronic anal fissure: subcutaneous or open technique? *British Journal of Surgery*, **71**, 360–362

DUTHIE. H. L. and BENNETT. R. C. (1964). Anal sphincter pressure in fissure in ano. *Surgery, Gynecology and Obstetrics*, **119**, 19–21

EISENHAMMER. S. (1953). The internal anal sphincter: its surgical importance. *South African Medical Journal*, **27**, 266–270

EISENHAMMER. S. (1959). The evaluation of the internal anal sphincterotomy operation with special reference to anal fissure. *Surgery, Gynecology and Obstetrics*, **109**, 583–590

GABRIEL. W. B. (1945). *The Principles and Practice of Rectal Surgery*, 3rd edn, pp. 129–145. London; H. K. Lewis

GRAHAM-STEWART. C. W.. GREENWOOD. R. K. and LLOYD-DAVIES. R. W. (1961). A review of 50 patients with fissure in ano. *Surgery, Gynecology and Obstetrics*, **113**, 445–448

HANCOCK. B. D. (1976). Measurement of anal pressure and motility. *Gut*, **17**, 645–651

HANCOCK. B. D. (1977). The internal sphincter and anal fissure. *British Journal of Surgery*, **64**, 92–95

HARDY. K. J. (1967). Internal sphincterotomy: an appraisal with special reference to sequelae. *British Journal of Surgery*, **54**, 30–31

HAWLEY. P. R. (1969). The treatment of chronic fissure-in-ano. A trial of methods. *British Journal of Surgery*, **56**, 915–918

HOFFMAN. D. C. and GOLIGHER. J. C. (1970). Lateral subcutaneous internal sphincterotomy in treatment of anal fissure. *British Medical Journal*, **3**, 673–675

HUGHES. E. S. R. (1953). Anal fissure. *British Medical Journal*, **2**, 803–806

JENSEN. S. L.. LUND. F.. NIELSEN. O. V. and TANGE. G. (1984). Lateral subcutaneous sphincterotomy versus anal dilatation in the treatment of fissure in ano in outpatients: a prospective randomised study. *British Medical Journal*, **289**, 528–530

KEIGHLEY, M. R. B., ARABI, Y. and ALEXANDER-WILLIAMS, J. (1976). Anal pressures in haemorrhoids and anal fissures. *British Journal of Surgery*, **63**, 665

KEIGHLEY, M. R. B., GRECA, F., NEVAH, E., HARES, M. and ALEXANDER-WILLIAMS, J. (1981). Treatment of anal fissure by lateral subcutaneous sphincterotomy should be under general anaesthesia. *British Journal of Surgery*, **68**, 400–401

LOCK, M. R. and THOMSON, J. P. S. (1977). Fissure-in-ano: the initial management and prognosis. *British Journal of Surgery*, **64**, 355–358

MARBY, M., ALEXANDER-WILLIAMS, J., BUCHMANN, P., ARABI, Y., KAPPAS, A., MINERVINI, S., GATEHOUSE, D. and KEIGHLEY, M. R. B. (1979). A randomised controlled trial to compare anal dilatation with lateral subcutaneous sphincterotomy for anal fissure. *Diseases of the Colon and Rectum*, **22**, 308–311

MARYA, S. K. S., MITTAL, S. S. and SINGLA, S. (1980). Lateral subcutaneous internal sphincterotomy for acute fissure in ano. *British Journal of Surgery*, **67**, 299

McDONALD, P., DRISCOLL, A. M. and NICHOLLS, R. J. (1983). The anal dilator in the conservative management of acute anal fissure. *British Journal of Surgery*, **70**, 25–26

MILES, W. E. (1919). Observations upon internal piles. *Surgery, Gynecology and Obstetrics*, **29**, 497–506

MILLAR, D. M. (1971). Subcutaneous lateral internal anal sphincterotomy for anal fissure. *British Journal of Surgery*, **58**, 737–739

MILLIGAN, E. T. C. (1942). The surgical anatomy and disorders of the perianal space. *Proceedings of the Royal Society of Medicine*, **36**, 365–378

NOTARAS, M. J. (1969). Lateral subcutaneous sphincterotomy for anal fissure—a new technique. *Proceedings of the Royal Society of Medicine*, **62**, 713

NOTARAS, M. J. (1971). The treatment of anal fissure by lateral subcutaneous internal sphincterotomy—a technique and results. *British Journal of Surgery*, **58**, 96–100

NOTARAS, M. J. (1983). Lateral subcutaneous internal anal sphincterotomy for fissure-in-ano, in *Rob and Smith's Operative Surgery—Alimentary Tract and Abdominal Wall*, vol. 3, *Colon, Rectum and Anus*, p. 512 (I. P. Todd and L. P. Fielding, Eds). London; Butterworths

NOTHMANN, B. J. and SCHUSTER, M. M. (1974). Internal anal sphincter derangement with anal fissures. *Gastroenterology*, **67**, 216–220

OH, C. (1982). The role of internal sphincterotomy. *Mount Sinai Journal of Medicine*, **49**, 484–486

PARKS, A. G. (1967). The management of fissure-in-ano. *British Journal of Hospital Medicine*, **1**, 737–739

RANKIN, F. W., BARGEN, J. A. and BUIE, L. A. (1932). *The Colon, Rectum and Anus*, pp. 584–593. Philadelphia; W. B. Saunders

RAVIKUMAR, T. S., SRIDHAR, S. and RAO, R. N. (1982). Subcutaneous lateral internal sphincterotomy for chronic fissure-in-ano. *Diseases of the Colon and Rectum*, **25**, 778–801

RAY, J. E., PENFOLD, J. C. B., GATHRIGHT, J. B. and ROBERSON, S. H. (1974). Lateral subcutaneous internal anal sphincterotomy for anal fissure. *Diseases of the Colon and Rectum*, **17**, 139–144

RUDD, W. W. H. (1975). Lateral subcutaneous internal sphincterotomy for chronic anal fissure, an outpatient procedure. *Diseases of the Colon and Rectum*, **18**, 319–323

Chapter 17

Constipation: pathophysiology, clinical features and treatment

J. E. Lennard-Jones

Definition

'You should say what you mean', the March Hare went on. 'I do', Alice hastily replied; 'at least—at least I mean what I say . . .'. (Lewis Carroll)

Doctors need to find out what their patients mean when they describe an unpleasant sensation or source of concern. Constipation has a double meaning; a person complaining of this symptom may mean that defaecation is difficult, that it is infrequent, or both (Moore-Gillon, 1984). Defaecation may be difficult because the stools are hard or difficult to expel, and there may be associated pain. Most people believe that a daily bowel action is a sign of health; if defaecation is less frequent, then symptoms such as abdominal distension or fulness, abdominal pain, flatulence, anorexia, nausea, or a bad taste in the mouth may be ascribed to constipation. Constipation has to be defined in the senses in which it is used. For example 'straining at stool for more than 25% of the time and/or two or fewer stools per week' (Drossman et al., 1982) or 'any patient who strains to defaecate and does not pass at least one soft stool daily, without effort, is constipated' (Painter, 1980). Having analysed the complaint, we can then seek to measure bowel function in various ways so that the symptom can be defined in quantitative terms.

Small hard stools

Hard stools contain little water; almost by definition they also tend to be small stools. Consistency is difficult to measure except in qualitative terms, although a device known as a penetrometer can give a figure (Exton-Smith, Bendall and Kent, 1975), but it is not generally used. A 'hard' stool is said to contain 40–60 per cent, a 'normal' stool about 70 per cent and a 'liquid' stool more than 95 per cent of water. Water content is thus the key to consistency.

Stool weight varies widely in an individual from day to day (Wyman et al., 1978), from person to person and from country to country. Mean daily weights among healthy people in the UK and the USA lie between 100 and 200 g daily, with frequent values below 100 g; in rural Uganda the mean observed was 470 g (Burkitt, Walker and Painter, 1974) and in healthy Indian adults it was 311 g (Tandon and Tandon, 1975). Larger stools tend to contain more water and are therefore softer.

350

Difficult defaecation

Many patients, particularly women, complain that they feel stool in the rectum but cannot expel it despite prolonged and repeated straining. Some patients use digital evacuation or the pressure of a finger in the vagina, or pressure with the fingers upwards on either side of the anus to try and help themselves. The problem appears to be largely one of a disordered defaecation mechanism, perhaps aggravated by small hard stools. Difficulty in the expulsion of stool must be distinguished from the sense of incomplete rectal emptying felt by patients with the descending perineum syndrome.

Infrequent defaecation

Surveys have shown that in Western countries most people do indeed pass a stool every day. Fewer than 1 per cent of a healthy British population said that they passed two or fewer stools a week and, interestingly, all these subjects were women (Connell *et al.*, 1965). In an American population sample, up to 5 per cent described themselves as having this bowel frequency (Drossman *et al.*, 1982). Bowel histories are fallible, but they have to be accepted unless a diary card is used (Manning, Wyman and Heaton, 1976). It seems reasonable for clinical purposes to accept a stated bowel frequency of two or fewer stools weekly as being at the lower limit of the normal range.

Stomach to caecum

Gastric and small intestinal transit rate

Studies with a radiotelemetering pill combined with an isotopically labelled marker have not shown any delay in gastric or small intestinal transit rate in constipated subjects (Waller, 1975). However, using exhaled breath hydrogen as a guide to the arrival of a meal residue in the right colon, small bowel transit time was a little longer, 5.4 ± 0.3 as compared with 4.2 ± 0.2 h, in constipated than in control subjects, although this time was a small fraction (< 10 per cent) of the whole gut transit time (Cann *et al.*, 1983). A decrease in transit time to the caecum has been demonstrated after treatment of hypothyroidism in 6 patients, 5 of whom were constipated (Shafer, Prentiss and Bond, 1984).

Ileal effluent as a bacterial substrate

The ileal effluent is fluid or semi-solid and contains water, electrolytes and unabsorbed food residue. The consistency of the stool in diarrhoea depends largely on the extent to which water and sodium are absorbed by the colon. However, in normal subjects and patients with constipation, most of the sodium is absorbed and stool water is largely incorporated within the solid component of stool. The unabsorbed residue which enters the right colon provides a metabolic substrate for the bacterial flora. These organisms partly digest cellulose (Cummings, 1984; Kelleher *et al.*, 1984), other unabsorbed carbohydrates of plant cell walls and some residual starch, to yield short chain fatty acids. In the process, the bacteria multiply and themselves provide a high proportion of the solid within the colon; recent estimates suggest 40–55 per cent (Cummings, 1983).

Diet and fibre

An inadequate oral intake of food, as in starvation or anorexia nervosa, or a low consumption of poorly absorbed carbohydrate therefore leads to small (and probably infrequent) stools. Different types of fibre increase faecal weight to a variable degree. Thus, under controlled conditions approximately 20 g of concentrated fibre derived from bran increased the stool weight by 127 per cent, as compared with 69 per cent on cabbage, 59 per cent on carrot and 40 per cent on apple fibre (Cummings *et al.*, 1978). These differences were related to the amount of pentose-containing polysaccharides in the fibre. On this standard fibre intake, healthy people showed widely different responses in terms of faecal weight, but in general the weight with the fibre supplement was proportional to the initial weight during a control period. The mean whole gut transit time decreased by almost half on 20 g of concentrated bran fibre and the mean stool weight more than doubled. Concentrated bran fibre is not generally available, and the efficacy of a given weight of bran for increasing stool weight is greatest if the particle size is large rather than small. However, coarse bran has a much greater volume than fine bran for a given weight and, for this reason, and the fact that it is more palatable, more fine than coarse bran tends to be added to the diet (Brodribb and Groves, 1978), thus compensating for the effect of particle size.

Colonic muscle

Deficient muscle

Disorders known to affect the structure of smooth muscle may be associated with constipation, and sometimes megacolon. Systemic sclerosis is characterized by a reduction in the number of smooth muscle cells in the gut and their replacement by collagen. The remaining muscle cells appear morphologically normal. In contrast, visceral myopathy is associated with vacuolar degeneration and loss of muscle cells; it seems likely that the fibrosis observed is a secondary event (Schuffler and Beegle, 1979). In some cases of megacolon treated surgically, the wall of the colon is described as very thin (Todd, 1971). No studies of the anatomy of the colonic muscle in such patients have been reported.

Movement of colonic contents

Methods of study

Contractions of the colonic smooth muscle may be divided into non-propulsive segmenting contractions, and propulsive (or retropulsive) movements. Transport of contents can be studied by the use of a radio-opaque or radioactive marker introduced into the lumen. Classic radiological observations, using bismuth or barium, early in the century demonstrated infrequent rapid movements of colonic contents over long segments of the colon. It is not known how often such movements occur physiologically and the prolonged observations necessary to observe them have become impossible now that the hazards of irradiation are appreciated. During recent years, investigation has been limited to sequential single radiographs taken at intervals after ingestion of appropriate solid markers (Hinton, Lennard-Jones and Young, 1969) or to surface mapping of a radioactive point source (Kirwan and Smith, 1974, 1977), sometimes incorporated in a telemetering capsule so that additional information about its site can be determined from characteristic pressure waves (Holdstock *et al.*, 1970; Waller, 1975).

Using either of these techniques, the whole gut transit time can be determined by observing either disappearance of markers from the abdomen or their appearance in the stool. If observations are restricted to collection of stools, the presence of markers can be detected either by sieving (Burkitt, Walker and Painter, 1974) or by X-ray, without hazard or inconvenience to the subject.

Forward and backward movements

If the colon is divided arbitrarily into segments, markers tend to pass progressively from one segment to another and to leave each segment at an exponential rate (Martelli *et al.*, 1978a). There is evidence both from radiographs (Halls, 1965) and from examination of stools (Wiggins and Cummings, 1976) that different shaped markers taken on successive days mix in the colon.

In constipated subjects, two types of abnormal transit through the colon may be seen. The usual pattern is a uniform delay in passage so that markers remain in each segment of the colon for longer than normal (Hinton and Lennard-Jones, 1968; Waller, 1975; Kirwan and Smith, 1974, 1977; Martelli *et al.*, 1978b). In some patients, especially younger patients with an enlarged rectum (Hinton and Lennard-Jones, 1968) and elderly patients (Eastwood, 1972; Melkersson *et al.*, 1983), there is normal transit of markers through the colon to the rectum, where they accumulate until infrequent rectal evacuation occurs.

Whether movement of markers in the colon is continuous or discontinuous is unknown. Studies by repeated radiographs, external mapping and telemetering pressure records suggested a series of discrete forward movements averaging about 10 cm each time towards the rectum (Holdstock *et al.*, 1970); on only one occasion was a rapid longer movement noted. In patients with diarrhoea, discrete forward movements were noted every few hours, but in constipated subjects the movements occurred only once every 24 h and almost always during the night (Waller, 1975).

Retrograde movements were noted only occasionally and only in those with constipation. In a study of the position of radio-opaque markers before and after defaecation in normal subjects, the whole of the left colon from the splenic flexure downwards was cleared in some whereas in others the rectum was only partially emptied. Repression of the urge to defaecate by one subject led to proximal movement of markers (Halls, 1965).

Total gut transit time

Normal range.   All but about 8 h of whole gut transit time is taken up by passage through the large intestine. A single value for transit time is obtained if a single solid marker is studied. If a liquid unabsorbed marker is given or a number of solid markers, some of the marker usually appears in different stools so that the first and last appearance, or any proportion, can be recorded. In constipation, the stools tend to be infrequent and it is most convenient to record the first appearance and passage of a large fraction of the markers. Because stools are infrequent and patients wish to limit the time without treatment, a method of giving markers daily over weeks to obtain a mean transit time (Cummings, Jenkins and Wiggins, 1976) is not applicable to the study of severe constipation.

In the original study, all 25 normal young male subjects had passed the first marker by the end of the third day and all but one had passed 80 per cent of the markers within 5 d (Hinton, Lennard-Jones and Young, 1969). The results in a series of elderly subjects aged 69–90 yr were the same (Eastwood, 1972). Similar observations were reported by Devroede and Soffié (1973) and none of their 26 control subjects had any marker remaining in the colon after 6 d and at 5 d fewer than 5 of 20 markers were present. In a larger series of 114 healthy subjects, about half of whom were children, every person passed all the markers within 7 d (Martelli *et al.*, 1978b). The presence of more than 20 per cent of markers within the colon 5 d after ingestion has been generally accepted as above the normal range.

Results in constipation.   In patients complaining of constipation, the whole gut transit time may be normal or prolonged (Hinton and Lennard-Jones, 1968; Eastwood, 1972). It is likely that those patients with a normal transit time are mainly complaining of difficult defaecation or abdominal symptoms, such as distension or pain, which they ascribe to abnormal bowel function. It is clearly very important to differentiate those with a normal or abnormal transit rate. In the latter, transit may be greatly prolonged (*Figure 17.1*), so that 80 per cent of markers may not be passed within 10 d. Similar observations have been made by others (Eastwood, 1972; Devroede and Soffié, 1973; Martelli *et al.*, 1978b; Watier *et al.*, 1983).

Pressure changes

Difficulties of interpretation

Pressure changes in the colon are very difficult to interpret. Perfused open-ended tubes record the absolute pressure in the lumen, but do not distinguish between local contraction against resistance, inflation, due to movement elsewhere, or external pressure. Furthermore, an open-ended tube may not record any change in pressure if movement leads to displacement of contents without resistance. Similar considerations apply to pressure-sensitive membranes. A miniature balloon records not only the surrounding pressure but also any extra tension in its wall from deformation due to contact with the gut wall or solid faeces. Correlation between movement of the gut wall and pressure changes by simultaneous measurements of pressure and cinematography are very difficult (Ritchie, Ardran and Truelove, 1962; Deller and Wangel, 1965). Increase in the gut lumen may indicate inflation or relaxation; no change may imply quiescence or isometric contraction; reduction can mean compression or contraction. Cine-films show that not all radiologically observed movements can be correlated with pressure changes in the same segment and vice versa. Contractions of the large intestine tend to be slow and cause little movement of contrast medium.

Is there an activity gradient in the colon?

For convenience, observations of pressure changes tend to be made in the rectum and sigmoid colon. A few studies have combined telemetering records of pressure from the proximal colon and direct pressure measurements from the distal colon. In one study (Wangel and Deller, 1965), the control subjects had more activity in the distal colon than the proximal colon while resting, but the reverse was true after food. In a single patient with constipation, the distal large intestine was more active throughout the recording. The concept of a reversible pressure gradient from proximal to distal colon in normal subjects is interesting and its presence or absence deserves further study in constipation. Pressure and movement records from the proximal colon have shown constant increases in motor activity and propulsion of contents after food, and

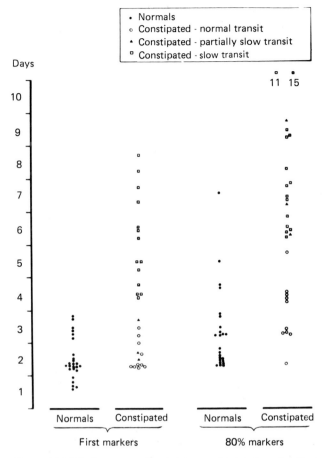

Figure 17.1. Whole gut transit rate in normal subjects and patients who complained of constipation, measured as the appearance of the first radio-opaque marker and 80 per cent of the markers in the stools. The normal subjects all passed the first marker within 3 d and all but one normal subject passed 80 per cent of the markers within 5 d. Some of the patients had a normal transit rate, others were abnormal by one criterion and not the other, whereas some showed prolonged transit by either criterion (J. M. Hinton and J. E. Lennard-Jones, unpublished data)

suggestive increases after physical activity (Holdstock *et al.*, 1970). Little data on these changes in constipated subjects is available.

Basal records from the distal colon

Pressure changes in the sigmoid colon under basal conditions vary greatly in one subject from minute to minute and week to week (Dinoso *et al.*, 1983). These variations make interpretation of records difficult unless the conditions are precisely recorded and recordings are prolonged or repeated. One of the earlier studies (Connell, 1962) in 33 patients with severe persistent constipation, most of whom defaecated once a week or less, showed that the sigmoid colon was active for a greater proportion of the time in constipated than in normal subjects, but the mean amplitude of the pressure waves was less among the patients. A difference was found between younger and older patients with constipation; those under 40 yr of age tended to have normal or hyperactive records whereas older persons had hypoactive traces. Whether this difference was due to a natural progression of the disorder or to prolonged use of laxatives could not be determined. In the upper rectum, the duration and mean amplitude of pressure waves was less in all the constipated subjects than normal. Other investigators (Meunier, Rochas and Lambert, 1979) were not able to demonstrate any difference between the basal records of normal and constipated subjects, after prolonged fasting. In another study, activity was not different from normal in patients with slow transit constipation, but was significantly increased in those with constipation and a normal transit rate (Preston and Lennard-Jones, 1985a).

Is there a zone of hyperactivity at the rectosigmoid?

Using a pull-through technique, a zone of complex wave activity 1.5–2 cm in length located 9–15 cm from the anal verge was identified in most of a group of constipated subjects, but not in healthy persons (Chowdhury, Dinoso and Lorber, 1976). In a later study using static pressure sensors, patients with mild constipation showed slightly greater pressure changes at 15 cm than normal subjects, but there were no differences at 20 and 25 cm (Dinoso et al., 1983). Further studies at different levels of the rectosigmoid would be of interest.

Stimulated pressure activity

Effect of a meal.   It has long been known that pressure changes in the sigmoid colon tend to increase with emotion, after a meal, or after prostigmine. Integrity of the nervous system appears important in the response to a meal because in patients with severe constipation due to complete traumatic transection of the spinal cord, the response to a meal was lost, but not the response to prostigmine (Glick et al., 1984). The response to a meal was also absent in diabetic patients with severe constipation, presumably due to autonomic neuropathy (Battle et al., 1980). In the absence of other disease, a comparative study showed similar mean increases after food or prostigmine in normal and constipated subjects. However, the variation, both decreased and increased responses, was greater in the constipated subjects, especially after food. On the basis of the response to a meal, constipated subjects could thus be divided into a relatively small group of 'hypomotor' responders, a majority of 'normomotor', and another small group of 'hypermotor' responders (Meunier, Rochas and Lambert, 1979). Other investigators have found little change in motor activity in constipated subjects during or after a meal (Waller and Misiewicz, 1972; Waller, Misiewicz and Kiley, 1972).

Peristaltic activity induced by laxatives.   Propulsive waves are very rarely identified in colonic or rectal pressure recordings and are not usually induced by distension (Hardcastle and Mann, 1970). Peristalsis can be regularly induced in the transverse or descending colon by topically acting laxatives such as bisacodyl, oxyphenisatin (Hardcastle and Mann, 1968), or rheinanthrone (Hardcastle and Wilkins, 1970) and once the bowel has been sensitized by one of these drugs physical stimuli may cause fresh waves of contraction. These drugs stimulated increased pressure waves in the rectum, usually fast low amplitude waves, but peristalsis was not seen.
    Since many patients with constipation complain that chemical laxatives appear to lose their effect, it seemed relevant to test the effect of bisacodyl introduced into the

sigmoid colon. In some constipated subjects, definite peristaltic waves were observed and in others no increase in activity, although some of the latter may develop pain and an urge to defaecate (Preston and Lennard-Jones, 1985a). It had been hoped that this effect of bisacodyl, which probably acts via the myenteric plexus because it can be blocked by the prior application of 4 per cent lignocaine, could be used as a test of myenteric nerve function. However, no correlation was found between the effect of bisacodyl preoperatively and the anatomy of the myenteric plexus shown by silver staining in a subsequent colectomy specimen. Failure to respond to bisacodyl did correlate with the duration of constipation, suggesting that this disorder may either be spontaneously progressive or that it becomes unresponsive to laxatives with long-continued use.

Electrical activity

Observations on the normal colon

In the stomach and small bowel there is a well-defined myogenic control system manifested by periodic depolarization and repolarization of smooth muscles—the so-called slow wave. Contractions of muscle are linked to the slow waves and are characterized electrically by a superimposed action spike potential. These potentials are best recorded by electrodes implanted in the muscle, but can be detected by luminal electrodes, particularly if closely applied to the mucosa by suction or a clip. Many investigators have studied the electrical activity of human colonic muscle, a few by implanting electrodes in the muscle at operation (Taylor et al., 1975) and most by recording from electrodes attached to the mucosa or lying free in the lumen. The subject has been reviewed by Daniel (1975). Observers appear to agree that slow waves are not present all the time, but are recorded for a greater proportion of the time near the anus than in the proximal colon. The slow waves may be associated with spike potentials which can occur at any phase of the slow wave. Gradients along the large bowel of both frequency and percentage electrical activity have been observed which may be related to transit (Taylor et al., 1975).

Recordings in constipated subjects

A simultaneous study using bipolar electrodes and a pressure recorder in the sigmoid colon of patients with constipation (defined by a slow whole gut transit rate) showed periods of slow waves, of irregular rhythm and variable configuration, appearing for only part of the time. Two groups of slow wave frequencies with a normal distribution were recorded both in patients and control subjects, a slower rhythm at about 3 c/min and a faster rhythm at about 6 c/min. The frequency of the slower rhythm was significantly higher (3.01 ± 0.8 vs. 2.65 ± 0.29 c/min) in the patients with constipation, whereas that of the faster rhythm was similar in patients and controls (Frieri et al., 1983). There was a suggestive increase in the proportion of time for which slow waves were recorded in the constipated subjects. Spike activity was occasionally recorded, but there was no fixed relationship between spikes and contractions.

In a study using 8 groups of bipolar luminal electrodes wound round a 150 cm probe which could be introduced as far as the transverse colon (Bueno et al., 1980), 2 categories of slow wave were recognized at frequencies of 2–3 and 10–12 c/min recorded during 16 and 28 per cent, respectively, of the recording time. Short and long spike bursts were recognized. Constipation with pain was characterized by an increase

there is a considerable depletion of VIP and substance-P containing nerves (Bishop *et al.*, 1981; Polak and Bloom, 1983).

Chagas' disease is an acquired form of denervation of the gut due to infection by *Trypanosoma cruzi* (Ferreira-Santos, 1961). Periganglionitis and degeneration of neurons are the main histological features, with dilatation of the affected segment of colon and consequent constipation. In this condition there is a reduction of regulatory peptides, as in Hirschsprung's disease. It is interesting that no such reduction occurs with an extrinsic autonomic neuropathy, as in chronic autonomic failure (Long *et al.*, 1980).

Idiopathic megabowel.   Evidence is accumulating that an anatomical abnormality of the myenteric plexus on silver staining may be present both in patients with 'idiopathic' megacolon and others with severe constipation but without megacolon. Progress has been delayed and data are scanty, because the histological technique is only applicable to large full-thickness biopsy or colectomy specimens, and because the technique of sectioning and staining has not been widely used. A patient with megarectum and intractable constipation was found to have a severe abnormality of the myenteric plexus on silver staining (Dyer *et al.*, 1969). Three other patients with megarectum, 2 with a megasigmoid, all with symptoms beginning in childhood, were treated surgically by colectomy, and in each case the myenteric plexus showed a similar abnormality. Only occasional normal argyrophil ganglion cells were present; most neurons were abnormal with small, dark nuclei without nucleoli or visible chromatin structure, ballooned cytoplasm and no stainable processes (Smith, Grace and Todd, 1977). Severe abnormalities of the myenteric plexus have been shown to affect the whole length of the gut in another patient treated by colectomy for severe constipation and megacolon (Schuffler and Jonak, 1982).

'Slow-transit' constipation.   Among 12 women treated by colectomy for severe intractable constipation, with an apparently normal colon on X-ray and on conventional pathological investigation, abnormalities of the myenteric plexus were found in all but one. Findings were a qualitative reduction in numbers of neurons in 8, abnormal appearance of neurons in 9, reduced neuronal processes in 10 and Schwannosis in 6 (Preston *et al.*, 1983). Similar changes have been described in 8 other women treated surgically for severe constipation (Krishnamurthy and Schuffler, 1983). It seems possible that this particularly severe type of constipation, usually seen only in women, may be due to an abnormality of the myenteric plexus, although it is also possible that the plexus damage could be secondary to long-continued use of laxatives.

Other disorders.   It is likely that other abnormalities of the myenteric plexus will be recognized as associated with constipation. For example, a diffuse abnormality may occur in neurofibromatosis and be associated with megacolon (Feinstat *et al.*, 1984). Similar findings have been reported in the multiple endocrine neoplasia syndrome.

Circulating hormones and regulatory peptides

Thyroid hormones.   The basic electrical rhythm of the human duodenum decreases in hypothyroidism and increases in thyrotoxicosis (Christensen, Schedl and Clifton, 1964), and decreased transit rate through the stomach and small intestine has been demonstrated in hypothyroidism (Shafer, Prentiss and Bond, 1984). It seems likely that the constipation of hypothyroidism is partly due to altered muscle function, although megacolon may also develop due to myxoedematous infiltration (Burrell *et al.*, 1980).

Reproductive hormones.   Constipation with greatly prolonged intestinal transit time but a normal-sized colon is a disorder seen almost entirely in women. The symptoms may be noted during childhood, but characteristically become progressively worse during the second and third decades. Such women tend to have irregular painful menstrual periods, find difficulty in starting a pregnancy, undergo ovarian cystectomy and hysterectomy, and experience galactorrhoea, more commonly than a control group. Abnormalities of sex hormones are found in some of these patients with raised serum prolactin, low urinary oestrogen and low plasma oestradiol levels (Preston, Rees and Lennard-Jones, 1983). Other investigators have also noted an increased frequency of galactorrhoea, but without raised prolactin levels (Watier *et al.*, 1983). At present, the significance of these gynaecological abnormalities is unknown. It is possible that they are secondary and due to an effect of the bowel disorder on the enterohepatic circulation of oestrogen, or that they are primary and the bowel disturbance is in some way related to reproductive hormone abnormalities.

Gastrin and motilin.   In normal subjects there is a rise in circulating blood levels of some regulatory peptides after drinking water given as a constant and reproducible stimulus. Patients with constipation, with or without megacolon, show a smaller rise of gastrin and motilin after this stimulus than normal, suggesting a widespread disorder affecting the upper gut as well as the colon (Preston *et al.*, 1985). It has been suggested that gastrin plays a part in the increased motor activity of the colon after meals (Kirwan and Smith, 1976). Studies in animals have suggested a relationship between circulating motilin levels and the peristaltic activity of the gut (Itoh, 1981). It has also been demonstrated that human colonic pressure activity can be stimulated by infusion of motilin (Rennie *et al.*, 1980), a hormone which accelerates gastric emptying (Christofides *et al.*, 1981) and possibly initiates the interdigestive motor complex (Vantrappen *et al.*, 1979). Reduced motilin levels have been reported in pregnancy, when there is reduced smooth muscle tone and a tendency to constipation (Christofides *et al.*, 1982). Whether the abnormal gastrin and motilin responses in constipation are a primary or secondary phenomenon is unknown, but further observations are needed.

Neurotensin.   Neurotensin is released from the small intestine by food, especially by fat, but its physiological role is unknown. Experimental infusions of neurotensin to give levels about three times higher than after meals led to increased abdominal noise and defaecation in five normal subjects (Calam, Unwin and Peart, 1983). Whether or not neurotensin has a role in normal defaecation or constipation remains to be determined.

Mucosal absorption

Absorption of water from the colonic contents presumably depends on the mucosal area, the time of contact between mucosa and the bowel contents, the degree of mixing, and perhaps on the avidity for water and sodium of the mucosa per unit area. Mucosal area is determined by the circumference and length of the colon. The time of contact is related to transit rate and thus, among other factors, to the volume of the colon and muscular propulsive activity. The degree of mixing of the contents is likely to depend on the consistency of the bowel contents and on movements of the colonic wall. A perfusion study showed that the total net absorption of water and sodium was greater in constipation than in health, but when rates of absorption were corrected for transit times there was no evidence for increased avidity of the mucosa for water and salt in constipated subjects (Devroede and Soffié, 1973). Theoretically, the concentration of bile salts unabsorbed from the distal ileum entering the colon could affect water and sodium absorption; there is at present no data available to suggest that deficiency of bile salts in the colon is a factor in constipation.

Size of the colon

The width of the colon along its length can be measured on barium enema films obtained by a standard technique (Patriquin, Martelli and Devroede, 1978). A normal range has been established for the width at various points and for rectal area, for example the upper limit of the rectosigmoid in a lateral view at the pelvic brim can be taken as 6.5 cm (Preston, Lennard-Jones and Thomas, 1984b). So far, no quantitative clinical technique has been developed for measuring the length or volume of the colon. Using continuous colonic perfusion and a dye dilution technique, colonic volumes were about 50 per cent greater in constipated than in control subjects (Devroede and Soffié, 1973). Most of these patients had an enlarged colon on barium enema and their symptoms were suggestive of megacolon. Qualitative examination of barium enema films suggests that in some patients the length of the colon rather than its width is greater than normal. A condition of 'redundant colon' has been defined as 'any case in which the enema-filled pelvic loop rises above a line joining the iliac crests' (Kantor, 1934). A comparison of constipated and non-constipated persons showed that about half of those with a history of constipation exceeding 10 yr had a 'redundant colon' as compared with 2 per cent in the control group; patients with a shorter history of constipation fell between these values (Brummer, Seppälä and Wegelius, 1962).

Increasing length of colon could prolong transit rate which in turn could promote water absorption and completeness of bacterial fermentation of unabsorbed carbohydrate. Increasing width of the colon could also prolong transit rate and perhaps decrease the effectiveness of muscular propulsive contractions. Increased capacity of the rectum impairs the sensory response to distension and possibly also the defaecation mechanism. The capacity of the rectum and the size of the colon are thus possible important factors in the pathophysiology of constipation.

Defaecation

Normal defaecation

The process of defaecation is incompletely understood. It is postulated that stool entering the rectum stimulates the nerve receptors involved in the act of defaecation. Halls (1965) administered markers to normal subjects and noted on X-ray their position in the colon and rectum before and after a normal urge to defaecate was felt. All but one of the 18 subjects had faeces in the rectum on the first X-ray, but without any sensation. No gross changes in the position of the markers could be detected on the second X-ray to account for the sense that stool was now present in the rectum. Further work is needed to define what initiates this sensation.

Experimentally, progressive distension of the rectum by a balloon first causes temporary relaxation of the internal anal sphincter, then greater and more sustained relaxation, and finally inhibition for as long as the distension persists (Martelli *et al.*, 1978a; Baldi *et al.*, 1982). Sensation is usually felt by normal subjects when relaxation of the internal sphincter first occurs, but in over half of subjects with constipation inhibition of the sphincter may occur without any conscious sense of distension at volumes up to 50 ml in the balloon (Baldi *et al.*, 1982). As the volume in the balloon increases, to about 150 ml in normal subjects, inhibition of the striated external sphincter muscle occurs (Porter, 1961; Parks, Porter and Melzack, 1962).

Physiologically, it is presumed that the pressure in the rectum rises before defaecation, with consequent relaxation of the internal sphincter and a sense of the need to defaecate. If convenient, the act is completed voluntarily by adoption of a suitable posture, contraction of the diaphragm and abdominal muscles to raise intra-abdominal pressure, and relaxation of the striated muscles of the pelvic floor (Phillips and Edwards, 1965). As the pelvic floor relaxes it descends and the anorectal angle widens (Fry, Griffiths and Smart, 1966; Tagart, 1966). The role, if any, of colonic or rectal contraction is unclear.

Abnormal defaecation

Failure of the defaecation mechanism can arise from deficient sensation, ignored sensation, failure of relaxation of the smooth or striated sphincters, laxity of the pelvic floor, inability to raise intra-abdominal pressure, or inappropriate posture.

Deficient sensation

Patients with constipation who have an enlarged rectum fail to appreciate normal volumes in a distending balloon, but usually appreciate larger volumes than normal (Callaghan and Nixon, 1964). Occasionally the rectum is so large that no sensation is induced, even by 1000 ml or more in the balloon. There is also suggestive evidence that many patients with constipation without obvious megarectum fail to appreciate small volumes of up to 50 ml in a balloon, whereas this volume is felt by all normal adults (Baldi *et al.*, 1982); similar results have been obtained in children (Meunier *et al.*, 1979). It seems likely that deficient sensation leading to impaction of stools in the rectum is an important cause of infrequent difficult defaecation when the rectum is enlarged. It is not known how often rectal enlargement is primary and congenital, or secondary to chronic distension of the rectum by faeces from some other cause of defaecatory failure.

If rectal sensation is deficient, the person has to rely on sensation from the upper anal canal or from the abdomen to know when the rectum is full. In a group of 64 women with severe constipation, but a normal barium enema, only half experienced rectal sensation before defaecation, as compared with 87 per cent in a control group; 6 of the patients felt no rectal or abdominal sensation at all (Preston and Lennard-Jones, unpublished data).

Ignored sensation

Distension of the rectum experimentally leads to a rapid rise in pressure, followed by a fall in pressure due to receptive relaxation. At appropriate volumes, the initial distension is perceived and then sensation decreases or disappears. It seems likely that a similar loss of sensation occurs if a physiological urge to defaecate is ignored or resisted. If recurrent calls to defaecate are ignored, stool will accumulate in the rectum until the bolus is so big that it is difficult and painful to pass. The commonest cause of repressed rectal sensation is social inconvenience, but psychological factors may also be important in some patients. Cerebral impairment for any reason can also lead to loss of perception of rectal fulness and faecal accumulation in the rectum.

Failure of inhibition of the internal sphincter

Relaxation of the internal anal sphincter on distension of the rectum is an involuntary myenteric reflex independent of the spinal cord (Denny-Brown and Robertson, 1935). This reflex is lost in aganglionosis of the rectum and its absence can be used as a diagnostic test (Aaronson and Nixon, 1972; Faverdin *et al.*, 1981). Tonic contraction of the distal rectum and failure of relaxation of the internal sphincter is presumed to be the cause of outlet obstruction in Hirschsprung's disease. There is evidence of increased resting pressure of the internal sphincter in some patients with constipation from other causes, but in these patients the recto-anal distension reflex is normal. It is unlikely that the excessive contraction of the sphincter in these patients causes difficulty in defaecation; it is rather a manifestation of a generalized increased colonic tone (Meunier, Marechal and De Beaujeu, 1979).

Failure to relax the striated muscles of the pelvic floor and external anal sphincter

Normal relaxation.   During normal defaecation, the external anal sphincter relaxes to allow passage of the stool and the puborectalis muscle permits widening of the anorectal angle so that progress of the stool is unimpeded by an acute angle at this point (Fry, Griffiths and Smart, 1966). Relaxation of these striated muscles can be induced by abdominal straining, attempted micturition and distension of the normal rectum above 150 ml, but not by distension of the sigmoid colon (Parks, Porter and Melzack, 1962; Rutter, 1974).

An experimental model.   A balloon model has been developed for the investigation of defaecatory function. Almost all normal subjects can expel from the rectum with ease an ovoid balloon containing 50 ml of water (Barnes and Lennard-Jones, 1985; Preston and Lennard-Jones, 1985b). Women with severe slow-transit constipation but a normal barium enema usually cannot expel the balloon, and no patients with a megarectum can expel it. Some patients with a complaint of constipation but a normal whole gut transit rate can expel the balloon and some are unable to do so. A few patients who cannot expel the balloon while lying on their left side can do so when sitting with the knees raised. No patient is able to expel a larger balloon who cannot expel one of 50 ml (Barnes and Lennard-Jones, 1985).

   This model of defaecation is not entirely physiological because there is no stimulus to contraction of the sigmoid colon and upper rectum, if such contraction plays a role in normal defaecation. However, as a model it does show that a disorder of defaecatory function is probably universal in some forms of constipation and common in others.

Resistance to passage of a balloon.   In the normal subject at rest, a tension of about 700 g has to be applied to a 50 ml balloon in the rectum to pull it through the anal canal. However, when a healthy person strains the balloon is extruded spontaneously without any need for external tension. In the constipated subject, an entirely different situation is observed because, not only is there a failure to expel the balloon on straining, but an external pull on the balloon, approximating to the pull needed at rest, is required to withdraw the balloon while vigorous straining efforts are being made. Electromyography shows that this resistance to passage of the balloon is due to continued contraction of the puborectalis and external anal sphincter muscles. The normal inhibition of these muscles on straining does not therefore occur, as first observed by Kerremans (1969) and Rutter (1974). It seems likely that it is this failure of striated muscle relaxation which prevents constipated subjects from expelling a balloon, and perhaps stool, normally (Preston and Lennard-Jones, 1985b).

Radiological observations.   Confirmatory evidence about this failure of muscular relaxation has been obtained by radiological observation. A balloon was inserted into the distal rectum and filled with 100 ml of barium suspension. A narrow extension of the balloon outlined the anal canal. The subjects attempted to pass the balloon in the normal sitting position and at the same time lateral radiographs were taken before and during straining. Normal subjects could expel the balloon without difficulty. In constipated subjects who could not expel it, the anorectal angle produced by the puborectalis muscle remained constant, the anal canal remained tightly closed and the pelvic floor did not descend (Preston, Lennard-Jones and Thomas, 1984a).

Is the failure to relax a behavioural response?   The reason for the failure of the pelvic floor muscles to relax is unknown. It has been suggested that downward pressure on the puborectalis muscle leads to an urge to defaecate, with a wave of rectal contraction that may lead to external sphincter relaxation (Scharli and Kiesewetter, 1970). However, pulling a balloon down against the puborectalis does not appear to result in sphincter relaxation either in normal subjects or in constipated patients. Normal people can learn to inhibit the contraction of the external sphincter which occurs when the rectum is distended, showing that the contraction is at least partly under voluntary control (Whitehead *et al.*, 1981). Failure of pelvic floor relaxation may be analogous to the spasm of the related muscles in vaginismus and the descriptive term 'anismus' has been suggested (Preston and Lennard-Jones, 1985b).

Lax pelvic floor

Some patients with marked descent of the pelvic floor on straining complain of difficulty in expelling stool. To extrude a solid stool through a relatively narrow anal canal, it may be essential that the orifice is supported by the pelvic floor muscles, otherwise the force of raised intra-abdominal pressure will be dissipated by ballooning of the lower rectum and pelvic floor. A weakened pelvic floor may therefore be both the result of persistent straining (Kiff, Barnes and Swash, 1984) and also a cause of further difficulty in expulsion of stool.

Failure to raise intra-abdominal pressure

Measurements of the rise in intrarectal pressure during attempted expulsion of a balloon show that failure to expel the balloon is not due to generation of less intra-abdominal pressure than normal (Barnes and Lennard-Jones, 1985). However, any condition which may prevent a rise in intra-abdominal pressure, such as lax muscles or pain on straining, for example in sciatic nerve compression, may impair the ability to defaecate.

Posture

Tagart (1966) has shown that the anorectal angle in normal volunteers averages about 80° when erect, 70° when the hips are flexed to a right-angle and 60° when the hips are fully flexed. The angle decreases further on straining with the hips fully flexed. The distance between markers placed on the anterior and posterior margins of the anus increased as the hips were flexed, suggesting that the walls of the anal canal tend to be drawn apart. Both factors, widening of the angle and the drawing forward of the anterior wall of the anal canal, appear likely to aid defaecation, and both are fulfilled in the squatting posture or when a person sitting on a lavatory seat leans forward to obtain full flexion of the hips.

Observations of intrarectal pressure during straining efforts while subjects were lying on their left side and then sitting erect showed no difference (Barnes and Lennard-Jones, 1985), although a difference might be observed in the full squatting posture.

Psychological and mental factors

Personality and bowel habit

Studies in 21 men, all volunteers selected for their normal physical health and psychological fitness, observed under closely supervised conditions for up to 6 months, showed that their stool weight and bowel frequency correlated as greatly with their personality as with variations of fibre intake. Results of rigorous metabolic studies and a detailed personality rating scale (the Minnesota Multiphasic Personality Inventory) showed that dietary and psychological variables each accounted for part of the variance in daily stool production. Heavier stools tended to be produced by the people who were more socially outgoing, more energetic and optimistic, less anxious, and who described themselves in more favourable terms than others (Tucker *et al.*, 1981).

It has long been recognized that, on a standard diet, daily stool weight varies greatly from person to person. The finding in this study that psychological factors seemed as important as dietary ones came as a surprise. The complex interactions already described between colonic transit time, bacterial action on the colonic contents and mucosal absorption perhaps show how this correlation might occur.

Withholding of stool as a possible cause of megabowel

Withholding of stool is thought to be a major cause in childhood rectal accumulation of faeces, with consequent soiling due to inhibition of the anal sphincters (Nixon, 1967; Oppé, 1967). The common factor among 30 children was conflict between parent and child over bowel function (Pinkerton, 1958). It has been postulated that chronic rectal distension due to voluntary repression of defaecation leads to megacolon. This explanation seems over-simple in those children who pass infrequent stools from the early months of life before toilet training and who are later found to have an enlarged rectum with deficient sensation. If, as has been suggested, many adults with severe constipation withhold stool involuntarily, it has to be explained why they do not develop a large rectum and wide colon.

Psychological factors in 'slow-transit' constipation

Among women with prolonged whole gut transit time but a normal barium enema, there often appears to be a childhood background of parental deprivation or cruelty.

Psychological rating scales do not reveal any significant abnormality, but suggestive contributory factors are found on psychiatric interview (Preston, Pfeffer and Lennard-Jones, 1984). Whether or not these factors are related to the abnormal contraction of the pelvic floor muscles on attempted defaecation is unknown.

Mental defect

Patients with severe mental defect are liable to the development of megacolon, possibly due to repeated faecal impaction (Watkins and Oliver, 1965).

Clinical features and treatment

Classification of constipation in adults

No structural abnormality of the anus, rectum or colon, and no associated physical disorder

1. Faulty diet or habit.
2. Pregnancy.
3. Old age.
4. Idiopathic 'slow-transit' constipation in women.
5. Symptom of the 'irritable bowel' syndrome.

With structural disease of the anus, rectum or colon

1. Anal pain or stenosis.
2. Colonic stricture.
3. Aganglionosis and/or abnormal myenteric plexus:
    (a) congenital—Hirschsprung's disease;
    (b) acquired—Chagas' disease;
    (c) East African megacolon;
    (d) 'pseudo-obstruction'.
4. Idiopathic megarectum, sometimes with megacolon.
5. Segmental megacolon with a normal rectum.

Secondary to abnormality outside the colon

1. Endocrine and metabolic:
    (a) hypothyroidism;
    (b) hypercalcaemia;
    (c) porphyria.
2. Neurological:
    (a) damage to sacral outflow or spinal cord;
    (b) central nervous disorders;
    (c) pain on straining, e.g. sciatic root compression.
3. Systemic sclerosis and other connective tissue disorders.
4. Psychological:
    (a) depression;
    (b) anorexia nervosa;
    (c) denied bowel action.
5. Drug side effect.

Discussion in this chapter will be limited to functional disorders of the colon or pelvic floor, many of unknown cause.

Faulty diet or habit

Fibre deficiency is probably the commonest cause of constipation in Western countries. Simple dietary advice about the addition of poorly absorbed carbohydrate to the diet in the form of wholemeal bread, fruit, vegetables and a bran supplement increases the daily weight and water content of the stool and benefits most such patients. Others lose the habit of daily defaecation because of a rushed life or poor toilet facilities. Explanation, usually combined with dietary advice, suffices to give relief.

Idiopathic 'slow-transit' constipation of women

Clinical features

This disorder of women is characterized by an apparently normal colon on barium enema and biopsy (except perhaps for melanosis coli), but a greatly prolonged whole gut transit time. Bowel actions usually become infrequent during adolescence, although some patients remember infrequent bowel actions as a child. The onset of constipation may date from an abdominal or pelvic operation. The interval between bowel actions steadily increases over several years until it is a week or more, and many patients say that they would never pass a stool without a laxative. Abdominal distension and pain are major symptoms. The disorder can become so severe that it dominates and restricts the patient's mode of life.

Medical treatment

An increase in dietary fibre is ineffective and often aggravates the abdominal distension. A wide variety of laxatives in bigger and bigger doses has usually been tried with diminishing success. Medical treatment is usually very unsatisfactory. Osmotic laxatives in small doses are ineffective and in large doses tend to produce liquid bowel actions which can be explosive and difficult to control. Some patients can be managed with large doses of osmotic or stimulant laxatives, or with a daily administered phosphate enema.

Surgical treatment

Sometimes symptoms become so severe, life so disrupted and medical measures so ineffective that colectomy is advised. Partial colonic resection is usually unhelpful, but total colectomy with ileorectal anastomosis often gives a satisfactory result. Caecorectal anastomosis has the drawback that constipation can recur with progressive distension of the caecal remnant. Even after ileorectal anastomosis, continued mild constipation or liquid stools with a tendency to incontinence can be a problem (Preston et al., 1984).

Anorectal myotomy or an anal stretch does not help this group of patients. Evidence that there is failure of relaxation of the puborectalis led to a trial of posterior division of this muscle as a treatment for intractable constipation, but without benefit (Barnes et al., 1985). Such operations have been reported as successful by other investigators

(Wasserman, 1963; Wallace and Madden, 1969) and it is possible that an effective surgical treatment directed to the pelvic floor may be developed.

Constipation as a symptom of the 'irritable bowel' syndrome

Constipation, often associated with abdominal pain and distension, and sometimes alternating with episodes of bowel frequency and looseness, is one symptom of the 'irritable bowel' syndrome. In such patients, the total gut transit rate tends to be normal. It is possible that idiopathic 'slow-transit' constipation is a variant of the 'irritable bowel' syndrome, but with constantly delayed passage of stool. Treatment consists in explanation, a high fibre diet and stool bulking agents, antispasmodics and psychotropic drugs as necessary (Lennard-Jones, 1983).

Aganglionosis of the rectum

Clinical features in adults

Congenital aganglionosis is usually diagnosed in infancy or childhood, but in a few patients it is recognized for the first time in adult life (Todd, 1977; Orr and Scobie, 1983; Rich, Lennard and Wilsdon, 1983). Such patients give a history of infrequent bowel actions from birth, complain of abdominal distension and need to use laxatives or enemas regularly. Retained faecal masses can cause stercoral ulceration of the colon with bleeding or perforation, or respiratory failure can occur due to the greatly distended abdomen and elevated left diaphragm with shift of the mediastinum.

Surgical treatment

In patients with short segment disease, an extended internal sphincterotomy may be adequate (Bentley, 1966; Martelli *et al.*, 1978b). Adults with more extensive aganglionosis are difficult to treat surgically because the proximal bowel is often enormously dilated and hypertrophied and the pelvis is relatively deep. The Duhamel operation is generally preferred, although older patients may need a stoma (Todd, 1977; McCready and Beart, 1980).

Idiopathic megarectum and megacolon

Aetiology

With the recognition in the late 1940s of the aganglionic segment in Hirschsprung's disease, it became clear that the majority of patients with megarectum and megacolon, both children and adults, had normal ganglia. In a series of 90 adults with megacolon, only 20 had aganglionosis (Todd, 1971). Unlike Hirschsprung's disease, which occurs predominantly in males, idiopathic megacolon occurs more equally in the sexes (Tobon and Schuster, 1974). Many believe that it is an acquired condition related to refusal during toilet training (Pinkerton, 1958; Nixon, 1967; Oppé, 1967). However, there is also the possibility that some cases are congenital.

Clinical features

Adult patients with idiopathic megacolon can be divided arbitrarily into two main groups: those who develop constipation, rectal impaction and faecal soiling in childhood, and those who present sporadically throughout later life with constipation and abdominal pain but no soiling (P. R. H. Barnes, unpublished data).

In both groups the major symptom is constipation and periods of weeks to months may elapse between bowel actions. Stools when passed are hard, large and often block the toilet; painful defaecation is common. Unlike patients with Hirschsprung's disease, these patients' general health is good and they are often strangely unperturbed about their lack of bowel function, and even soiling. In an adult series, 7 of 42 patients were mentally subnormal and 2 had a personality disorder (Lane and Todd, 1977).

A hard faecal mass rising out of the pelvis is often palpable and on digital examination the rectum contains a large mass of stool immediately above the anal canal. The anus is often patulous and may gape due to inhibition of the internal and external sphincters (Porter, 1961). Faecal soiling on the perianal skin is common and the buttocks may be held tightly together to improve continence.

Investigation

Contrast X-ray examination should be performed without previous bowel preparation and using a small quantity of water-soluble contrast to avoid impaction of barium. Such X-rays frequently show gross faecal loading of the enlarged rectum, and possibly of the colon also for a variable distance proximally. A lateral view of the pelvis should be taken, for it is only in this view that the narrow distal rectal segment of aganglionosis can be seen; in anteroposterior views it tends to be obscured by the enlarged proximal rectum.

It is important in all such cases to demonstrate the recto-anal inhibition reflex by balloon distension of the rectum. Sometimes the reflex cannot be elicited because the rectum is so much larger than the distending balloon, or the internal sphincter is already fully inhibited as a consequence of a faecal mass in the rectum, or the internal sphincter has recently been stretched during manual disimpaction of the rectum. When the reflex cannot be elicited after these sources of error have been excluded, a full thickness biopsy of the lower rectum is indicated. Thus biopsy can conveniently be combined with an extended sphincterotomy if short segment Hirschsprung's disease seems likely.

Medical treatment

Treatment is directed to emptying the rectum and keeping it empty. As a first step, disimpaction by enemas and washouts is necessary, and often manual removal of faeces under anaesthetic is required. Thereafter, the patient should be encouraged to develop a regular habit of attempted defaecation at a regular time each day, even though no urge to defaecate is felt. Regular and continuous laxatives are generally needed, as whenever treatment is stopped impaction recurs. Magnesium sulphate, in a dose of 10–20 ml of the crystals daily dissolved in water, is often a satisfactory regimen. Some patients prefer lactulose or take this preparation in addition to magnesium sulphate. A few patients need to give themselves evacuant suppositories or enemas at the first sign of impaction.

Surgical treatment

Medical treatment is often successful, provided that the patient understands the problem and adheres to a regular regimen. Surgical treatment is sometimes needed if a medical regimen fails. Sigmoid resection tends to give unsatisfactory results unless there are features suggesting recurrent sigmoid volvulus. A Duhamel procedure is often successful, otherwise subtotal colectomy with ileorectal or caecorectal anastomosis is performed. However, results of such operations are unpredictable and recurrent faecal retention in the rectum or diarrhoea with urgency and a tendency to incontinence (sometimes due to previous anal operations) may occur (Lane and Todd, 1977; Belliveau *et al.*, 1982).

Psychological disorders

Constipation may be a presenting symptom of a depressive illness. Patients with anorexia nervosa often develop intractable constipation, presumably due in part to inadequate food intake, although other aspects of the constipation may resemble the idiopathic 'slow-transit' type seen in women with normal diet and nutrition.

Rarely, a patient may deny the passage of stool, although studies with insoluble radio-opaque markers clearly show that defaecation is occurring (Hinton and Lennard-Jones, 1968). This unusual psychological disorder may present as apparently intractable constipation unresponsive to any drug therapy. The occurrence of this disorder emphasizes the need to obtain objective evidence of a prolonged intestinal transit rate before any surgical treatment of constipation is proposed.

References

AARONSON, I. and NIXON, H. H. (1972). A clinical evaluation of anorectal pressure studies in the diagnosis of Hirschsprung's disease. *Gut*, **13**, 138–146

BALDI, F., FERRARINI, F., CORINALDESI, R., BALESTRA, R., CASSAN, M., FENATI, G. P. and BARBARA, L. (1982). Function of the internal anal sphincter and rectal sensitivity in idiopathic constipation. *Digestion*, **24**, 14–22

BARNES, P. R. H., HAWLEY, P. R., PRESTON, D. M. and LENNARD-JONES, J. E. (1985). Experience of posterior division of the puborectalis muscle in the management of chronic constipation. *British Journal of Surgery* (in press)

BARNES, P. R. H. and LENNARD-JONES, J. E. (1985). Balloon expulsion from the rectum in constipation of different types. *Gut*, **26** (in press)

BATTLE, W. M., SNAPE, W. J. Jr, ALAVI, A., COHEN, S. and BRAUNSTEIN, S. (1980). Colonic dysfunction in diabetes mellitus. *Gastroenterology*, **79**, 1217–1221

BELLIVEAU, P., GOLDBERG, S. M., ROTHENBERGER, D. A. and NIVATVONGS, S. (1982). Idiopathic acquired megacolon: the value of subtotal colectomy. *Diseases of the Colon and Rectum*, **25**, 118–121

BENTLEY, J. R. F. (1966). Posterior excisional ano-rectal myotomy in management of chronic faecal accumulation. *Archives of Disease in Childhood*, **41**, 144–147

BISHOP, A. E., POLAK, J. M., LAKE, B. D., BRYANT, M. G. and BLOOM, S. R. (1981). Abnormalities of the colonic regulatory peptides in Hirschsprung's disease. *Histopathology*, **5**, 679–688

BRODRIBB, A. J. M. and GROVES, C. (1978). Effect of bran particle size on stool weight. *Gut*, **19**, 60–63

BRUMMER, P., SEPPÄLÄ, P. and WEGELIUS, U. (1962). Redundant colon as a cause of constipation. *Gut*, **3**, 140–141

BUENO, L., FIORAMONTI, J., RUCKEBUSCH, Y., FREXINOS, J. and COULOM, P. (1980). Evaluation of colonic myoelectrical activity in health and functional disorders. *Gut*, **21**, 480–485

BURKITT, D. P., WALKER, A. R. P. and PAINTER, N. S. (1974). Dietary fiber and disease. *Journal of the American Medical Association*, **229**, 1068–1074

BURRELL, M., CRONAN, J., MEGNA, D. and TOFFLER, R. (1980). Myxedema megacolon. *Gastrointestinal Radiology*, **5**, 181–186

CALAM, J., UNWIN, R. and PEART, W. S. (1983). Neurotensin stimulates defaecation. *Lancet*, **i**, 737–738

CALLAGHAN, R. P. and NIXON, H. H. (1964). Megarectum: physiological observations. *Archives of Disease in Childhood*, **39**, 153–157

CANN, P. A., READ, N. W., BROWN, C., HOBSON, N. and HOLDSWORTH, C. D. (1983). Irritable bowel syndrome: relationship of disorders in the transit of a single solid meal to symptom patterns. *Gut*, **24**, 405–411

CHOWDHURY, A. R., DINOSO, V. P. and LORBER, S. H. (1976). Characterization of a hyperactive segment at the rectosigmoid junction. *Gastroenterology*, **71**, 584–588

CHRISTENSEN, J., SCHEDL, H. P. and CLIFTON, J. A. (1964). The basic electrical rhythm of the duodenum in normal human subjects and in patients with thyroid disease. *Journal of Clinical Investigation*, **43**, 1659–1667

CHRISTOFIDES, N. D., GHATEI. M. A., BLOOM, S. R., BORBERG, C. and GILLMER, M. D. G. (1982). Decreased plasma motilin concentrations in pregnancy. *British Medical Journal*, **285**, 1453–1454

CHRISTOFIDES, N. D., LONG, R. G., FITZPATRICK, M. L., McGREGOR, G. P. and BLOOM, S. R. (1981). Effect of motilin on the gastric emptying of glucose and fat in humans. *Gastroenterology*, **80**, 456–460

CONNELL, A. M. (1962). The motility of the pelvic colon. Part II. Paradoxical motility in diarrhoea and constipation. *Gut*, **3**, 342–348

CONNELL, A. M., HILTON, C., IRVINE, G., LENNARD-JONES, J. E. and MISIEWICZ, J. J. (1965). Variation of bowel habit in two population samples. *British Medical Journal*, **2**, 1095–1099

CUMMINGS. J. H. (1983). Fermentation in the human large intestine: evidence and implications for health. *Lancet*, **i**, 1206–1208

CUMMINGS. J. H. (1984). Cellulose and the human gut. *Gut*, **25**, 805–810

CUMMINGS. J. H., JENKINS, D. J. A. and WIGGINS, H. S. (1976). Measurement of the mean transit time of dietary residue through the human gut. *Gut*, **17**, 210–218

CUMMINGS. J. H., SOUTHGATE, D. A. T., BRANCH, W., HOUSTON, H., JENKINS, D. J. A. and JAMES, W. P. T. (1978). Colonic response to dietary fibre from carrot, cabbage, apple, bran, and guar gum. *Lancet*, **i**, 5–8

DANIEL, E. E. (1975). Electrophysiology of the colon. *Gut*, **16**, 298–329

DELLER, D. J. and WANGEL, A. G. (1965). Intestinal motility in man. 1. A study combining the use of intraluminal pressure recording and cineradiography. *Gastroenterology*, **48**, 45–57

DENNY-BROWN, D. and ROBERTSON, E. G. (1935). An investigation of the nervous control of defaecation. *Brain*, **58**, 256–309

DEVROEDE, G. and LAMARCHE, J. (1974). Functional importance of extrinsic parasympathetic innervation to the distal colon and rectum in man. *Gastroenterology*, **66**, 273–280

DEVROEDE, G. and SOFFIÉ, M. (1973). Colonic absorption in idiopathic constipation. *Gastroenterology*, **64**, 552–561

DINOSO, V. P. Jr, MURTHY, S. N. S., GOLDSTEIN, J. and ROSNER, B. (1983). Basal motor activity of the distal colon: a reappraisal. *Gastroenterology*, **85**, 637–642

DROSSMAN, D. A., SANDLER, R. S., McKEE, D. C. and LOVITZ, A. J. (1982). Bowel patterns among subjects not seeking health care. *Gastroenterology*, **83**, 529–534

DYER, N. H., DAWSON, A. M., SMITH, B. F. and TODD, I. P. (1969). Obstruction of bowel due to lesion in the myenteric plexus. *British Medical Journal*, **1**, 686–689

EASTWOOD. H. D. H. (1972). Bowel transit studies in the elderly: radio-opaque markers in the investigation of constipation. *Gerontology Clinics*, **14**, 154–159

EXTON-SMITH, A. N., BENDALL, M. J. and KENT, F. (1975). A new technique for measuring the consistency of faeces: a report on its application to the assessment of Senokot therapy in the elderly. *Age and Ageing*, **4**, 58–62

FAVERDIN, C., DORNIC, C., ARHAN, P. et al. (1981). Quantitative analysis of anorectal pressures in Hirschsprung's disease. *Diseases of the Colon and Rectum*, **24**, 422–427

FEINSTAT, T., TESLUK, H., SCHUFFLER, M. D. et al. (1984). Megacolon and neurofibromatosis: a neuronal intestinal dysplasia. *Gastroenterology*, **86**, 1573–1579

FERREIRA-SANTOS, R. (1961). Megacolon and megarectum in Chagas' disease. *Proceedings of the Royal Society of Medicine*, **54**, 1047–1053

FERRI, G-L., ADRIAN, T. E., GHATEI, M. A. et al. (1983). Tissue localization and relative distribution of regulatory peptides in separated layers from the human bowel. *Gastroenterology*, **84**, 777–786

FRIERI, G., PARISI, F., CORAZZIARI, E. and CAPRILLI, R. (1983). Colonic electromyography in chronic constipation. *Gastroenterology*, **84**, 737–740

FRY, I. K., GRIFFITHS, J. D. and SMART, P. J. G. (1966). Some observations on the movement of the pelvic floor and rectum with special reference to rectal prolapse. *British Journal of Surgery*, **53**, 784–787

GLICK, M. E., MESHKINPOUR, H., HALDEMAN, S., BHATIA, N. N. and BRADLEY, W. E. (1982). Colonic dysfunction in multiple sclerosis. *Gastroenterology*, **83**, 1002–1007

GLICK, M. E., MESHKINPOUR, H., HALDEMAN, S., HOEHLER, F., DOWNEY, N. and BRADLEY, W. E. (1984). Colonic dysfunction in patients with thoracic spinal cord injury. *Gastroenterology*, **86**, 287–294

GUNTERBERG, B., KEWENTER, J., PETERSEN, I. and STENER, B. (1976). Anorectal function after major resections of the sacrum with bilateral or unilateral sacrifice of sacral nerves. *British Journal of Surgery*, **63**, 546–554

HALLS, J. (1965). Bowel content shift during normal defaecation. *Proceedings of the Royal Society of Medicine*, **58**, 859–860

HARDCASTLE, J. D. and MANN, C. V. (1968). Study of large bowel peristalsis. *Gut*, **9**, 512–520

HARDCASTLE, J. D. and MANN, C. V. (1970). Physical factors in the stimulation of colonic peristalsis. *Gut*, **11**, 41–46

HARDCASTLE, J. D. and WILKINS, J. L. (1970). The action of sennosides and related compounds on human colon and rectum. *Gut*, **11**, 1038–1042

HINTON, J. M. and LENNARD-JONES, J. E. (1968). Constipation: definition and classification. *Postgraduate Medical Journal*, **44**, 720–723

HINTON, J. M., LENNARD-JONES, J. E. and YOUNG, A. C. (1969). A new method for studying gut transit times using radio-opaque markers. *Gut*, **10**, 842–847

HOLDSTOCK, D. J., MISIEWICZ, J. J., SMITH, T. and ROWLANDS, E. N. (1970). Propulsion (mass movements) in the human colon and its relationship to meals and somatic activity. *Gut*, **11**, 91–99

HOWARD, E. R. (1972). Hirschsprung's disease: a review of the morphology and physiology. *Postgraduate Medical Journal*, **48**, 471–477

ITOH, Z. (1981). Effect of motilin on gastrointestinal tract motility, in *Gut Hormones*, pp. 280–289 (S. R. Bloom, Ed.). London; Churchill Livingstone

KANTOR, J. L. (1934). Anomalies of the colon: their roentgen diagnosis and clinical significance. *Radiology*, **23**, 651–662

KELLEHER, J., WALTERS, M. P., SRINIVASAN, T. R., HART, G., FINDLAY, J. M. and LOSOWSKY, M. S. (1984). Degradation of cellulose within the gastrointestinal tract in man. *Gut*, **25**, 811–815

KERREMANS, R. (1969). *Morphological and Physiological Aspects of Anal Continence and Defaecation*. Brussels; Editions Arscia

KIFF, E. S., BARNES, P. R. H. and SWASH, M. (1984). Pudendal neuropathy in chronic constipation and perineal descent. *Gut*, **25**, 1279–1282

KIRWAN, W. O. and SMITH, A. N. (1974). Gastrointestinal transit estimated by an isotope capsule. *Scandinavian Journal of Gastroenterology*, **9**, 763–766

KIRWAN, W. O. and SMITH, A. N. (1976). Post prandial changes in colonic motility related to serum gastrin levels. *Scandinavian Journal of Gastroenterology*, **11**, 145–149

KIRWAN, W. O. and SMITH, A. N. (1977). Colonic propulsion in diverticular disease, idiopathic constipation, and the irritable colon syndrome. *Scandinavian Journal of Gastroenterology*, **12**, 331–335

KRISHNAMURTHY, S. and SCHUFFLER, M. D. (1983). Severe idiopathic constipation is caused by a distinctive abnormality of the colonic myenteric plexus. *Gastroenterology*, **84**, 1218

LANE, R. H. S. and TODD, I. P. (1977). Idiopathic megacolon: a review of 42 cases. *British Journal of Surgery*, **64**, 305–310

LENNARD-JONES, J. E. (1983). Functional gastrointestinal disorders. *New England Journal of Medicine*, **308**, 431–435

LONG, R. G., BISHOP, A. E., BARNES, A. J. *et al.* (1980). Neural and hormonal peptides in rectal biopsy specimens from patients with Chagas' disease and chronic autonomic failure. *Lancet*, **1**, 559–562

MANNING, A. P., WYMAN, J. B. and HEATON, K. W. (1976). How trustworthy are bowel histories? Comparison of recalled and recorded information. *British Medical Journal*, **2**, 213–214

MARTELLI, H., DEVROEDE, G., ARHAN, P., DUGUAY, C., DORNIC, C. and FAVERDIN, C. (1978a). Some parameters of large bowel motility in normal man. *Gastroenterology*, **75**, 612–618

MARTELLI, H., DEVROEDE, G., ARHAN, P. and DUGUAY, C. (1978b). Mechanisms of idiopathic constipation: outlet obstruction. *Gastroenterology*, **75**, 623–631

McCREADY, R. A. and BEART, R. W. (1980). Adult Hirschsprung's disease: results of surgical treatment at Mayo Clinic. *Diseases of the Colon and Rectum*, **23**, 401–407

MELKERSSON, M., ANDERSSON, H., BOSAEUS, I. and FALKHEDEN, T. (1983). Intestinal transit time in constipated and non-constipated geriatric patients. *Scandinavian Journal of Gastroenterology*, **18**, 593 597

MEUNIER, P., MARECHAL, J. M. and DE BEAUJEU, M. J. (1979). Rectoanal pressures and rectal sensitivity studies in chronic childhood constipation. *Gastroenterology*, **77**, 330–336

MEUNIER, P., ROCHAS, A. and LAMBERT, R. (1979). Motor activity of the sigmoid colon in chronic constipation: comparative study with normal subjects. *Gut*, **20**, 1095–1101

MOORE-GILLON, V. (1984). Constipation: what does the patient mean? *Journal of the Royal Society of Medicine*, **77**, 108–110

NIXON, H. H. (1967). Megarectum in the older child. *Proceedings of the Royal Society of Medicine*, **60**, 3–5

OPPÉ, T. E. (1967). Megacolon and megarectum in older children. *Proceedings of the Royal Society of Medicine*, **60**, 5–7

ORR, J. D. and SCOBIE, W. G. (1983). Presentation and incidence of Hirschsprung's disease. *British Medical Journal*, **287**, 1671

PAINTER, N. S. (1980). Constipation. *Practitioner*, **224**, 387–391

PARKS, A. G., PORTER, N. H. and MELZACK, J. (1962). Experimental study of the reflex mechanism controlling the muscles of the pelvic floor. *Diseases of the Colon and Rectum*, **5**, 407–414

PATRIQUIN, H., MARTELLI, H. and DEVROEDE, G. (1978). Barium enema in chronic constipation: is it meaningful? *Gastroenterology*, **75**, 619–622

PHILLIPS, S. F. and EDWARDS, D. A. W. (1965). Some aspects of anal continence and defaecation. *Gut*, **6**, 396–406

PINKERTON, P. (1958). Psychogenic megacolon in childhood: the implications of bowel negativism. *Archives of Disease in Childhood*, **33**, 371–380

POLAK, J. M. and BLOOM, S. R. (1983). Regulatory peptides: key factors in the control of bodily functions. *British Medical Journal*, **1**, 1461–1466

PORTER, N. H. (1961). Megacolon: a physiological study. *Proceedings of the Royal Society of Medicine*, **54**, 1043–1047

PRESTON, D. M., ADRIAN, T. E., CHRISTOFIDES, N. D., LENNARD-JONES, J. E. and BLOOM, S. R. (1985). Positive correlation between symptoms and circulating motilin, pancreatic polypeptides and gastrin levels in functional bowel disorders. *Gut*, **26** (in press)

PRESTON, D. M., BUTLER, M. G., SMITH, B. and LENNARD-JONES, J. E. (1983). Neuropathology of slow transit constipation. *Gut*, **24**, A997

PRESTON, D. M., HAWLEY, P. R., LENNARD-JONES, J. E. and TODD, I. P. (1984). Results of colectomy for severe idiopathic constipation in women (Arbuthnot Lane's disease). *British Journal of Surgery*, **71**, 547–552

PRESTON, D. M. and LENNARD-JONES, J. E. (1985a). Pelvic colon motility and response to intraluminal bisacodyl in slow transit constipation. *Digestive Diseases and Sciences* (in press)

PRESTON, D. M. and LENNARD-JONES, J. E. (1985b). Anismus in chronic constipation. *Digestive Diseases and Sciences* (in press)

PRESTON, D. M., LENNARD-JONES, J. E. and THOMAS, B. M. (1984a). The balloon proctogram. *British Journal of Surgery*, **71**, 29–32

PRESTON, D. M., LENNARD-JONES, J. E. and THOMAS, B. M. (1984b). Towards a radiological definition of idiopathic megacolon. *Gastrointestinal Radiology* (in press)

PRESTON, D. M., PFEFFER, J. M. and LENNARD-JONES, J. E. (1984). Psychiatric assessment of patients with severe constipation. *Gut*, **25**, A582–583

PRESTON, D. M., REES, L. H. and LENNARD-JONES, J. E. (1983). Gynaecological disorders and hyperprolactinaemia in chronic constipation. *Gut*, **24**, A480

RENNIE, J. A., CHRISTOFIDES, N. D., MITCHENERE, P., JOHNSON, A. G. and BLOOM, S. R. (1980). Motilin and human colonic activity. *Gastroenterology*, **78**, A1243

RICH, A. J., LENNARD, T. W. J. and WILSDON, J. B. (1983). Hirschsprung's disease as a cause of chronic constipation in the elderly. *British Medical Journal*, **287**, 1777–1778

RITCHIE, J. A., ARDRAN, G. M. and TRUELOVE, S. C. (1962). Motor activity of the sigmoid colon of humans: a combined study by intraluminal pressure recording and cineradiography. *Gastroenterology*, **43**, 642–668

RUTTER, K. R. P. (1974). Electromyographic changes in certain pelvic floor abnormalities. *Proceedings of the Royal Society of Medicine*, **67**, 53–56

SCHARLI, A. F. and KIESEWETTER, W. B. (1970). Defecation and continence: some new concepts. *Diseases of the Colon and Rectum*, **13**, 81–107

SCHUFFLER, M. D. and BEEGLE, R. G. (1979). Progressive systemic sclerosis of the gastrointestinal tract and hereditary hollow visceral myopathy: two distinguishable disorders of intestinal smooth muscle. *Gastroenterology*, **77**, 664–671

SCHUFFLER, M. D. and JONAK, Z. (1982). Chronic idiopathic pseudo-obstruction caused by a degenerative disorder of the myenteric plexus: the use of Smith's method to define the neuropathology. *Gastroenterology*, **82**, 476–486

SCOTT, H. W. Jr and CANTRELL, J. R. (1949). Colonmetrographic studies of the effects of section of the parasympathetic nerves of the colon. *Bulletin of the Johns Hopkins Hospital*, **85**, 310–319

SHAFER, R. B., PRENTISS, R. A. and BOND, J. H. (1984). Gastrointestinal transit in thyroid disease. *Gastroenterology*, **86**, 852–855

SMITH, B. (1972). *The Neuropathology of the Alimentary Tract*. London; Edward Arnold

SMITH, B., GRACE, R. H. and TODD, I. P. (1977). Organic constipation in adults. *British Journal of Surgery*, **64**, 313–314

TAGART, R. E. B. (1966). The anal canal and rectum: their varying relationship and its effect on anal continence. *Diseases of the Colon and Rectum*, **9**, 449–452

TANDON, R. K. and TANDON, B. N. (1975). Stool weights in North Indians. *Lancet*, **ii**, 560–561

TAYLOR, I., DUTHIE, H. L., SMALLWOOD, R. and LINKENS, D. (1975). Large bowel myoelectrical activity in man. *Gut*, **16**, 808–814

TOBON, F. and SCHUSTER, M. M. (1974). Megacolon: special diagnostic and therapeutic features. *Johns Hopkins Medical Journal*, **135**, 91–105

TODD, I. P. (1971). Some aspects of adult megacolon. *Proceedings of the Royal Society of Medicine*, **64**, 561–565

TODD, I. P. (1977). Adult Hirschsprung's disease. *British Journal of Surgery*, **64**, 311–312

TUCKER, D. M., SANDSTEAD, H. H., LOGAN, G. M. Jr et al. (1981). Dietary fiber and personality factors as determinants of stool output. *Gastroenterology*, **81**, 879–883

VANTRAPPEN, G., JANSSENS, J., PEETERS, T. L., BLOOM, S. R., CHRISTOFIDES, N. D. and HELLEMANS, J. (1979). Motilin and the interdigestive migrating motor complex in man. *Digestive Diseases and Sciences*, **24**, 497–500

WALLACE, W. C. and MADDEN, W. M. (1969). Experience with partial resection of the puborectalis muscle. *Diseases of the Colon and Rectum*, **12**, 196–200

WALLER, S. L. (1975). Differential measurement of small and large bowel transit times in constipation and diarrhoea: a new approach. *Gut*, **16**, 372–378

WALLER, S. L. and MISIEWICZ, J. J. (1972). Colonic motility in constipation or diarrhoea. *Scandinavian Journal of Gastroenterology*, **7**, 93–96

WALLER, S. L., MISIEWICZ, J. J. and KILEY, N. (1972). Effect of eating on motility of the pelvic colon in constipation or diarrhoea. *Gut*, **13**, 805–811

WANGEL, A. G. and DELLER, J. D. (1965). Intestinal motility in man. III. Mechanisms of constipation and diarrhea with particular reference to the irritable colon syndrome. *Gastroenterology*, **48**, 69–84

WASSERMAN, I. F. (1963). Puborectalis syndrome (rectal stenosis due to anorectal spasm). *Diseases of the Colon and Rectum*, **7**, 87–98

WATIER, A., DEVROEDE, G., DURANCEAU, A. *et al.* (1983). Constipation with colonic inertia: a manifestation of systemic disease? *Digestive Diseases and Sciences*, **28**, 1025–1033

WATKINS, G. L. and OLIVER, G. A. (1965). Giant megacolon in the insane: further observations on patients treated by subtotal colectomy. *Gastroenterology*, **48**, 718–727

WHITE, J. C., VERLOT, M. G. and EHRENTHEIL, O. (1940). Neurogenic disturbances of the colon and their investigation by the colonmetrogram. *Annals of Surgery*, **112**, 1042–1057

WHITEHEAD, W. E., ORR, W. C., ENGEL, B. T. and SCHUSTER, M. M. (1981). External anal sphincter response to rectal distension: learned response or reflex. *Psychophysiology*, **19**, 57–62

WIGGINS, H. S. and CUMMINGS, J. H. (1976). Evidence for the mixing of residue in the human gut. *Gut*, **17**, 1007–1011

WYMAN, J. B., HEATON, K. W., MANNING, A. P. and WICKS, A. C. B. (1978). Variability of colonic function in healthy subjects. *Gut*, **19**, 146–150

Chapter 18

Sphincter sparing colo-anal surgery

R. J. Nicholls

Introduction

The increasing use of sphincter saving surgery has been one of the most important developments in the treatment of colorectal disease. In this chapter only those operations which involve the particular consideration of pelvic floor anatomy and function will be described. These include procedures which result in an anastomosis between the proximal bowel and anal canal itself requiring a perineal approach to the rectum. The type of operation is determined by the nature of the disease. When it is only necessary to remove the rectum and distal colon as, for example, in rectal carcinoma, it will be possible to carry out a colo-anal anastomosis. When, however, the entire large bowel is removed as in ulcerative colitis or familial adenomatosis, an ileo-anal anastomosis will be necessary. The types of operation will be considered separately owing to different pathological considerations, but they are based equally on the physiological fact that the rectum is not necessary for continence, which will be preserved provided the skeletal musculature of the pelvic floor and visceral internal sphincter are functioning adequately (Parks, 1966).

General technical considerations

In most cases the anastomosis is carried out using a per-anal endo-anal technique and the development of this type of surgery has been made possible by instruments especially designed for the purpose. Exposure of the anal canal and lower rectum by adjustable anal specula of Parks or Eisenhammer design is the most necessary requirement. Lighting is equally important and a high intensity headlight is strongly recommended. Adequate mobility of proximal bowel to enable the anastomosis to be fashioned without tension is essential. Careful dissection with division of selected mesenteric vessels may be necessary in some cases, but it is important to avoid producing ischaemia of the bowel.

Sphincter saving operations can be divided into two types, namely anterior resection and restorative proctocolectomy. With anterior resection only those operations involving a colo-anal anastomosis are considered.

Anterior resection with colo-anal anastomosis

The first surgical approaches to the rectum were posterior, either through or lateral to the sacrum (Kraske, 1885; Hochenegg, 1888) owing to the greater safety of an extraperitoneal approach. Anterior resection via the peritoneal cavity only became practicable as surgical and anaesthetic technique and postoperative care improved. Initially, the operation was used for carcinomas in the rectosigmoid and upper rectum, but gradually anterior resection was increasingly applied to tumours of the middle rectum as it became appreciated that cure was not vitiated by extending the scope of the operation to lower seated carcinomas (Waugh, Bluck and Gage, 1955; Slanetz, Herter and Grinnell, 1972; Nicholls et al., 1979). Anterior resection is divided into high anterior resection where the anastomosis is made above the peritoneal reflection and low anterior resection in which it is made below. By definition, an anterior resection involving a colo-anal anastomosis is low in type.

Indications

The greatest application of low anterior resection is in the treatment of carcinoma of the upper and middle thirds of the rectum or in patients with an extensive rectal adenoma. Less commonly, it may be used in some patients with a rectal stricture, for example due to Crohn's disease, and in cases of radiation proctitis, rectovaginal and rectoprostatic fistulae, haemangioma of the rectum and rectal prolapse.

A competent anal sphincter is a prerequisite of the operation and manometric assessment may be a useful addition to clinical examination in cases where there is apparent weakness. In treating cancer, the surgeon's first duty is to cure the disease and criteria for choosing anterior resection over total rectal excision are now reasonably established. In both operations, proximal and lateral clearance of the tumour is similar and it is in the length of rectum removed below the tumour that there is a difference. Pathological examination of resected specimens has shown that spread within the bowel wall of more than 2 cm below the lower border of the rectal carcinoma is rare, occurring in less than 5 per cent of cases (Dukes, 1930; Westhues, 1930; Quer, Dahlin and Mayo, 1953), and clinical retrospective studies have suggested that adequate local clearance is achieved by a resection margin of 3 cm (Wilson and Beahrs, 1975; Pollett and Nicholls, 1983). It seems reasonable at the present time to regard 3 cm as safe, which in practice means that anterior resection is justifiable for tumours down to a minimum distance of 7 cm from the anal verge. The diagnosis of poorly differentiated carcinomas as assessed from histological examination of preoperative biopsy material is generally regarded as a contraindication to anterior resection if the growth is situated in the middle third of the rectum, although there was no apparent difference in survival when the results of anterior resection and total rectal excision for these lesions were compared (Elliot, Todd and Nicholls, 1982).

Survival and local recurrence rates can be related to the local extent of the tumour (Dukes and Bussey, 1958; Morson, Vaughan and Bussey, 1963). Low anterior resection is therefore inadvisable where there is extensive perirectal spread or where local clearance is considered at operation to be inadequate or of doubtful completeness. While some local failures are due to the presence of involved pelvic wall nodes (Sauer and Bacon, 1952), it may be that others are due to inadequate clearance of the rectal mesentery (Heald, Husband and Ryall, 1982).

Types of operation

The operations in use at present are distinguished by the method of anastomosis. Those involving a perineal approach are derived from techniques described in the late nineteenth century (Kraske, 1885; Hochenegg, 1888; Maunsell, 1892; Weir, 1901), which enabled a segment of rectum to be excised and an anastomosis at the level of the upper anal sphincter to be carried out either via a posterior approach or directly to the everted rectal stump. Those in which the anastomosis is constructed per abdomen are an extension of conventional anastomotic technique, most recently modified by the development of circular stapling devices.

In all cases the abdominal dissection is the same. Adequate mobility of the left colon is achieved by mobilization of the splenic flexure and division of the inferior mesenteric artery which, if left intact, will tether the colon and reduce its mobility when it is brought down to the anal canal.

There have been no prospective trials randomizing patients to have different operations, and comparison can be made only through results of series obtained by retrospective analysis. Other variables such as the accuracy of follow-up and differences in surgical technique must apply and make it difficult to draw conclusions as to the relative merits of various procedures.

Mortality, morbidity and survival rates are easier to monitor than other important aspects of outcome such as local recurrence rates and function. It is, however, clear in the case of function, that the frequency, urgency and incontinence is more likely, the shorter the rectal stump (Goligher et al., 1965). Further, it is well recognized that function improves with the passage of time up to about 18 months postoperatively (Bennett, 1976) and thus the time at which any assessment has been made is an important factor to consider when comparing results.

Pull-through operations

There are several modifications of the original operation of Babcock (1939). In all, however, the proximal colon is brought through the anal sphincter to protrude beyond the anus, where it is left for 10 d. After this time, union between the colon and anal canal is anticipated to have occurred and the redundant bowel is excised. Babcock's operation, in which the mucosa of the anal canal is not excised, was modified by Bacon (1945) who cored out the anorectal stump. In the Cutait–Turnbull modification, a direct sutured anastomosis between the colon and everted anorectal stump was performed at 10 d, immediately after excision of the redundant pulled-through colon.

The reported operative mortalities ranged from 1 to 10 per cent (Goligher et al., 1965; Bennett, 1976; Kirwan et al., 1978), and anastomotic dehiscence usually with pelvic abscess formation occurred in 10 to 30 per cent. Necrosis of the colon has been a feared complication and has been reported in 5 to 22 per cent of cases (Black and Botham, 1958; Goligher et al., 1965; Kennedy et al., 1970; Kirwan et al., 1978). Five-year survival rates of cancer patients treated by apparently curative operations ranged from 50 to 65 per cent (Bacon, 1956; Black and Botham, 1958; Waugh and Turner, 1958; Kirwan et al., 1978). Functional results have been variable. Waugh and Turner (1958) reported that only about 10 per cent of patients had normal continence after the Bacon procedure, while Black and Botham (1958) obtained perfect continence in 90 per cent. More careful assessment of patients having the Cutait–Turnbull operation revealed that 75 per cent had some degree of disturbed continence, although it was tolerable in 90 per cent (Goligher *et al.*, 1965; Kennedy *et al.*, 1970; Bennett, Hughes and Cuthbertson, 1972; Kirwan *et al.*, 1978).

Abdominosacral procedures

These originated from the posterior operation of Kraske which was subsequently modified by D'Allaines (1956) to incorporate an abdominal dissection. Modern examples include the operations used by Localio (Localio and Stahl, 1969) and York Mason (1972). In the former, the patient is placed in the right lateral position to give simultaneous access to the abdomen and sacrum. After a radical abdominal dissection and removal of the specimen, a trans-sacral approach to the pelvis with excision of the coccyx is made and a colo-anal anastomosis is carried out leaving the pelvic floor undisturbed. In the latter, the patient is turned to the jack-knife position after the abdominal dissection and access to the pelvis is obtained by a posterior approach involving division of the anal sphincter, puborectalis and levator plate. After the anastomosis has been made, the sphincter and pelvic floor are repaired.

Localio *et al.* (1978) reported an operative mortality of 2 per cent, with anastomotic complications in at least 12 per cent and a 5-year survival rate of 58 per cent in 36 patients treated for cure. Local recurrence occurred in 16.7 per cent. Continence both to flatus and faeces was normal in all cases. Mortality was 12 per cent in 39 patients after a mixture of palliative and curative operations (A. York Mason, 1980, personal communication) and 18 per cent developed pelvic sepsis. Survival and local recurrence rates are not yet available, but continence was normal in 60 per cent of patients in this series and a further 30 per cent had very slight impairment. In the remainder there was a significant disturbance.

Endo-anal colo-anal anastomosis

Parks (1972) first described this operation (*Figure 18.1*), which permits an anastomosis between the colon and anal canal under direct vision and without eversion of the latter. The patient is placed in the Trendelenberg position with the legs elevated on crutches, and the operative specimen is removed following an abdominal dissection. An anal retractor is passed by the perineal operator and the colon is delivered into the anal lumen. Between 12 and 20 interrupted sutures are then placed between the colon and anal stump. This technique may be modified to produce an overlapped anastomosis, whereby the colon is enclosed within a sleeve of anorectal circular muscle after removal of the mucosa down to the dentate line by sharp scissor dissection. This is facilitated by the submucosal injection of saline containing adrenaline (1:300 000). The operation is covered by a temporary colostomy, which is closed after satisfactory healing.

Operative mortality in a series of 76 patients was 4 per cent and pelvic sepsis occurred in 14 per cent (Parks and Percy, 1982). There was some selection of patients for the operation, usually on the basis of histological grade of tumour. Only 12 per cent of this series had a poorly differentiated carcinoma, compared with 18 per cent among all cases treated by total rectal excision at the same hospital. As far as Dukes's stage was concerned, there was no difference in the proportion of cases (colo-anal anastomosis A 14.5 per cent, B 39.5 per cent, C 46 per cent; all rectal cancers A 14.3 per cent, B 35.6 per cent, C 49.8 per cent).

Three-year survival and local recurrence rates in 37 patients followed for this period

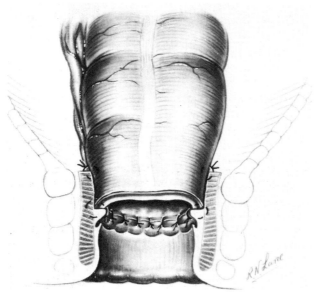

Figure 18.1. Endo-anal colo-anal anastomosis

TABLE 18.1. Anterior resection with colo-anal anastomosis: survival and local recurrence at 3 yr, 37 patients

	No.	*Cancer deaths*	*Local recurrence*	*Alive without recurrence*
Palliative	7	7	0	0
Curative	30	9	4 (13 per cent)	21 (70 per cent)

are shown in *Table 18.1.* Overall, local recurrence occurred in 6 of the 73 patients who survived the original operation, a rate of 8 per cent. These figures indicate that cancer cure is as likely after this operation as for any other for rectal cancer. Function was assessed in 70 patients followed postoperatively. Thirty-nine (56 per cent) were continent, with a frequency of 1–3 evacuations per 24 h, and 30 experienced minor occasional leakage with a frequency of 4–6 times per 24 h. Only 1 patient had significant faecal leakage. It is clear that function can be related to the physiological performance of the pelvic floor musculature, but is satisfactory in the majority of cases.

Restorative proctocolectomy

Stoma prevention in surgery of inflammatory bowel disease and familial adenomatosis has been one of the chief aims for more than 40 years. Of various operations developed, two involve an ileo-anal anastomosis. These include proctocolectomy with ileo-anal anastomosis, described by Ravitch and Sabiston (1947), and restorative proctocolectomy with ileal reservoir developed in man by Parks (Parks and Nicholls, 1978), but first reported in dogs by Valiente and Bacon (1955).

General considerations

The aim of both operations is to remove all disease-prone tissue while preserving the anal sphincter. The pathology of ulcerative colitis makes this possible, since only the large bowel is affected and the disease is confined to the mucosa. Adenomatosis is also a mucosal disease, but all parts of the gastrointestinal tract are potentially involved. The colon is the most common site of malignant disease, however, and is therefore amenable to restorative proctocolectomy on the same principle of complete removal of the entire large bowel mucosa by combining a conventional colectomy and removal of the majority of the rectum, with stripping of mucosa from the remaining rectal stump down to the dentate line.

Such operations are only acceptable in practice if function is satisfactory afterwards. Careful follow-up to monitor frequency, urgency, continence, the need for medication, the metabolic state of the patient and the state of the small bowel 'neorectum' must be maintained and results reported in detail.

The belief that the rectum is necessary for continence and defaecation sensation is erroneous, since both are preserved even after division of the gut tube at the anorectal junction. Mucosal proctectomy of a long rectal stump is therefore unnecessary and time consuming.

Proctocolectomy with ileo-anal anastomosis (Ravitch)

Technique

Nevertheless, a long rectal stump with mucosal stripping by sharp scissor dissection has been recommended by Ravitch and Sabiston (1947) and subsequently by others (Martin, LeCoultre and Schubert, 1977; Telander and Perrault, 1981). This follows a colectomy and the divided terminal ileum is then brought down to the anal canal where an anastomosis is carried out. The operation is covered by an ileostomy which is closed some weeks later after healing has occurred.

Results

Failure, defined by conversion to a permanent ileostomy, has occurred in 10 to 15 per cent of cases and there has been a high morbidity with complications occurring in 11 out of 17 patients reported by Martin, LeCoultre and Schubert (1977), anastomotic or cuff abscess formation being the commonest and intestinal obstruction occurring in about 15 per cent. Telander and Perrault (1981) had a similar experience.

A review of functional results by Valiente and Bacon (1955) revealed that a high proportion of patients had an unsatisfactory outcome. About 50 per cent were troubled by frequency and urgency and many developed peri-anal skin soreness ascribable to diarrhoea. Incontinence was, however, uncommon. After a period of disuse, the operation was revived by Martin, LeCoultre and Schubert (1977), who claimed satisfactory function in 11 children who had had the ileostomy closed, although precise details were not given. Telander and Perrault (1981) reported a series of 25 children and young adults of whom 19 out of 22 available for assessment had a frequency of more than 5 times per 24 h, with a mean frequency in the whole group of 7.3 times. They claim that this could be reduced by the balloon dilatation of the neorectum before closure of the ileostomy.

It is clear, however, that function is related to capacitance of the neorectum, and balloon distension studies have shown poorer expansion after the simple ileo-anal procedure than after construction of an ileal reservoir (Taylor *et al.*, 1983). The operation has consequently not been favoured by most surgeons working in the field.

Restorative proctocolectomy with ileal reservoir (Parks)

This operation (*Figure 18.2*) is an advance upon the simple ileo-anal anastomosis by the incorporation of an ileal reservoir to improve function. The experience of Kock with a continent ileostomy demonstrated that a small bowel reservoir could function satisfactorily in practice (Kock, 1973).

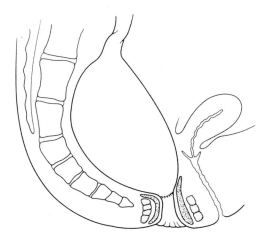

Figure 18.2. Restorative proctocolectomy with ileal reservoir

Indications

Indications can be divided into medical and personal. The patient must not have Crohn's disease (thus those with ulcerative colitis and polyposis are suitable), the anal sphincter must be competent and proctocolectomy with a permanent ileostomy should be the only therapeutic alternative. Provided medical indications are satisfactory, all depends on the desires and motivation of the patient. The drawbacks as well as the advantages should be pointed out. Results, including failures, must be given and possible functional problems discussed. The duration of treatment, which includes the time necessary for closure of the temporary ileostomy, is likely to be several months before normal life can be resumed.

The operation should not be carried out in severely ill patients or in those taking steroids. Under these circumstances a colectomy with ileostomy and preservation of the rectal stump will result in restoration of health, after which a reservoir operation can be carried out as a second stage. This approach has the added advantage of supplying the pathologist with a specimen of colon to exclude Crohn's disease. Patients with adenomatosis must have the diagnosis confirmed by histological examination of the biopsy from an adenoma, before undertaking restorative proctocolectomy. The presence of cancer has not been considered a contraindication, provided adequate clearance on conventional principles for radical surgery is possible.

Technique

After a conventional mobilization of the colon, the rectal mesentery is divided close to the bowel wall to mobilize the rectum to within 5–7 cm of the anal verge. The bowel is divided at this level and the specimen removed. The remaining mucosa lining the anorectal stump is then stripped by scissor dissection to the level of the dentate line via a per-anal approach. This is facilitated by elevating the mucosa from the muscularis propria by the submucosal injection of saline containing diluted adrenaline (1:300 000). The reservoir is then constructed from the terminal 40–50 cm of ileum and joined to the anal canal at the level of the dentate line via a per-anal approach using a similar suture technique to colo-anal anastomosis. In the original Parks model, the reservoir is formed by 3 loops of terminal ileum, each 15 cm long, with a short spout of intact small bowel projecting 3–5 cm distally. The ileo-anal anastomosis is consequently carried out end-to-end. The two-loop design described by Utsunomiya *et al.* (1980) avoids the distal ileal segment altogether and requires a side-to-end ileo-anal anastomosis. This is also necessary in the larger four-loop reservoir, in which each limb measures 12 cm. The operation is covered by a loop ileostomy which is closed some 8 weeks later, provided healing of suture lines is satisfactory.

Three technical aspects require emphasis. The close rectal dissection avoids damage to pelvic autonomic nerves and creates a small pelvic cavity which reduces the opportunity for haematoma formation. Where, however, a cancer in the upper rectum is present, a conventional dissection should be used. Removal of mucosa should be complete; hence the need to continue the submucosal excision to the dentate line. Adequate mobility of the small bowel is essential if tension on the ileo-anal anastomosis is to be avoided. Tension is usually due to vessels within the mesentery, which should itself be mobilized on the right side to the level of the duodenum. Before constructing the reservoir, a trial of mobility should be made. The small bowel site for the future anastomosis is selected and passed down into the pelvis to a perineal operator who has inserted an anal speculum. The intestine is then drawn through the anorectal muscle tube and adequate mobility, when it is at the level of the dentate line, can be verified. If there is too much tension, it is necessary to divide selected vessels in the mesentery, taking care to maintain adequate blood flow to the small bowel.

Results

Several hundred operations have now been performed throughout the world and there is therefore considerable experience in the immediate mortality and morbidity and the functional results after closure of the ileostomy. In a series of 105 patients treated at St Mark's Hospital between 1976 and 1984, there was 1 postoperative death (1 per cent) and 2 late deaths, one of which was related to the treatment. Others reporting large series have also experienced a low operative mortality (Rothenberger *et al.*, 1983; Metcalf *et al.*, 1984). Failure, as defined by removal of the reservoir and creation of a permanent ileostomy, occurred in 6 of 104 operations at St Mark's (6 per cent) and 10 of 188 patients treated at the Mayo Clinic (5.3 per cent) (Metcalf *et al.*, 1984). Reasons have been due to misdiagnosis of Crohn's disease, pelvic sepsis and unsatisfactory function.

The most common postoperative complications after restorative proctocolectomy are pelvic sepsis, usually with a degree of breakdown of the ileo-anal anastomosis, and intestinal obstruction due to adhesions requiring laparotomy with reported rates of 17–21 per cent and 9–11.5 per cent, respectively (Metcalf *et al.*, 1984; Nicholls and Pezim, 1984). In our experience, 61 per cent of patients had no complications following

TABLE 18.2. Restorative proctocolectomy with ileal reservoir function in 88 patients: follow-up 2–65 months (mean 18.2)

	Type of reservoir		
	Three-loop $n=58$	Two-loop $n=12$	Four-loop $n=18$
Evacuation/24 h	3.7 ± 1.6	5.5 ± 1.6	4.1 ± 1.3
Night evacuation	15 (26)*	7 (58)	4 (22)
Antidiarrhoeal medication	11 (19)	7 (58)	6 (33)
Continence:			
normal	39 (67)	9 (75)	16 (89)
minimal leak	16 (28)	3 (25)	2 (11)
troublesome leak	3 (5)	0 (0)	0 (0)

* Figures in parentheses are percentages.

the pouch operation, although closure of the ileostomy has resulted in further complications in 11 out of 98 cases (11 per cent).

Immediately after closure of the ileostomy, some patients experience frequency and urgency of defaecation and some episodes of incontinence which improve spontaneously over subsequent weeks in most cases. The duration of follow-up is therefore a very important factor when assessing function.

In the St Mark's series, 88 of 104 patients are available for functional assessment, the difference of 16 being accounted for as follows: ileostomy not closed (6), reservoir removed (6), late death (2, including 1 patient who had the reservoir removed), loss to follow-up (2).

The functional results are shown in *Table 18.2*. Three reservoir types have been used, with the longest follow-up in patients having the triple loop design. Evacuation by catheterization has been necessary in over 50 per cent of these patients, although this was needed in only 2 (8 per cent) of the 24 patients reported by Rothenberger *et al.* (1983). However, all cases having two- or four-loop reservoirs are able to defaecate spontaneously, and it is the presence of the distal ileal segment which is probably responsible for the need to catheterize in those with three-loop reservoirs (Pescatori, Manhire and Bartram, 1983). Frequency of defaecation is significantly greater for two-loop compared with three- or four-loop reservoirs, as is the need for night evacuation and antidiarrhoeal medication. A mean frequency in a much larger series of two-loop reservoirs of 6.0 ± 2.6 per day and 1.2 ± 1.3 per night (Metcalf *et al.*, 1984) is similar to the small group of 12 two-loop reservoirs in this series. There is every indication that frequency is related to the volume of the reservoir, as shown in *Figure 18.3*. The inverse relationship is good evidence that the reservoir is acting as a capacitance organ and suggests that a reservoir volume of 350 ml or more is necessary to achieve frequencies of 5 or less. Frank faecal incontinence is uncommon but minimum disturbances, usually with the passage of small amounts of mucus every 2–3 d, occur in about 25 per cent of patients. Mucus leakage can be related to resting anal canal pressure (*Table 18.3*). Anal soreness is related to frequency and leakage.

There is some indication that function is better in patients with familial adenomatosis compared with those who originally had ulcerative colitis. This may be related to a possible difference in the prevalence of microscopic mucosal inflammation in biopsy material from the reservoirs. It seems that 80 per cent of those from patients

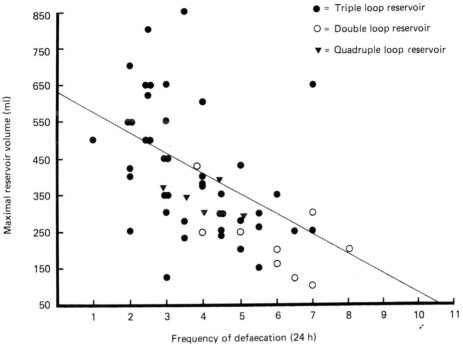

Figure 18.3. Relationship between frequency of defaecation and maximal tolerated reservoir volume after ileostomy closure

TABLE 18.3. Restorative proctocolectomy with ileal reservoir: resting anal canal pressure in patients with and without mucus leakage

Patient	Resting pressure (cmH$_2$O)	Patient	Resting pressure (cmH$_2$O)
2	60	1	50
4	60	3	40
6	90	5	40
7	100	8	36
10	60	9	20
13	100	11	30
14	80	12	40
Mean	78.6		36.6
±s.d.	18.6		9.4

$P < 0.05$.

with ulcerative colitis compared with 20 per cent from adenomatosis patients show inflammation, although more data are required to be certain of any difference. A few patients have developed clinically overt inflammation, producing symptoms identical to proctitis. Further investigation of the clinical manifestations of pouch inflammation and its possible causes is in progress.

Vitamin B$_{12}$ absorption and low serum iron levels have been observed in 5–10 per cent of patients, but no serious metabolic disturbances have yet occurred.

While continued long-term follow-up is clearly necessary, the results so far have been encouraging, and restorative proctocolectomy with ileal reservoir would seem to have an important place in the surgical treatment of diffuse mucosal large bowel disease.

References

BABCOCK, W. W. (1939). Experiences with resection of the colon and the elimination of colostomy. *American Journal of Surgery*, **46**, 186–203

BACON, H. E. (1945). Evolution of sphincter muscle preservation and re-establishment of continuity in the operative treatment of rectal and sigmoidal cancer. *Surgery, Gynecology and Obstetrics*, **81**, 113–127

BACON, H. E. (1956). Abdomino-perineal proctosigmoidectomy with sphincter preservation. Five-year and ten-year survival after pull-through operation for cancer of the rectum. *Journal of the American Medical Association*, **160**, 628–634

BENNETT, R. C. (1976). The place of pull-through operations in the treatment of carcinoma of the rectum. *Diseases of the Colon and Rectum*, **19**, 420–424

BENNETT, R. C., HUGHES, E. S. R. and CUTHBERTSON, A. M. (1972). Long-term review of function following pull-through operations of the rectum. *British Journal of Surgery*, **59**, 723–725

BLACK, B. M. and BOTHAM, R. J. (1958). Combined abdomino-perineal resections for lesions of the mid and upper parts of the rectum. *Archives of Surgery*, **76**, 688–696

D'ALLAINES, F. (1956). *Die Chirurgische Behandlung des Rektumcarzinoms*. Leipzig; Barth

DUKES, C. E. (1930). The spread of cancer of the rectum. *British Journal of Surgery*, **17**, 643–648

DUKES, C. E. and BUSSEY, H. J. R. (1958). The spread of rectal cancer and its effect on prognosis. *British Journal of Cancer*, **12**, 309–320

ELLIOT, M. S., TODD, I. P. and NICHOLLS, R. J. (1982). Radical restorative surgery for poorly differentiated carcinoma of the mid rectum. *British Journal of Surgery*, **69**, 273–275

GOLIGHER, J. C., DUTHIE, H. L., DeDOMBAL, F. T. and McK. WATTS, J. (1965). The pull-through abdominoanal excision for carcinoma of the middle third of the rectum: a comparison with low anterior resection. *British Journal of Surgery*, **52**, 323–335

HEALD, R. J., HUSBAND, E. M. and RYALL, R. H. D. (1982). The mesorectum in rectal surgery—the clue to pelvic recurrence. *British Journal of Surgery*, **69**, 613–617

HOCHENEGG, J. (1888). Die Sakrale Methode der extirpation von Mastdarm Krebsen nach Prof. Kraske. *Wiener Klinische Wochenschrift*, **1**, 254–257

KENNEDY, J. T., McOMISH, D., BENNETT, R. C., HUGHES, E. S. R. and CUTHBERTSON, A. M. (1970). Abdomino-anal pull-through resection of the rectum. *British Journal of Surgery*, **57**, 589–596

KIRWAN, W. O., TURNBULL, R. B., FAZIO, V. W. and WEAKLEY, F. L. (1978). Pull-through operation with delayed anastomosis for rectal cancer. *British Journal of Surgery*, **65**, 695–698

KOCK, N. G. (1973). Continent ileostomy, in *Progress in Surgery*, ch. 12, p. 180 (M. Allgöwer, S. E. Bergentz and R. Y. Calne, Eds). Basel; Karger

KRASKE, P. (1885). Zur Extirpation hoch sitzender Mastdarm Krebse. *Verhandlungen Deutscher Gesellschaft für Chirurgie*, **14**, 464

LOCALIO, A. S., ENG, K., GOUGE, T. H. and RANSON, J. H. C. (1978). Abdominosacral resection for carcinoma of the mid rectum: ten years experience. *Annals of Surgery*, **188**, 475–480

LOCALIO, A. S. and STAHL, W. M. (1969). Simultaneous abdominosacral resection and anastomosis for mid rectal cancer. *American Journal of Surgery*, **117**, 282–289

MARTIN, L. W., LeCOULTRE, C. and SCHUBERT, W. K. (1977). Total colectomy and mucosal proctectomy with preservation of continence in ulcerative colitis. *Annals of Surgery*, **188**, 245–248

MAUNSELL, H. W. (1892). A new method of excising the two upper portions of the rectum and the lower segment of the sigmoid flexure of the colon. *Lancet*, **2**, 473–476

METCALF, A., BEART, R. W., DOZOIS, R. R. et al. (1984). Ileal-pouch anal anastomosis: the procedure of choice? *Proceedings of the 83rd Annual Meeting of the American Society of Colon and Rectal Surgeons*, New Orleans

MORSON, B. C., VAUGHAN, E. G. and BUSSEY, H. J. R. (1963). Pelvic recurrence after excision of the rectum for carcinoma. *British Medical Journal*, **2**, 13–17

NICHOLLS, R. J. and PEZIM, M. (1984). Restorative proctocolectomy with ileal reservoir for ulcerative colitis and familial adenomatous polyposis: a comparison of three reservoir designs (in press)

NICHOLLS, R. J., RITCHIE, J. K., WADSWORTH, J. and PARKS, A. G. (1979). Total excision or restorative resection for carcinoma of the middle third of the rectum. *British Journal of Surgery*, **66**, 625–627

PARKS, A. G. (1966). In *Clinical Surgery*, vol. 10, p. 541 (C. Rob, R. Smith and C. N. Morgan, Eds). London; Butterworths

PARKS, A. G. (1972). Transanal technique in low rectal anastomosis. *Proceedings of the Royal Society of Medicine*, **65**, 975–976

PARKS, A. G. and NICHOLLS, R. J. (1978). Proctocolectomy without ileostomy for ulcerative colitis. *British Medical Journal*, **2**, 85–88

PARKS, A. G. and PERCY, J. P. (1982). Resection and sutured colo-anal anastomosis for rectal carcinoma. *British Journal of Surgery*, **69**, 301–304

PESCATORI, M., MANHIRE, A. and BARTRAM, C. I. (1983). Evacuation pouchography in the evaluation of ileo-anal reservoir function. *Diseases of the Colon and Rectum*, **26**, 365–368

POLLETT, W. G. and NICHOLLS, R. J. (1983). The relationship between the extent of distal margin and survival and local recurrence rates after curative anterior resection for carcinoma of the rectum. *Annals of Surgery*, **198**, 159–163

QUER, E. A., DAHLIN, D. C. and MAYO, C. W. (1953). Retrograde intramural spread of carcinoma of the rectum and rectosigmoid: a microscopic study. *Surgery, Gynecology and Obstetrics*, **96**, 24–30

RAVITCH, M. M. and SABISTON, D. C. (1947). Anal ileostomy with preservation of the sphincter. A proposed operation in patients requiring total colectomy for benign lesions. *Surgery, Gynecology and Obstetrics*, **84**, 1095–1099

ROTHENBERGER, D., VERMENLEN, F. D., CHRISTENSEN, C. E. et al. (1983). Restorative proctocolectomy with ileal reservoir and ileoanal anastomosis. *American Journal of Surgery*, **145**, 82–88

SAUER, I. and BACON, H. E. (1952). A new approach for excision of carcinoma of the lower portion of the rectum and anal canal. *Surgery, Gynecology and Obstetrics*, **95**, 229–242

SLANETZ, C. A., HERTER, F. P. and GRINNELL, R. S. (1972). Anterior resection versus abdomino-perineal resection for carcinoma of the rectum and rectosigmoid. *American Journal of Surgery*, **123**, 110–117

TAYLOR, B. M., CRANLEY, B., KELLY, K. A., PHILLIPS, S. F., BEART, R. W. and DOZOIS, R. R. (1983). A clinico-physiological comparison of ileal pouch-anal and straight anal ileo-anal anastomosis. *Annals of Surgery*, **198**, 462–468

TELANDER, R. L. and PERRAULT, J. (1981). Colectomy with rectal mucosectomy and ileoanal anastomosis in young patients. *Archives of Surgery*, **116**, 623–629

UTSUNOMIYA, J., IWAMA, T., IMAGO, M., MOTSUO, S., SAWAI, S., YAEGASHI, K. and HIRAYAMA, R. (1980). Total colectomy, mucosal proctectomy and ileoanal anastomosis. *Diseases of the Colon and Rectum*, **23**, 459–466

VALIENTE, M. A. and BACON, H. E. (1955). Construction of pouch using 'pantaloon' technique for pull-through of ileum following colectomy. *American Journal of Surgery*, **90**, 742–750

WAUGH, J. M., BLUCK, M. A. and GAGE, R. P. (1955). Three and five year survivals following combined abdomino-perineal resection, abdomino-perineal resection with sphincter preservation and anterior resection for carcinoma of the rectum and lower part of the sigmoid colon. *Annals of Surgery*, **142**, 752–757

WAUGH, J. M. and TURNER, J. C. (1958). Abdomino-perineal resection with preservation of the anal sphincter for carcinoma of the mid rectum. *Surgery, Gynecology and Obstetrics*, **107**, 777–783

WEIR, R. F. (1901). An improved method of treating high-seated cancers of the rectum. *Journal of the American Medical Association*, **37**, 801–803

WESTHUES, A. (1930). Über die Entstehung und Vermeidung des lokalen Rektum Karzinom-Rezidivs. *Archiv für Klinische Chirurgie*, **161**, 582–624

WILSON, S. M. and BEAHRS, O. H. (1975). The curative treatment of carcinoma of the sigmoid, rectosigmoid and rectum. *Annals of Surgery*, **183**, 556–565

YORK MASON, A. (1972). Transsphincteric exposure for low rectal anastomosis. *Proceedings of the Royal Society of Medicine*, **65**, 974–976

Chapter 19

Chronic perianal pain

M. Swash

Introduction

Few complaints produce such mixed reactions among family, friends and physicians as chronic anal or perianal pain without evident cause. Pain in the anal canal or perineum is usually the result of common and easily recognized disorders such as anal fistula, intersphincteric abscess, thrombosed haemorrhoids or anorectal cancer, but when no cause can be found management is difficult. Patients are then often referred from one specialist to another and a variety of different but ineffective treatments are tried.

What is the cause of this idiopathic perianal pain and how can it be relieved? Several syndromes have been described.

Syndromes

The first reference to anal pain appeared in 1859 when Simpson described the syndrome which he called *coccygodynia* (Simpson, 1859). Since then, however, a number of different terms have been used, leading to confusion as to the definition of this syndrome. Coccygodynia is said to consist of a vague tenderness or ache in the region of the sacrum and coccyx, and in the adjacent muscles and soft tissues. It is often associated with similar rectal and perianal discomfort. Sometimes the pain radiates to the back of the thighs or buttocks. In Thiele's (1963) series of 324 cases, 85 per cent were women. The syndrome usually presents in the fifth and sixth decades and symptoms often persist for many years. Thiele noted that sitting seemed to induce or exacerbate the pain, and suggested that it was referred from chronic spasm of the levator ani muscles either because of infection or trauma to these muscles. This suggestion led to the use of the term 'levator syndrome' (Grant, Salvati and Rubin, 1975), and to treatment by digital massage of the pelvic floor musculature.

Proctalgia fugax, described by Thaysen (1935), is a relatively well-defined syndrome of obscure causation. It is commoner in men than women, beginning in early adult life and ceasing spontaneously in late middle life (Abrahams, 1935). A curiously large number of reports have concerned doctors. It occurs at any time, but is particularly common at night. It begins suddenly and progresses to a cramp-like pain which may be very severe, but which usually resolves after less than 30 min. The pain is felt at a constant site in the anal canal or rectum, above the level of the external anal sphincter. It may sometimes be relieved by flexing the extended legs as far as possible onto the abdominal wall, as when sitting on the floor, a feature which suggests that it may be due to a cramp-like spasm of the muscles of the pelvic floor. The pain itself is not accompanied by an acute bowel disturbance, but there is a high incidence of symptoms of 'irritable bowel' syndrome in patients with proctalgia fugax (Bensaude, 1965; Thompson and Heaton, 1980).

Perianal pain is also a feature of some patients with the *descending perineum syndrome* (Parks, Porter and Hardcastle, 1966). In these patients a dull aching pain in the posterior perineum is associated with abnormal descent of the perineum during straining at defaecation, and sometimes with prolapse of the anterior rectal mucosa. The pain is prominent after defaecation, or after prolonged standing, and it is usually relieved by lying down. Examination reveals that the perineum descends below the plane of the ischial tuberosities at rest, or during straining (Parks, Porter and Hardcastle, 1966). The pain sometimes improves when the abnormal defaecation habit is modified, but pelvic floor repair may be necessary.

The classification of anal pain syndromes given in *Table 19.1* summarizes the main clinical features of the syndromes, and introduces the concept of chronic idiopathic perianal pain. The latter is an ill-defined and perhaps heterogeneous clinical syndrome. In many cases there are strong indications that psychiatric disturbances are important.

Patients

In a study of 35 patients, aged 36–78 years (mean 58 yr), 28 (80 per cent) were women (Neill and Swash, 1982). All presented with continuous anal and perianal pain of at least several months' duration. Twenty-eight (80 per cent) were able to localize their pain to a definite point in the anal canal, but no site was significantly more frequent. Twenty-six (74 per cent) patients described radiation of their pain away from its point of maximum intensity in the anal canal. In 21 (60 per cent), the pain radiated into the sacrum and to the back of the thighs, and in 5 (14 per cent), it radiated into the pelvis and abdomen. In all but one patient, the pain was aggravated by sitting. Nineteen (54 per cent) were relieved by lying down and 14 (40 per cent) by standing. Defaecation had no constant effect. A characteristic description of the pain was that it was 'like sitting on a ball' in the anal canal. The pain was usually intense, sometimes throbbing or burning, but never sharp in character, although its radiating component was often prickly. The pain was invariably described as continuous and the patients were distressed and often tearful in giving their account of it. Sleep, however, was often not interrupted by pain, since the pain was usually relieved by lying down.

Twenty (57 per cent) gave a history of surgery to the pelvic viscera, lumbar spine or anal canal prior to the onset of chronic anal pain. This included hysterectomy, vaginal repair for anterior perineal prolapse, pelvic floor procedures for rectal prolapse, haemorrhoidectomy, and lumbosacral laminectomy for sciatica.

Thirteen (37 per cent) gave a history of sciatica and 4 (11 per cent) had been investigated by myelography in the 4 years before the onset of anal pain. Eight (23 per cent) patients described difficult childbirth some years before their anal pain commenced. Most patients had been investigated elsewhere and many had been treated by minor surgical procedures to the anal canal and rectum, such as removal of anal tags, partial haemorrhoidectomy or maximal anal dilatation, in ineffective attempts to

TABLE 19.1. Types of anal and perineal pain

Disorder	Mean age of onset	Sex predom-inence	Nature of pain	Site	Radiation	Time of onset	Aggravating factors	Relieving factors	Associated features
Proctalgia fugax	Young adults	M	Sudden, crescendo, lasts minutes, stops spon-taneously	Upper anal canal, constant site	Nil	Mostly at night	Anxiety	Stretching anus, flexing thighs	Tense, introspective personality; 'irritable bowel' syndrome
Coccygo-dynia	Adults	F	Continuous vague ache with exacerbations	Lower sacrum, perineum and anal canal	Thighs and coccyx	Any time, more during the day	Sitting posture?, defaecation, ? trauma to coccyx	—	Tender spots in sacro-coccygeal region, levator muscle spasm
Descending perineum syndrome	Any age?	F	Constant heavy dull perineal ache, sometimes with brief sharp pain	Perineum and anal canal	Nil, possibly to lower abdomen	Usually late in the day	Standing, walking, after defaecation	Lying down	Irregular bowel habit, straining at stool
Chronic idiopathic anal pain	58 yr	F	Continuous dull throb-bing, burning likened to a ball in the anal canal, intermittent or continuous	Mid-anal canal, well localized, may be unilateral	Sacrum, thighs, lower abdomen, anterior perineum and vagina	Any time, usually late in the day	Sitting	Lying down	Pelvic or spinal surgery, myelography, perineal descent

relieve their pain. Two patients reported that a maximal anal stretch procedure seemed to have made their pain worse.

In each patient, examination of the perineum, anal canal and rectum, including endoscopy of the upper anal canal and rectum, revealed no cause for the pain. Gynaecological examination was normal. The coccyx and the levator ani muscles were not tender to digital examination per rectum. Twenty-one (60 per cent) patients showed a significant degree of perineal descent on straining. No patient was incontinent. There was slight impairment of sensation to pinprick in the perineum in one patient, and in the buttocks (lower sacral dermatomes) in another. Both these patients gave a history of previous sciatica, with myelography and lumbar laminectomy. Neurological examination was otherwise normal in all the patients, apart from asymmetry of the ankle jerks in 11 of the 13 patients with a previous history of sciatica.

Investigations were largely uninformative. Most of these patients had normal anorectal manometric studies; the minor changes in contraction pressures observed in the external anal sphincter region in 20 per cent of the patients were probably the result of previous surgical procedures. Single fibre electromyography studies showed an increased fibre density in 17 of the 24 patients in whom this investigation was performed; 6 of these patients had radiological evidence of marked lumbosacral spondylosis.

All the patients had been treated without success before referral. In most cases this included tricyclic antidepressants, benzodiazepines, phenothiazines, paracetamol, codeine, dihydrocodeine, and stronger narcotic analgesics. Local measures such as local anaesthetic creams, and surgical approaches such as maximal anal stretch procedures, removal of anal mucosal tags, haemorrhoidectomy or pelvic floor repair were also unsuccessful.

Some patients were considered to be suffering from pain of psychogenic origin and in several of them psychiatric opinion had been sought before referral, but without therapeutic success. In the absence of evidence as to causation, it is difficult to devise appropriate treatment. Percutaneous vibration was tried without effect in 3 patients and pudendal nerve block relieved the pain on the treated side for a few hours in 2 patients. Carbamazepine was ineffective or only partially effective in 8 patients. Six were treated with diflunisal: 5 of these claimed partial benefit during periods of 6 weeks to 8 months. Treatment thus remained unsatisfactory. Massage of the pelvic floor musculature was uniformly ineffective.

Conclusions

The 35 patients in the study by Neill and Swash (1982) presented a consistent clinical syndrome of chronic perianal pain. The pain was usually likened to a feeling 'like sitting on a ball' in the anal canal. In most of the patients it was precipitated by sitting. It was usually relieved, if only partially, by standing or lying on one side. The clinical features overlap those of coccygodynia, but differ from those of proctalgia fugax. We have no evidence of chronic spasm of the pelvic floor musculature in our patients and thus discount this as a cause of such long-lasting and severe pain.

In some patients, the radiation of the pain into a partial sciatic distribution, together with the slight sensory disturbance in the sacral dermatomes and the radiographic features of lumbosacral spondylosis, suggest that the disorder represents a form of radiculopathy due to sacral nerve root compression or fibrosis. That chronic perianal pain might be neuralgic was also considered by Boisson, Debbasch and Bensaude (1966). The pain is often predominantly pudendal in distribution, although it usually radiates more widely.

The high incidence of previous sciatica in these patients may be relevant, but studies using translumbar spinal stimulation at L1 and L4 vertebral levels have not revealed consistent abnormalities in patients with this syndrome of chronic perianal pain (see Chapter 7). Nevertheless, some patients ascribe their pain to a delayed complication of myelography (Neill and Swash, 1982).

The innervation of the external anal sphincter muscle derives from the pudendal nerve, and the puborectalis muscle, the component of the pelvic floor musculature largely responsible for the maintenance of faecal continence, is probably innervated by branches of the sacral plexus situated on the peritoneal surface of the pelvic floor, and not by the pudendal nerve (Percy et al., 1981). Faecal incontinence would thus not be expected to occur in patients with perineal pain due to pudendal nerve damage, unless there was also damage to the sacral nerves innervating the puborectalis muscles. These findings therefore suggest that if chronic perianal pain is neuralgic, the lesion lies either in the pudendal nerves or in the sacral roots more proximally. If the lesion is situated in the latter site, it must be insufficiently severe to lead to marked weakness of the puborectalis muscle. A number of patients with perianal pain, 60 per cent in the series of Neill and Swash (1982), have weakness of the pelvic floor musculature (Parks, Porter and Hardcastle, 1966).

Treatment of chronic anal pain is disappointing, as is apparent from the multiplicity of treatments tried by our patients. In our experience, pudendal block with lignocaine relieved the pain for only a few hours. Non-steroidal anti-inflammatory analgesics, especially diflunisal, seemed to improve some patients in uncontrolled trials. Treatment with other analgesics was only partially successful, and percutaneous vibration of the perianal skin was ineffective. It is unlikely that treatment will be effective in the absence of clearer understanding of the cause of the syndrome. The complaint is rare in men, and chronic prostatitis must always be considered.

In many patients, there are overt depressive symptoms with insomnia and marked disruption of family life. Most are elderly and many describe abnormal or unfulfilled sexual behaviour. In many, the disorder seems to intensify when the husband retires from work and comes to spend all day at home, perhaps without meaningful occupation. The perianal pain then is used as a diversion into invalidism, perhaps representing a substituted conversion symptom in the face of emotional conflict. Psychiatric help may be rewarding in such patients.

References

ABRAHAMS, A. (1935). Proctalgia fugax. Lancet, 2, 444

BENSAUDE, A. (1965). Proctalgies fugaces. Acta Gastro-Enterologica Belgica, 28, 594–604

BOISSON, J., DEBBASCH, L. and BENSAUDE, A. (1966). Les algies ano-rectales essentielles: étude clinique, étiologique, pathogenique et thérapeutique. Archives Françaises des Maladies Appareil Digestique (Paris)

GRANT, S. R., SALVATI, E. P. and RUBIN, R. J. (1975). Levator syndrome: an analysis of 316 cases. Diseases of the Colon and Rectum, 18, 161–163

NEILL, M. E. and SWASH, M. (1982). Chronic perianal pain: an unsolved problem. Journal of the Royal Society of Medicine, 75, 96–101

PARKS, A. G., PORTER, N. H. and HARDCASTLE, J. D. (1966). The syndrome of the descending perineum. Proceedings of the Royal Society of Medicine, 59, 477–482

PERCY, J. P., NEILL, M. E., PARKS, A. G. and SWASH, M. (1981). Electrophysiological study of motor nerve supply of pelvic floor. Lancet, 1, 16–17

SIMPSON, J. Y. (1859). Coccygodynia and diseases and deformities of the coccyx. Medical Times and Gazette, 40, 1009–1010

THAYSEN, Th. E. H. (1935). Proctalgia fugax: a little known form of pain in the rectum. Lancet, 2, 243–246

THIELE, G. H. (1963). Coccygodynia: cause and treatment. Diseases of the Colon and Rectum, 6, 422–436

THOMPSON, W. G. and HEATON, K. W. (1980). Proctalgia fugax. Journal of the Royal College of Physicians, London, 14, 247–248

Index